T0323354

Deep Brain Stimulation Programming

Deep Brain Stimulation Programming

Mechanisms, Principles, and Practice

SECOND EDITION

ERWIN B. MONTGOMERY JR., MD

MEDICAL DIRECTOR
GREENVILLE NEUROMODULATION CENTER
GREENVILLE, PA

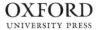

OXFORD

UNIVERSITY PRESS

Oxford University Press is a department of the University of Oxford. It furthers
the University's objective of excellence in research, scholarship, and education
by publishing worldwide. Oxford is a registered trade mark of Oxford University
Press in the UK and certain other countries.

Published in the United States of America by Oxford University Press
198 Madison Avenue, New York, NY 10016, United States of America.

© Oxford University Press 2017

First Edition published in 2010

Second Edition published in 2017

Library of Congress Cataloging-in-Publication Data
Names: Montgomery, Erwin B., Jr., author.
Title: Deep brain stimulation programming : mechanisms, principles, and practice / by Erwin B. Montgomery Jr.
Description: Second edition. | Oxford ; New York : Oxford University Press,
[2017] | Includes bibliographical references and index.
Identifiers: LCCN 2016014328 | ISBN 9780190259600
Subjects: | MESH: Deep Brain Stimulation—methods | Brain Diseases—therapy | Neurologic Manifestations
Classification: LCC RC350.B72 | NLM WL 368 | DDC 616.8/4—dc23 LC record available at http://lccn.loc.gov/2016014328

DISCLAIMER

The information in this monograph on deep brain stimulation (DBS) is advisory only and is not meant to direct the specific management of any individual patient. Physicians and other healthcare providers must use their own professional judgement when evaluating this information and must consider the unique circumstances of each patient when providing therapy. Patients and their caregivers are strongly advised not to change patient care without approval from the treating physician or healthcare professional.

The field of DBS is continually evolving, and physicians and other healthcare providers are strongly advised to keep abreast of developments that could alter the information and advisories contained here. They should review the appropriate operation and safety manuals from the manufacturers of the equipment they use. When in doubt, they should consult the manufacturer directly. While the information provided in this monograph will help the physician in deciding which specific DBS systems to use, the decision in each case must be based on the treatment team's own assessment of the relative advantages and disadvantages of each system and the unique circumstances of their practice and each particular patient.

This monograph should not be construed as an endorsement, either explicit or implicit, of any particular medical device or treatment. Information that may not conform to federal Food and Drug Administration guidelines is explicitly noted in the text.

The author has no conflicts of interest related to the preparation of this monograph.

Erwin B. Montgomery, Jr., MD

To Lyn Turkstra, who makes all things possible

and to Rachael (Shirley) Turkstra, whose smile brightens the darkest places

CONTENTS

Preface to the Second Edition • xiii
Preface to the First Edition • xvii
Abbreviations • xxi

1. Introduction • 1
    The Fundamentals Still Pertain • 2
    Principles of Effective and Efficient
        Programming • 2
    The Basis of DBS Effects • 3

2. Principles of Electricity and Electronics • 5
    Electricity • 5
    Electronics • 10
    Note Regarding Impedances • 14

3. Principles of Electrophysiology • 15
    Therapeutic Mechanisms versus Delivery
        of Therapy • 15
    The Neuron • 16
    Neuronal Electronics • 17
    Voltage-Gated Ionic Conductance
        Channels and Action Potentials • 22
    Downstream Secondary Issues • 24

4. Controlling the Flow of Electrical
    Charges • 27
    Orientation of the Lines of Electrical
        Force • 27
    Orthodromic and Antidromic Conduction
        of Action Potentials • 28
    Axon Diameter • 30
    Electrode Configurations • 31

Current Intensity in Monopolar and
    Bipolar Electrode Configurations • 36
Segmented DBS Leads • 43

5. DBS Safety • 45
    The Range of Safety Concerns • 45
    Injury Secondary to Electricity • 45
    Medical Complications • 47
    Adverse Effects Related to Activation
        of Neural Networks • 48
    The Potential Psychosocial Consequences
        of DBS • 48

6. Nervous System Responses to DBS • 49
    Knowledge of Nervous System Responses
        versus Knowledge of Therapeutic
        Mechanisms • 49
    Effects Mediated by Voltage-Gated Ionic
        Conductance Channels in the Neuronal
        Membrane • 51
    Post-Hyperpolarization Rebound
        Excitation, Depolarization
        Blockade, and Neurotransmitter
        Exhaustion • 52
    Dissociation of Effects on Action-
        Potential-Initiating Segment, Dendrites,
        and Cell Bodies • 54
    Network Effects of DBS • 55
    Critically Important Caveats Concerning
        Interpretation of Nervous System
        Responses to DBS • 57

Reentry Propagations
and Resonance • 59
Synchronization Among Neurons • 62
Interactions Between DBS Pulses in
Intrinsic Neuronal Mechanisms • 71
Effects on Behaviorally Related Intrinsic
Neuronal Dynamics • 73
Temporal Evolution of Nervous
System Responses • 77

7. DBS Effects on Motor Control • 81
Orchestration of Motor Unit
Activities • 81
Orchestration of Motor Unit Recruitment
and De-Recruitment over Different
Time Scales • 87
Lessons to Be Learned • 87

8. Pathophysiological Mechanisms • 89
The Globus Pallidus Interna
Rate Theory • 90
Excessively High Beta Oscillations • 90
Excessive Synchronization of Neuronal
Activities • 90
Excessive Bursting • 91
The Systems Oscillators Theory • 93

9. Approaches to Programming • 99
Battery Life • 99
DBS Contact Nomenclature • 100
Prior to DBS Programming • 102
When to Program DBS • 103
Conceptual Approaches • 105
The Growing Importance of Monopolar
Surveys • 107
Detection of a Response is Critical • 114
Programming for Optimal Benefit in
the Absence of Adverse Effects • 114
Programming to Prevent Adverse
Effects • 117
Exiting the DBS Programming
Session • 119

10. Clinical Assessments • 121
Clinical Assessments by Disease • 121
Clinical Evaluation of Parkinson's
Disease • 122
Clinical Assessment of Corticospinal and
Corticobulbar Stimulation • 128

Clinical Assessment of Speech, Language,
and Swallowing • 129
Hints for Clinical Evaluations • 130

11. Approach to DBS in the Vicinity of the
Subthalamic Nucleus • 131
DBS Regional Anatomy of the Subthalamic
Nucleus (STN) • 131
Adverse Effects Created by the
Position of the DBS Lead Relative to
the STN • 131
Approach to DBS in the Vicinity of the
STN for Parkinson's Disease • 136
Approach to DBS in the Vicinity of the
STN for Other Disorders • 141

12. Approach to DBS in the Vicinity of the
Globus Pallidus Interna • 143
Regional Anatomy of the Globus Pallidus
Internal (GPi) • 143
Adverse Effects Resulting from the
Position of the DBS Lead Relative to
the GPi • 143
Approaches to DBS in the Vicinity of the
GPi for Parkinson's Disease • 146
Treating Dystonia with DBS in the Vicinity
of the GPi • 148
Treating Hyperkinetic Disorders • 148

13. Approach to DBS in the Vicinity of the
Ventral Intermediate Nucleus of the
Thalamus DBS • 149
Regional Anatomy of the Ventral
Intermediate Thalamus (Vim) • 149
Adverse Effects Resulting from the
Position of the DBS Lead Relative to
the Vim • 149
Effects of DBS on Speech, Language,
and Swallowing • 154
An Approach to DBS in the Vicinity of Vim
for Tremor • 155

14. Algorithm for Selecting Electrode
Configurations and Stimulation
Parameters • 157

15. Helpful Programming Hints • 165
Use of Constant Voltage DBS (To Be
Discouraged) • 165

Conduct a Monopolar Survey • 166

Always Increase the Current/Voltage to
Clarify Any Side Effects • 166

Check Therapeutic Impedances on IPGs
in Accordance with the Manfacuturer's
Recommendations • 166

Confirm That the Parameters Under Patient
Control Are Within Safe Limits • 166

Systematically Document All Clinical
Responses to All DBS Stimulation
Parameters and Electrode
Configurations • 166

Always Reset Counters and Troubleshoot
Inconsistent Responses • 167

Advise Patients, Family Members,
and Caregivers to Take Their
DBS Controlling Devices with
Them to Emergency Rooms or
Doctor's Visits • 167

Be Patient and Persistent! • 167

When in Doubt, Turn the Pulse Generator
Off and Wait • 168

Troubleshooting • 168

16. Oscillator Basics • 171

17. Discrete Neural Oscillators • 179
Importance of Neural Oscillators in
Nervous System Function • 179
Continuous Harmonic Oscillators • 180
Discrete Oscillators • 184
Single Reentrant Discrete
Oscillator • 188
Interactions Among Discrete
Oscillators • 189
Discrete Neural Oscillators • 191
Oscillators with Multiple Realistic
Neurons • 195
The Systems (Discrete) Oscillators
Theory • 198

Appendix of Supplemental Material • 203

Glossary • 205

References • 209

Index • 213

PREFACE TO THE SECOND EDITION

The years since the publication of the first edition have seen remarkable advances in the technology related to deep brain stimulation (DBS). New commercially available implanted pulse generators (IPGs) have greatly increased DBS functionality, and in doing so, have also increased the tools programmers have at their disposal for helping patients. One such advance is that of constant current stimulation, which improves on the original constant-voltage IPGs because current relates more directly to stimulation effects, allowing more direct comparison of experiences within a patient and between patients. Furthermore, constant current stimulation is more effective than constant voltage stimulation. Another advance is the possibility of simultaneous (or nearly so) interleaving of stimulation to produce different currents and voltages on different electrical stimulating contacts. (Readers should associate "contacts" with *electrodes* rather than with *DBS leads*, which carry an array of electrodes.) This new capability affords programmers greater flexibility in shaping an electrical field to a patient's unique regional anatomy around a DBS lead.

Research currently under way is looking at different DBS frequencies and patterns of stimulation pulse trains. It is also looking at closed-loop stimulation, in which the DBS system measures a signal in the brain in order to determine a stimulus's proper moment and duration. In development are DBS leads that feature a greater number of electrodes, as well as leads whose electrodes provide direct stimulation current to a specific region of the brain orthogonal to the long axis of the lead rather than sending it over the entire circumference of the DBS lead.

With increased functionality and complexity come decreases in other areas. More numerous and variegated types of DBS increase the chance of maximum benefit. Yet, absent any clear and simple algorithm, sorting through all possibilities becomes inordinately time-consuming from a programmer's viewpoint. Though constant current and interleaved stimulation have come onto the market, relatively few programmers are taking advantage of them. A cursory perusal of the literature on variance in stimulation parameters reveals that few programmers venture far from the reported mean or median values.

Computer-based algorithms for facilitating DBS programming are on the market or under development. Some of these, are image-based such as Magnetic Resonance Imaging (MRI); they identify regional anatomy relevant to DBS lead placement. Such systems are capable of precisely modeling and displaying the spread of electrical currents in the brain. A programmer then presumably selects electrode configurations and stimulation parameters that best fit regional anatomy. Methods of this sort depend on a presumption of prior knowledge of the best anatomical site for stimulation. Yet the target for stimulation to improve movement disorders, which constitutes the majority of DBS use, is defined physiologically rather than anatomically; and no current imaging method enables precise identification of the physiological target. Nevertheless, such anatomy-based techniques may be capable of revealing sites—corticospinal and corticobulbar fibers, for example—whose stimulation must be avoided.

Other attempted automations of DBS programming are based on the belief that, with detailed study of enough patients, the determination of optimal electrode configurations and stimulation parameters becomes an empirical matter. Admittedly, it is relatively simple to reduce a vast amount data on a very large number of patients to a mean, or median, and standard deviation. The error lies in thinking that somehow knowledge of a mean, or median, and standard deviation applies sufficiently well to an individual patient who sees a programmer. An analogy is that of a shoe company that only manufactures men's size 9 shoes because 9 is the average male shoe size.

What constitutes a manageable approach to DBS programming will not be determined by the technology that can be brought to bear. The pace of recent advances suggests that the new technologies that can be conceived and implemented are quite numerous, perhaps astronomically so. Needed is a set of heuristics that guides the programmer through all implementations of available technologies in an efficient manner and, most importantly, enables her or him to tailor these technologies to an individual patient's particulars needs. Such heuristics will not come from randomized controlled trials or other empirical studies. The very information-processing manipulations that allow inferences to be drawn from randomized controlled trials reduce the inferences that may be made about an individual patient. This is because information, which may be defined as the opposite of entropy, is governed by something akin to the Second Law of Thermodynamics in physics.

What is needed for the heuristics for a manageable approach to DBS programming is a set of fundamental principles that fosters an understanding of the nervous system effects of DBS. Knowledge of these fundamental principles may enable one to reconstruct a specific electroneurophysiological instantiation, which in turn may enable the programmer to gain clinical understanding of an individual patient. The available technologies may then be judged and utilized according to their relationship to the fundamental principles.

The first edition of this text essentially ended with the principles that underlie action potential generation in the axonal elements of the neuron. These principles remain necessary for an understanding of the clinical effects of DBS and for effective and efficient DBS programming. And they possibly remain sufficient for understanding and managing adverse effects of DBS, which are created by the unintended spread of electrical current to structures associated with adverse effects. However, recent advances suggest that principles that only address generation of action potentials are insufficient. The observations of the effects of DBS frequency (or rate) on motor manifestations alone, for example, indicate a far more complex situation.

In light of the realization that heuristics for therapeutic effects must include more than action potential generation, more extensive discussion of the nervous system responses to DBS is needed. This second edition addresses this need. Though the catalog of nervous system responses has increased greatly, there is as yet no understanding of how some combination of these responses results in a therapeutic effect. In large part, this is due to the failure to understand what it is that DBS corrects. The inescapable fact is that knowledge of the problem to be corrected has behind it a presupposition of theories about the pathophysiology of the disorders to be treated with DBS. Needed, then, is a thorough critique of various theories of pathophysiology.

As will be shown, these theories require enabling assumptions, and presuppositions that are untenable. These assumptions and presuppositions result in quite specific ways of framing questions, which are determined by specific perspectives. Unfortunately, the failure of these theories necessitates a reevaluation of the perspectives and the creation of novel metaphors that may seem foreign. This reevaluation is undertaken in this second edition.

This edition focuses on DBS for movement disorders. It does so in the recognition that DBS is used to treat disorders other than those affecting movement—obsessive-compulsive disorder (OCD), for example. It is also guided by the recognition that, in theory, there is no limit to the range of neurological and psychiatric disorders to which DBS may be applied. The reason for our focus here is that the use of DBS for disorders other than movement disorders is beyond the direct knowledge and experience of this author. Yet he is optimistic that the nature of nervous system responses to DBS is universal, or at least common. Indeed, with respect to the basal ganglia-thalamic-cortical system, the basic architecture is similar for structures underlying emotional (limbic), cognitive, and motor functions. In this regard, the second edition's efforts regarding the therapeutic mechanisms of action and pathophysiological mechanisms for the motor aspects of movement disorders may serve as a metaphor for investigating and understanding these other conditions.

An important, if underappreciated, advance is the increase in battery efficiency, which has reduced the importance of conserving battery life in the programming algorithms and approaches presented in the first edition. The advances in rechargeable systems also enable a programmer to better optimize programming according to a patient's responses. Thus, wasted electricity in DBS programming has become much less of a concern. Consequently, the perceived need for preserving battery life is now less of a justification for DBS methods that exact a price for their greater efficiency. For example, one rationale for closed loop stimulation, beyond its scientific-engineering appeal, is a need for conserving battery life. In the era of rechargeable systems, this rationale seems less convincing, particularly if the use of closed loop DBS introduces initially daunting complexities in programming that would lead a most programmers to avoid them. This is not to discount the potential of closed loop DBS for greater clinical efficacy. Indeed, preliminary evidence appears to support it.

On one hand, reduction of battery drainage as the first order of business conveniently reduced the complexities of DBS programming. The main effort, then, went into finding the lowest effective frequency, current (or voltage), and pulse width; as noted in the first edition, efficacy was almost a secondary issue. At first glance, freedom from the need to conserve battery life and the increased functionality of both IPG and leads appear to be wholly beneficial developments. Yet they may not be so. Despite the introduction of constant current stimulation, for example, far more programmers, in this author's experience, continue to use constant voltage. Their failure to adopt constant current stimulation attests to the power of habit.

It is most important that the individuals who are responsible for postoperative programming be those with the most influence on the choice of DBS system to be implanted. These individuals may not necessarily be those who implant IPGs. Those involved in postoperative programming need to be included in any preoperative decision. It must not be left to surgeons alone, unless they also happen to be responsible for postoperative DBS programming. If a particular device's price affects her terms of reimbursement, a surgeon may find herself with a significant conflict of interest. The availability of various devices at various prices creates serious ethical issues, which are addressed in this second edition.

Because the pace of technology development is unlikely to slow, it is difficult to elaborate an algorithmic approach to programming and, more importantly, choosing among future DBS systems. Thus, greater understanding of the mechanisms of action and the principles underlying effectiveness of DBS, tempered by clinical experience, will help in the choice of optimal DBS systems.

One may say that the current state of understanding about how DBS works is at best largely nonexistent, any reluctance to admit this fact notwithstanding. And no amount of wishful thinking to the contrary is likely to improve the clinical situation. If one wishes to avoid excessive pessimism, one must bear in mind that, whatever the state of our current understanding, DBS is the most remarkably successful therapy for patients with movement disorders since the introduction of levodopa therapy for Parkinson's disease, and it is no less remarkably successful in the treatment of other neurological disorders. If one brackets from consideration the risks, DBS is superior to levodopa and just about any other symptomatic therapy for Parkinson's disease and other movement disorders. In Parkinson's disease, for example, the mechanisms of DBS are different from those of levodopa; and, for those with eyes to see it, the former reveals another way of understanding the disease's pathophysiology and, by extension, the therapy itself.

It would be quite counterproductive to suggest that concerns about any aspect of DBS amounts to slights that somehow diminish DBS's value. The concerns raised in this edition are solely those for future improvement. Some individuals measure themselves by what they have done; others, by what they need to do. To those prone to the former tendency, criticism of what was done in the past is received as a personal rebuke—an all too human reaction, yet no less counterproductive for being so.

Despite uncertainty and the lack of definitive knowledge that drives a single simple solution to the complex problem of DBS programming, programmers must collaborate with each patient in order to discover the best benefit for that patient. There persists a temptation to retreat to what is familiar when confronted with bewildering situations and putative facts. This author, for instance, has seen programmers retreat from DBS and return to prescribing the same failed medications that led their patients to seek DBS in the first place. The purpose of this edition is to enable programmers to sort through various facts, real and purported, on DBS for the purpose of developing their best approaches. This applies not only to present putative facts but to future ones as well. This text cannot render DBS intuitively obvious. But it can perhaps render it a bit more understandable and manageable.

Even though knowledge, experience, and technical advances have greatly increased, the size of this text is fixed. However, there are topics, tools, forms, and other documentation that are not primary to the goals of this text but that readers may find valuable. These have been placed in a website (http://www.greenvilleneuromodulationcenter.com/DBS_Programming_forms/ and http://www.greenvilleneuromodulationcenter.com/DBS_Programming_essays/) for consultation by the interested reader.

As with the first edition, this author continues to owe a debt of gratitude to computer scientist and neurophysiologist He Huang, a collaborator and friend for many years. For supporting the creation of the second edition, the author is grateful to Fred Haer, founder and chief executive officer of the Greenville Neuromodulation Center in Greenville, Pennsylvania. Also, gratitude is owed Erwin B. Montgomery III, Ph.D., who translated the poor grammar of this author (who suffers from severe dyslexia) to prose that is understandable. Finally, the author wishes to thank all those readers who have been so complimentary of the first edition.

Erwin B. Montgomery, Jr.

PREFACE TO THE FIRST EDITION

Deep brain stimulation (DBS) is a remarkable therapy. For many neurological and psychiatric disorders, DBS is more effective than the best medical therapy. For other disorders, DBS may be the only therapy (*see Commentary 1.1, The Case for Deep Brain Stimulation* [in the first edition]).

It is difficult to convey the impact on the patients, family members, caregivers, and healthcare professionals of the nearly miraculous effect of DBS on some patients. Patients severely disabled for years are suddenly able to function nearly normally. The only comparable experience might be that which followed the introduction of levodopa for Parkinson's disease. But unlike the effects of levodopa, for some patients, the improvement with DBS is present at the click of a switch. For neurologists, the nearly immediate improvement of many neurological disorders provides a gratification not usually afforded in the discipline.

The adoption of DBS by neurologists lags far behind its promise. Several factors may explain this lag, including vicissitudes in financial reimbursement, but a potentially critical factor is that DBS appears foreign to many people in the field. Most healthcare professionals have never been exposed to the technology and so do not fully appreciate it. Most medical and professional schools no longer teach, or at least teach to a degree appropriate, the neuro- and electrophysiological principles that would facilitate the greater appreciation and acceptance of the technology, particularly in this era of molecular neurobiology. One purpose of this monograph is to redress this dearth of understanding of electrophysiological principles.

The lack of understanding of neuro- and electrophysiological principles makes it difficult for the physician or healthcare professional to feel comfortable using DBS. Many times, the lack of familiarity creates the impression that DBS is "magical." In such cases, the investment in time, effort, and resources needed to learn DBS programming appears to be too great to justify, particularly when healthcare professionals are already overworked. Lack of knowledge and skills often result in programmers' resorting to the "average" stimulation configurations and parameters and rarely venturing beyond, thereby potentially denying patients the benefit that unusual or atypical settings might provide. This is an increasing danger, as some devices may offer "cookbook" guides to DBS programming, which potential programmers may take too literally. The result is that many healthcare providers are giving up on the therapy too early (Moro, Poon, et al. 2006). Often they revert to a reliance on medications that previously failed, leading to the DBS surgery in the first place.

Knowing the electrophysiology and the neuroanatomy near the DBS electrodes would make DBS far less foreign. DBS programming does not need to be "magical" or involve blindly trying every one of the thousands of different DBS parameters. The premise of this monograph is that treating patients with DBS can be made more efficient and effective by understanding the principles on which it is based. An understanding of the fundamental principles will stand the programmer in good stead, regardless of future technical developments. The knowledge will never become obsolete.

Deep brain stimulation is more than a remarkable therapy. It also provides a unique opportunity to probe brain function and dysfunction. Already, DBS-related research has made obsolete several cherished notions of physiology and pathophysiology. The history of DBS also provides remarkable insight into the strengths and weaknesses of how we conduct research and deliver clinical care. For example, in response to case reports of rare conditions responding to DBS, some physicians have called for randomized controlled clinical trials, but the statistical sample size required would exceed the number of potential cases in any reasonable time frame. DBS is a symptomatic, not a disease-specific, therapy. And just as it would be unreasonable to require separate randomized clinical trials of a pain-relief medication for every conceivable cause of pain, similar judgements should apply to DBS.

In surveying the clinical and scientific responses to DBS, one is struck by how DBS is seen as intruding on more traditional therapies. The risks of DBS often are exaggerated, and that sometimes discourages its use or further research. The excitement about DBS pales in comparison to that surrounding stem cell treatment, despite the failure of fetal cell transplants and the lack of a cogent argument that dopamine-replacement therapy with stem cells will fare any better. Interest in DBS also pales in comparison with interest in gene therapy and despite the fact that the clinical benefits of DBS exceed those of gene therapy. And curiously missing from the discussions of both stem cell and gene therapy are mentions of their surgical risks, which are probably equal to or even exceed those of DBS, as the risk is proportional to the number of times the brain is penetrated.

Assuming this apparently poorer risk-to-benefit ratio of dopamine, stem cell, and gene therapy, why, then, is there greater interest in them? The likely answer is that scientists and healthcare professionals are more predisposed to stem cell and gene therapy because these therapies more closely resemble current concepts of disease pathogenesis, and because of the mistaken notion that treatment is synonymous with reversal of the pathogenesis. What could be more intuitive than the notion of dopamine cell replacement when Parkinson's disease is thought to be synonymous with dopamine cell loss? What could make more sense than converting the subthalamic nucleus (STN) neurons, which excite an already overactive

globus pallidus internal segment (GPi), to inhibit the overactive GPi? The intuitive appeal notwithstanding, these notions are misleading (*see Chapter 12, What DBS Is Tells Us about Physiology and Pathophysiology* [in the first edition]).

Current research suggests that the therapeutic mechanisms of DBS action are not related to direct effects on dopamine neurotransmission. This clearly implies that there are non-direct dopaminergic mechanisms involved, and, consequently, other potential therapeutic targets. It is likely that dopamine depletion sets up a cascade of effects throughout the basal ganglia-thalamic-cortical system, and each of these effects could be a potential therapeutic target. But the lesson is clear. Pathogenesis of the disease is not synonymous with the pathophysiology, and it is the pathophysiology that leads to the disabilities associated with the disease. Failure to recognize that pathogenesis is not the same as pathophysiology is likely to lead to failure to develop alternative and potentially better treatments. One could argue that the success of DBS is a case against the claims made above. That would be the case if the development of DBS were the result of the deliberate application of reason and science. The truth of the matter is that the origins of DBS were serendipitous. DBS followed from the demonstration of therapeutic effects during test electrical stimulation preceding surgical ablation (Cooper, Upton, et al. 1980).

Unfortunately, the mechanisms of action of DBS are largely unknown. However, this knowledge is increasing (Montgomery and Gale 2008). For example, DBS at any frequency excites various neuronal elements, such as axons and presynaptic terminals, which project to neurons in the stimulated target. In addition to generating action potentials that run down the axon to presynaptic terminals in the usual (orthodromic) direction, these action potentials travel upwards to the cell body in the reverse (antidromic) direction from the usual. DBS activates axons near the stimulated target, and activation of these axons may have more to do with the therapeutic benefit of DBS than stimulation of neurons within the stimulated target. Unfortunately, none of these neuronal responses maps conveniently onto preconceived notions of pathophysiology, and consequently, they seem to be given little credence or attention. It is human nature to discount observations that are counter to current theories (Johnson-Laird 2006), but these new observations can be the source of new and better theories. DBS-related research could revolutionize theories of brain function if given a chance. So far, the chances do not look good, but like Pascal's Wager, one tries to be optimistic.

The use of DBS also challenges how new therapies are justified and approved. As is the case with other complex, expensive, and less-commonly used technologies, DBS has not fared well under the current preoccupation with Evidence-Based Medicine, where randomized, placebo, and blinded trials are the preferred and often the exclusive form of evidence (Montgomery and Turkstra 2003). Case reports of DBS for rare disorders have been greeted by demands for randomized clinical trials requiring sample sizes that may exceed the numbers of candidate patients. Whereas in the past, these patients might still benefit from the "off-label" use of FDA-approved (US Food and Drug Administration) devices, such "off-label" use is under increasing attack. Compounding the problem, the costs of such studies and the low likelihood of finding financial sponsors mean that "off-label" uses are not likely to become "on-label" uses, and patients with "off-label" disorders clearly responding to DBS will not be treated. The increasing FDA censorship of physicians who speak of using their own judgement in the use of long-respected "off-label" use of FDA-approved therapies increasingly may endanger these patients.

The importance of DBS for understanding brain function cannot be overstated. In this era of remarkable advances in molecular neurobiology, we forget that the brain is essentially an electrical device. Although the prevailing view is that neurological disease is caused by a deficiency or surplus of neurotransmitters, DBS reminds us that the brain processes information electrically. Thus, neurological and psychiatric disorders can be seen as "misinformation" related to the patterns of electrical activities in and among neurons. The old saw of clinical neurology that there are "positive" symptoms, abnormal gain of function; "negative" symptoms, loss of function; and "disconnection" symptoms needs to be updated based on symptoms related to "misinformation." The information and misinformation in the brain most likely is primary and proximately represented in the electrical activities of neural systems. The brain has more in common with a computer circuit board than with a stew of chemicals.

The history of DBS also reflects much about the good and bad of research and clinical care. Personal accounts related to DBS have been both inspiring and disheartening. They include accounts of scientist-physicians who have displayed great perseverance and courage, such as Dr. Nicholas Schiff and his colleagues in New York in their work with DBS and minimally conscious patients, as well as physicians who have shamelessly exploited DBS for personal gain and compromised the scientific and clinical contributions that could have been made. But these accounts are for another time and place.

The primary goal of this monograph was to provide an aid to the many healthcare professionals who volunteered to care for patients receiving DBS therapies, but at the same time to enlarge the scope of the discussion as befits a truly revolutionary approach to the understanding and treatment of neurological disorders. There will be others disagreeing with the approaches and recommendations made here. That is fine; we learn more when we disagree. However, it is important to recognize what is the basis of disagreements, and the problem is that, many times, they appear to be based on habits and uncritical imitations of others. These do not represent knowledge. Even that fact is important to recognize and discuss. We should not be shy or coy about it.

Writing this monograph made clear to me how lucky I have been. My experiences range from the outpatient clinic, to the operating room, to the human and non-human primate laboratory, to computational modeling and simulations. This led me to value the unique opportunities for cross-fertilization of ideas, particularly through interactions with colleagues representing these different areas. There is no question that insights gained in the clinic and operating room greatly facilitated work in the human, non-human primate, and computer laboratories. Similarly, the insights gained in the labs enhanced my abilities as a physician. This experience reinforced my belief in the unique and valuable position of an academic neurologist/scientist fully immersed in the ethos of a true university. Unfortunately, such neurologist/scientists are increasingly an endangered species. The habitat for neurologist/scientists is shrinking, and it is a pity that some universities do not recognize, or cynically deny, the potential for the unique contributions possible by academic neurologists/scientists, perhaps as an excuse for their failure to support neurologists/scientists.

It is not possible here to recognize the many scientists whose work has greatly influenced DBS. Most of the citations in this monograph are to reviews or perspective papers, and I hope that interested readers will refer to those papers for citations of much of the original work.

The writing of this monograph was greatly aided by numerous discussions with esteemed colleagues and friends. I wish to acknowledge discussions with John Gale, PhD, who started as an employee, became a student, then a colleague, and was always a friend. I also acknowledge a great debt to Cameron McIntyre, PhD; Jerrold Vitek, MD, PhD; He Huang, MS; Frank Moss, PhD; and the National Primate Research Center of the University of Madison–Wisconsin, directed by Joseph Kemnitz, PhD.

The science reported here, and that not reported but that nevertheless was a basis for much of the work, was made possible by grants from the University of Wisconsin–Madison, ST/Dystonia Inc., Medtronic Inc., and the American Parkinson Disease Association.

Finally, I express my gratitude to St. Jude Medical Neuromodulation Division (formally Advanced Neuromodulation Systems, Inc.) for financially supporting the preparation of a white paper that was subsequently expanded into this book. While their participation ended with the completion of the white paper, throughout that process, their direction was clear: write a white paper that would be used as a basis to help healthcare professionals provide the best care, irrespective of the commercial products available or anticipated.

Some of the research described in this publication was made possible in part by Grant Number P51 RR000167 from the National Center for Research Resources (NCRR), a component of the National Institutes of Health (NIH), to the Wisconsin National Primate Research Center, University of Wisconsin–Madison. This research was conducted in part at a facility constructed with support from the Research Facilities Improvement Program, grant numbers RR15459-01 and RR020141-01. This publication's content is solely the responsibility of the author and does not necessarily represent the official views of NCRR or NIH.

Erwin B. Montgomery, Jr.

ABBREVIATIONS

AC-PC line	anterior and posterior commissure line	μC	Microcoulombs
DBS	deep brain stimulation	ma	Milliamperes
DC	Direct Current	Ω	Ohms
FDA	Food and Drug Administration of the United States	PPN	pedunculopontine nucleus
		pps	(electrical) pulses per second
GABA	gamma amino butyric acid	SNc	substantia nigra pars compacta
GPe	globus pallidus, external segment	SNr	substantia nigra pars reticulata
GPi	globus pallidus, internal segment	STN	subthalamic nucleus
Hz	Hertz, a measure of frequency; here, of electrical waveforms	Vim	ventrointermediate thalamus
		v	Volts
INS	implanted neurostimulator	Vop	ventral thalamus pars oralis
IPG	implanted pulse generator		

INTRODUCTION

Since the first description of deep brain stimulation (DBS) as we know it for movement disorders, by Cooper in 1980, DBS has rapidly expanded, both in the numbers of patients treated and in the range of approved indications (Cooper et al. 1980). Patients with marked disabilities who have experienced no relief from any alternatives often have remarkable improvements with DBS (*see Commentary 1.1, The Case for Deep Brain Stimulation, at http://www.greenvilleneuromodulationcenter.com/DBS_Programming_essays/*).

As will be demonstrated, the brain is basically an electronic device. Information is encoded, processed, and transmitted electronically. The neurotransmitters, which are the basis for most pharmacology, are just the messengers between neurons; they are not the message. Any information encoded in the pulsatile release of the neurotransmitters is determined by the sequence of electronic action potentials that are transmitted to the synaptic terminal. Consequently, it only makes sense that DBS should be effective and that the future for DBS and other electrophysiologically based therapies is bright (*see Commentary 1.2, The Future of Deep Brain Stimulation, at* http://www.greenvilleneuromodulationcenter.com/DBS_Programming_essays/). Indeed, remarkable advances have been made since the first edition of this text, particularly in expanding treatments based on electrophysiological principles, such as the artificial retina and brain–machine interfaces.

Even by the standards at the time of the first edition, programming DBS for some patients can be a challenge. Even with the old systems, there are literally thousands of possible combinations of stimulator parameters. The increases in functionality, such as multiple stimulation patterns and interleaved electrode configurations, have exponentially increased the number of combinations of DBS setting. Fortunately, most patients respond to a similar and narrow range of combinations, provided that the DBS-stimulating leads are optimally placed. For other patients, however, dedicated effort is required to identify the optimal combination. The greatest danger for these patients is that the practitioner will give up too soon. The premise of this text is that post-operative DBS programming can be made more effective and efficient by knowing some basic electrophysiological principles and some details of neuroanatomy.

Rapid advances in technology have created momentum in the field, and its future direction and achievements can only be guessed. Thus, any author is challenged with attempting to anticipate the needs of future programmers. Future technologies will increasingly be directed at pathophysiological mechanisms, and consequently, they are likely to be more disease- and disability-specific. Therefore, the programmers will need to have a grasp of pathophysiology and the mechanisms by which the nervous system responds to DBS in order to optimally treat their patients.

As knowledge of how the nervous system responds to DBS and increasing dependency of future DBS on understanding pathophysiological mechanisms, it is critical to understand exactly what DBS is supposed to correct or improve. For example, the rapid advances in the knowledge base of nervous system responses already demonstrate how current notions of pathophysiology of Parkinson's disease fail to provide insight and thus guidance to DBS treatment.

A new paradigm or approach to understanding the mechanisms of action of DBS in light of the pathophysiology of the disease being treated is needed. Parkinson's disease will be used as a model to develop important conceptual approaches and methodologies that will serve to improve our understanding of other neurological and psychological disorders. There are two important reasons to choose this disease as a model. First, our knowledge of patient clinical responses and neuronal responses to widely varied types of DBS is most advanced in Parkinson's disease. Furthermore, theories of pathophysiology probably are most explicit, at the neuronal level, for Parkinson's disease. Second, the anatomical organization of the basal ganglia-thalamic-cortical system related to motor control parallels the architecture of the basal ganglia-thalamic-cortical system thought to underlie cognitive and limbic functions, particularly as abnormalities of these parallel architecture are thought to be relevant to psychiatric disorders. How DBS relates to neuronal responses and clinical responses in patients with Parkinson's disease and in the context of several theories of its pathophysiology is addressed in this second edition as a model for similar approaches to other neurological and psychiatric disorders.

THE FUNDAMENTALS STILL PERTAIN

In this text, I first explain the principles of electrophysiology and the details of regional anatomy and show how this information can guide effective and efficient DBS programming. Often, you can visualize in your mind the orientation of the DBS contacts to the patient's unique regional anatomy on the basis of the patient's responses to test stimulations. You can also visualize the electrical fields generated by the DBS. Matching these visualized electrical fields to the regional anatomy can quickly suggest the DBS options most, and least, likely to be effective.

Some programmers are adept at visualization; others are not. Some programmers find it easier to follow a specific step-by-step algorithm, so the second part of this book provides such algorithms based on anatomical and electrophysiological principles. Following these algorithms provides some assurance that you have tried the most reasonable combinations of stimulation parameters.

Two major approaches underlie the programming methods described in this text. The first is to determine how to affect the intensity of the electrical fields, thereby exciting different neural elements in the field. This is accomplished by exploiting the electrophysiological principles that underlie the effects of pulse width, electrical current or voltage, and the configuration of active electrical contacts. This first approach is generally aimed at improving the efficacy of DBS for symptomatic control.

The second approach is to affect the shape, size, and anatomical location of the electrical field by exploiting the electrophysiological principles underlying the effects of electrical current or voltage and the configuration of active electrical contacts. Varying the intensity of the electrical field generally affects efficacy, whereas varying the size, shape, and anatomical location of the electrical fields generally allows you to avoid side effects and complications. These general principles of electrical stimulation of neural elements provide a context for understanding how you can exploit electrophysiological principles for effective and efficient DBS programming.

PRINCIPLES OF EFFECTIVE AND EFFICIENT PROGRAMMING

As more patients receive DBS implanted pulse generators (IPGs), the need for healthcare professionals who are capable of providing the post-operative management of these systems will increase. Currently, the relative lack of such trained healthcare professionals complicates the lives of these patients and makes getting emergency care difficult. Many physicians are reluctant to become involved in post-operative DBS management. The reasons are multiple and varied, but they include apprehension based on unfamiliarity with the treatment. Often, the healthcare professional's only exposure to electrophysiology was a short, rudimentary lecture in medical, nursing, or physician assistant school. Consequently, some healthcare professionals look at DBS programming as though it were "magical." Alternatively, others may believe that the complexity of DBS programming reduces the cost-effectiveness of the therapy. Neither belief is true.

Effective DBS programming is guided by biological and electrical principles. In many ways, these principles are analogous to the principles of pharmacokinetics and pharmacodynamics that underlie rational pharmacological treatments. These pharmacological principles can be used explicitly, although more often they are used implicitly by being embedded in clinical algorithms. However, in problem patients, explicit consideration of pharmacological principles is often necessary to provide effective treatment. The same is true for the principles of electrophysiology that underlie DBS.

THE BASIS OF DBS EFFECTS

Although the precise mechanism of therapeutic action of DBS is unknown, it is increasingly clear that it depends on the electrical excitation of neural elements and not on their suppression. To date, most evidence suggests that DBS effects rely on the electrical excitation of axons, particularly at the synaptic terminals, because they have the lowest threshold to stimulation. How stimulating axons improves neurological and psychiatric disorders is unclear. Indeed, research into the mechanisms of DBS has revealed more about how the brain works (or does not work) than about how DBS works. DBS has already proven that the present notions of pathophysiology, particularly of disorders of the basal ganglia, are simply wrong (Montgomery 2007a) (*see Chapter 8—Pathophysiological Mechanisms*).

The key to successful DBS is to excite the intended neural elements while preventing the unintended excitation of other elements. As discussed later, stimulating the neural elements effectively depends on changing the distribution of electrical charges on the cell membrane. The control of electrical charges is determined by the principles of electricity and electronics; consequently, an explanation of these principles is in order.

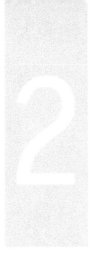

PRINCIPLES OF ELECTRICITY AND ELECTRONICS

The clinical effects of deep brain stimulation result from depositing or moving electrical charges in brain tissue. How the electrical charge is deposited or moved depends on the electronics of the DBS implanted pulse generators (IPGs), which is what you manipulate to deliver the electrical charge. Consequently, you need to know how controlling the electronics controls the deposition of the electrical charge into the brain.

ELECTRICITY

The physics of the electron is fundamental to the effects of DBS, as it is fundamental of the operations of the nervous system. In order to effect DBS, it is necessary to precisely control electrons; consequently, it is important to understand what forces operate on electrons. The electron has a negative electrostatic charge. The familiar experience of walking on a carpeted floor and then getting an electrical shock when touching a metal door knob is an example of electrostatic charge. When you walk across the carpet, electrons are stripped from the carpet and accumulate in your body. When your hand reaches for an electrical conductor, such as a metal door knob, the accumulated electrons on your body repel each other, therefore, there is an electrostatic force driving the excessive electrons away from each other (Figure 2.1). Touching the metal door knob gives the excess electrons a path

to escape. DBS utilizes electrostatic forces to move negative electrical charges into the nervous system or move charges onto neurons in order to excite the neurons (Figure 2.2).

Electrostatic forces contribute to the phenomenon of *capacitance*, which occurs when there is an abrupt obstacle in the path of the flow of electrical charges such as electrons (Figure 2.3). Electrical charges begin to pile up on one side of the obstacle, and as the charges continue to accumulate, there is a buildup of electrostatic charges. These electrostatic charges push electrical charges off the other side of the obstacle as well as resist the accumulation of any more electrical charges until the flow of electrical charges stops. This phenomenon is called *capacitive reactance*. Once the original force that was moving the electrical charges towards the obstacle is removed, the accumulated electrical charges move in the opposite direction, as they repel each other. This phenomenon in electrical terms is shown in Figure 2.3.

Capacitance is an important factor with DBS of the nervous system. The electrical contacts are highly conductive, but the surrounding nervous tissue is much less conductive of electrical charges. Just as described above, there is a buildup of electrical charges at the interface of the DBS electrode and the nervous system—in other words, the nervous system–electrode interface is charging and increasingly opposing the flow of electrical charges from the DBS lead into the nervous system (Figure 2.4). In the

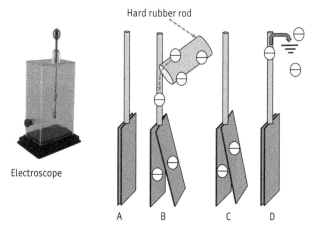

Hard rubber rod

Electroscope

A   B   C   D

Figure 2.1: Schematic representation of an electroscope to demonstrate electrostatic forces. The electroscope consists of two pieces of metal foil suspended from a metal rod. In the unaffected state, the force of gravity pulls the leaves of metal foil downward so that they lie next to each other (A). When a source of electrons, such as a hard rubber rod that has been vigorously rubbed against a piece of fur, is brought into contact with the metal rod from which the metal foil leaves are suspended, electrons are transferred to the metal foil leaves (B). As the electroscope has a relative excess of negative electrical charges including the two metal leaves. As like electrical charges repel, the two negatively charged foil leaves repel each other to move apart (C). Even after the hard rubber rod is moved away, excessive electrons remain on the metal foil leaves. Touch the metal rod allows the excessive electrons to escape, a process called *grounding* (D). As the metal foil leaves are now longer electrically charged, gravity pulls the two leaves to lie next to each other.

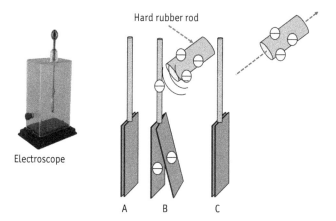

Hard rubber rod

Electroscope

A   B   C

Figure 2.2: Schematic representation of an electroscope to demonstrate electrostatic forces, as described in Figure 2.1. Unlike the situation described in Figure 2.1, the electrically charged hard rubber rod does not make physical contact and is not close enough to allow electrons to jump onto the metal rod of the electroscope (B). However, just as in Figure 2.1, the metal foil leaves repel each other, demonstrating a net negative electrical charge on both of the metal foil leaves. Unlike the case represented in Figure 2.1, the leaves fall back together when the hard rubber rod is moved away (C). In this case, there is no transfer of electrons to the electroscope. However, the excessive electrons on the hard rubber rod create a force or field that moves electrons from the metal rod into the metal foil leaves to cause the leaves to repeal each other (B). Once the electrostatic field is moved away, the electrons redistribute themselves so that the metal foil leaves are neutral, and gravity is able to pull the leaves down and thus, together.

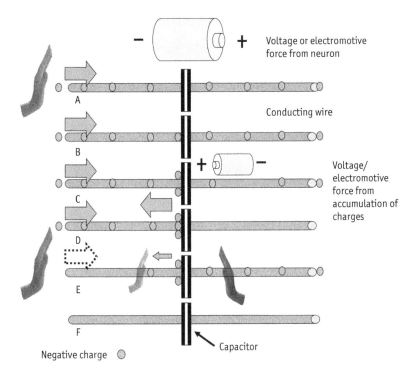

Negative charge ◯

Figure 2.3: Schematic representation of capacitance. A conductor is connected to the capacitor, which consists of two conductors separated by a non-conductive material. As electrons or other electrical charges are pushed onto the conductor leading to the capacitor (A–C), the electrons cannot get through the capacitor and begin to accumulate on one plate of the capacitor. The capacitor is said to be *charging*. As the electrons accumulate, they create a electrostatic force that pushes electrons off the other plate to move away from the capacitor by the conductor, analogous to the mechanisms described in Figure 2.2. Thus, initially there is a flow of electrical current through the capacitor. However, as the electrical charges continue to accumulate, the buildup of electrostatic charge opposes the initial voltage that originally was pushing electrons through the conductor, and the flow of electrical current through the capacitor diminishes. Eventually, the electrostatic forces prevent any flow of electrons (C), and the capacitor is said to be *saturated*. When the initial voltage is reduced to zero, the electrons that have built up on the capacitor now push the electrons in the opposite direction. The capacitor is said to be *discharging* (E) until there is no electrical current (F).

case of constant-voltage stimulation, there will be a progressive decrease in electrical charges or electrostatic fields injected into the nervous system, which is the primary means for the therapeutic effect of DBS. Constant-*current* stimulation counters the increased opposition to the delivery of electrical charges by increasing the voltage in the DBS lead, and thus maintains flow of electrical charges into the nervous system (Figure 2.4).

Electrons spin on their axis. Any time an electrical charge moves, it creates a magnetic field; the electron is no exception (Figure 2.5). Thus, electrons are magnetic as well as electric. This means that electrons can be moved by a magnetic field as well as by an electrostatic field. Furthermore, when an electrical charge,

such as an electron, moves at a constant speed, it creates a static magnetic field. When an electron accelerates or decelerates, such as in a conductor, it creates a magnetic field that moves. This moving magnetic field will cause electrons in the conductor to move as well, typically in a direction opposite to the movement of the electrons that created the magnetic field in the first place. Moving electrons by moving magnetic fields is called *induction*.

A practical benefit of magnetic induction is seen in flashlights like the one shown in Figure 2.6. The user rapidly shakes the flashlight up and down so as to rapidly move a permanent magnet back and forth through a coil of conducting wire. As the magnet moves through the coil, it drags electrons with it to

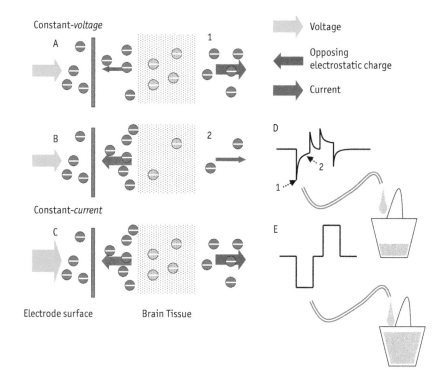

Figure 2.4: Schematic representation of the effects of capacitance on stimulation of the nervous system. The conductivity of the DBS contacts is much greater than the nervous tissue's, in this case the brain. As a consequence, electrical charges, in this case negative charges, build up (A and B) and oppose further injections of electrical charges. In other words, the force driving electrical charges into the nervous system is the voltage on the DBS lead minus the electrostatic charges that are building up. In the case of constant voltage stimulation, the net effect is to reduce the voltage, driving electrical charges into the nervous system. In the case of constant current stimulation, as the countering electrostatic charges build, the voltage applied to the DBS electrode is increased to compensate; thus, a constant amount of electrical charges is injected into the nervous system. Consider a DBS biphasic pulse with a negative square wave pulse followed by a positive square wave pulse. In the case of constant voltage stimulation, the actual current injected into the nervous system is shown in D, whereas with constant current stimulation, the actual current is shown in E. The total electrical charge delivered is the area under the curve (shown by the buckets). Thus, for the same DBS pulse, constant current stimulation will deliver more electrical charges than constant voltage stimulation; thus, constant current stimulation is more effective. (D and E are modified from Miocinovic et al. 2009, page 16).

produce an electrical current. This current is stored in a capacitor, which then passes the electrical current through the light-emitting diode (LED) to produce light.

Some rides in an amusement park use magnetic induction as a brake: for example, in rides where the rider in a car plummets, it stops the car. Before the car reaches the bottom, a braking mechanism slows it. Often this braking mechanism is a large permanent magnet sliding along an electrical conductor. The magnet induces an electrical current in the conductor, which in turn generates a magnetic field in the opposite direction from the way the car is moving. In this way,

the car slows down. The advantage of this system is that there are no moving parts that could fail and result in a catastrophe.

Another example of this effect is called the *Lenz tube* (Figure 2.7). A pipe or tube of electrically conducting material, such as copper, is held vertically, and a small pellet is dropped through the tube. The pellet falls quickly in increasing acceleration due to gravity. However, if a magnetic pellet with exactly identical properties (other than magnetism) is placed in the tube, it falls slowly at the same rate. There must be a force that is countering the effects of gravity, and that force must be magnetic.

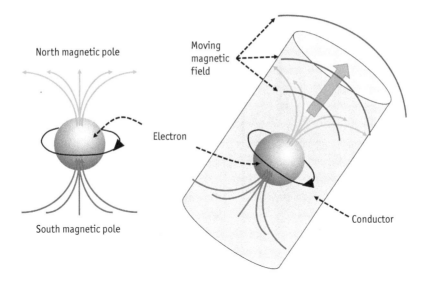

Figure 2.5: Schematic representation of a spinning electron that produces a magnetic field. Thus electrons act as tiny magnets and as such can be moved by an external magnetic field. For example, the figure on the right shows a magnetic field moving through an electrical conductor. As the magnetic field moves, it pulls the electron along with it, producing an electrical current. The process is called *induction*.

The Lenz effect can be extended to any movement of electrical charges, such as electrons through the DBS lead. As the electrons are also magnetic, their movement through the conductor will generate moving magnetic forces that will result in a magnetic force driving the electrons in the opposite direction. The faster the electrical current, the stronger the induced magnetic fields that oppose the movement

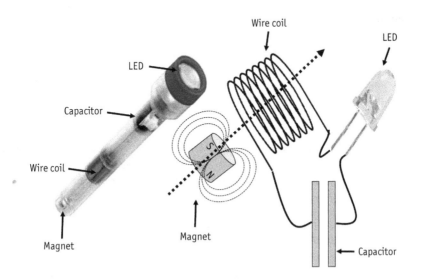

Figure 2.6: Example of a flashlight that utilizes magnetic induction. The user vigorously shakes the flashlight up and down to rapidly move a permanent magnet through the coil of an electrical conductor. As the magnet moves through the coil, it drags electrons (which are magnetic) with it to generate an electrical current. The current is fed to a capacitor, which stores the electrical energy to power a light-emitting diode to produce light.

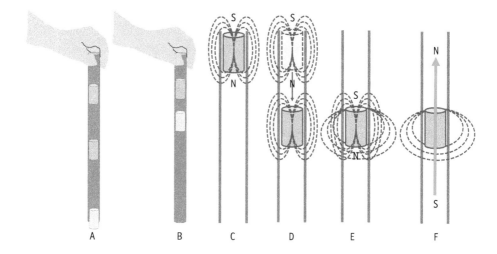

Figure 2.7: Schematic illustration of the Lenz effect. A tube made of an electrically conducting material is held upright. Pellets are dropped through the tube. A non-magnetic pellet will fall through the tube with an accelerating velocity due to gravity (A). When another pellet is dropped that is exactly the same shape and weight but is magnetic, the pellet falls slowly and at a constant rate (B). As the magnetic pellet falls through the tube, its magnetic force field moves through tube, dragging electrons in the tube along with it (C and D). These dragged electrons are moving and thereby create another magnetic field (E) that is in the direction opposite to the gravitational force (F). This induced second magnetic force causes the magnetic pellet to fall slowly.

of the electrons. This phenomenon is called *inductive reactance*. In DBS, inductive reactance opposes the flow of electrical charges or electrostatic fields into the nervous system and would reduce the efficacy of the DBS if constant-voltage stimulation were used, rather than constant-current stimulation.

From the preceding discussion, it can be appreciated that there are three forces that oppose the flow of electrical charges. These include *resistance*, which is a type of friction related to how tightly the atoms are holding onto their electrons; *capacitive reactance*, due to the buildup of electrostatic charges where there is a change in the conductivity, and *inductive reactance*. Together, these oppositional forces are called *impedance*. Capacitive reactance, and particularly inductive reactance, depend greatly on how fast the flow of electrical charges is fluctuating. In direct current (DC) electronics, the flow of electrical charges is constant; therefore, inductive reactance are negligible, and the main opposition to the flow of electrical charges is resistance. However, when the current is rapidly changing, such as the rapid pulses of electrical current in DBS, reactance is a significant factor. It is nevertheless important to understand that the frequency at

which the pulses are delivered is not a major determinant of impedance. Rather, impedance is determined by how fast the voltage on the DBS pulse goes from 0 to maximum voltage, down to the minimum voltage, and then back to 0 volts. These frequencies are very high in DBS; thus, reactance is a major factor influencing the ability of DBS to inject electrical charges into the nervous system.

ELECTRONICS

Electronics relates to the purposeful control of the flow of electrical charges. In typical electronic devices, the flow is in terms of electrons. In the nervous system, the flow of electrical charges is carried by ions. In a sense, ions are essentially determined by electrons. An atom with more electrons than protons (positively charged subatomic particles) will have a net negative charge and is called an *anion*. An atom with fewer electrons than protons will have a net positive charge and is called a *cation*.

The flow of negative charges is called *cathodal* or *negative current*. This could be due to the flow of electrons, as is typical of electronic devices such as radios, or it could be due to the flow of negatively charged ions, such as occurs in the body. *Positive* or *anodal current* could be due to the flow of positively charged ions, as occurs in the body, but the term can also be applied to the flow of electrons. In this case, an anodal current is the opposite of a cathodal current. One can think of it as the "wake" left behind by the moving electrons.

Likening the flow of electrical charge (current) to the flow of water is helpful. Imagine the situation shown in Figure 2.8. You have to put out a fire using a hose connected to a water tank. The amount of water coming out of the hose per unit of time corresponds to the *flow of electrical charge* or the *amount of charge per unit time*. In the case of DBS, current is usually expressed in units of *milliamperes (ma)*. The total

amount of water coming out of the hose corresponds to the total amount of electrical charge, measured in *coulombs*. The amount of charge in DBS typically is measured in *microcoulombs (μC)*. The amount of water flowing from the hose depends on the diameter of the hose: the smaller the hose, the more opposition there is to the flow of water. Think of the difference between drinking through a small soda straw and through a larger one. The diameter of the water hose corresponds to the *resistance*, which is one component of *impedance*, of the DBS electrodes. In the brain, the electrical properties of the tissue between the negative and positive contacts determine the resistance to electrical flow in the brain. In electronics, the relationship between electrical current, voltage, and impedance is given by *Ohm's law* (Figure 2.8).

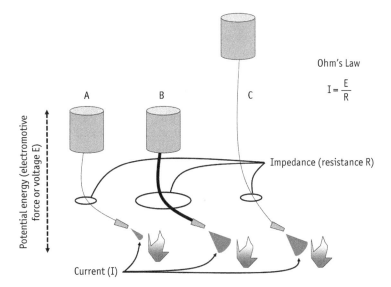

Figure 2.8 content labels: A   B   C

Ohm's Law

$$I = \frac{E}{R}$$

Impedance (resistance R)

Potential energy (electromotive force or voltage E)

Current (I)

Figure 2.8: Schematic representation of the factors involved in electronics using the flow of water as an analogy to the flow of electrical charges. The analogy consists of a water reservoir and hose that exits the bottom of the reservoir. The flow of water per unit of time is the *current* and in electricity is termed *current* or *electrical current*. The total amount of water depends on the current and how long the current was applied. In electronics, the measure of the total amount of electrical charge delivered is expressed in *coulombs*, and the range typically used in DBS is in *microcoulombs*. The amount of current or water to be delivered per unit of time depends on the force used to drive the flow. In the water analogy, the force is hydrostatic pressure and is related, in this example, to the relative height of the reservoir. In electronic devices, the force is referred to as *electromotive force* and is measured in *volts*. Often this force is just referred to as *voltage*. The hydrostatic force must push the water through the hose, which provides resistance to the flow of water. In this case, the narrower the diameter of the hose, the greater the resistance. If one wants to deliver the same amount of water through a wider hose (B) as when using a using a narrower hose (C), one just needs to increase the hydrostatic pressure by raising the height of the reservoir (C). Thus there is a specific relationship between the flow per unit of time of water, the hydrostatic pressure, and the resistance afforded by the hoses. Similarly, the amount of current that can be delivered with constant voltage depends on the *impedance*, and there is a relationship between voltage, current, and impedance (this case is analogous to direct current [DC] electronics [see text] in whose case the impedance is mostly due to resistance). This relationship is called *Ohm's law*.

The opposition to the flow of electrical charges, be they carried by electrons or ions, is due to several mechanisms. First, there is resistance that can be thought of as "friction" that opposes the movement of the particles, be they electrons or ions. In metal conductors of electrons, the friction is created by how strongly the nuclei of the metal atoms bind the electrons. The electrons in the outer orbit of a metal atom are very mobile; hence, there is little friction to oppose the movement of the electrons. In the case of ions, the opposition is created by having other atoms or ions getting in the way.

There are additional mechanisms that afford resistance to the flow of electrical charges, and they are related to capacitance related electrostatic forces and to magnetic induction. These oppositional mechanisms are referred to as *reactance*, as described above. Thus, the total opposition to the flow of electrical charges is the impedance and it is measured in *ohms (Ω)*.

You can adjust the amount of water coming out of the hose by changing the water pressure through raising or lowering the height of the water tank. In this case, the water pressure corresponds to *electromotive force* or *voltage* (Figure 2.8), which corresponds to the force that moves the electrical charges, and it is measured in *volts (V)*. Electrical charge flows from the negative DBS contact (also called the *cathode*) as an administered negative electrical charge. Electrical charge flows towards, and is returned by, the positive contact (also called the *anode*). Flow of negative electrical charge is termed *cathodal current*, and the return flow is called the *anodal current*. The distinction between cathode—an electrical contact, and cathodal—the flow of negative electrical charges, should be kept in mind.

Electrical current (*amperage*) and voltage are not the same; thus, constant current IPGs and constant voltage IPGs are not the same. The same voltage (corresponding to the height of the water tank) will not produce the same water flow (current) when the impedance (the diameter of the hose) is different. Constant current IPGs compensate for different impedances by automatically adjusting the voltage. The water analogy can also illustrate the difference between constant-*current* stimulation and constant-*voltage* stimulation (Figure 2.9).

Another useful analogy to understand the advantage of a constant current stimulator is driving a car over a hilly road (Figure 2.10). Stepping on the gas pedal is analogous to increasing the voltage. The speed of the car is analogous to the electrical current, which is the prime determinant of neuronal responses. The height of the hill and the effects of gravity on the car represent the impedance. If you keep the gas pedal at the same point (constant voltage), the car will slow down (less electrical current and possibly loss of effectiveness) when going up the hill and speed up (more electrical current and possibly more side effects) when going down the hill. Cruise control (a constant current stimulator) automatically adjusts the gas pedal (voltage) with the up and down of the hills (impedance) to keep the car going at the same speed (electrical current and clinical response). Furthermore, even in patients whose impedances stabilize some period of time after DBS lead implantation, different contacts on the same DBS lead can have widely varying impedances. This means that generalizations based on the stimulation voltage necessary for an effect or side effects on one electrode contact often cannot be applied to a different contract on the same DBS lead in the same patient.

There are three main drawbacks to constant voltage stimulation. First, because of capacitance, the waveform of the DBS pulse is distorted relative to the waveform using constant current stimulation (Figure 2.4). The second disadvantage of the constant-voltage stimulation is that unpredictable or uncontrolled changes in impedance can have a marked clinical effect, as there may be unpredictable or uncontrolled changes in the electrical current delivered. However, evidence suggests that, after a few weeks, impedances are generally stable. The third disadvantage is the considerable variability in impedances in different patients. Thus, it is highly unlikely that patients receiving DBS with the exact same electrode configurations and stimulation parameters in constant-voltage stimulation will have the same clinical response. It is not the voltage that determines the clinical response, but rather the amount of electrical charges injected into the nervous system, which is proportional to the electrical current times the pulse width. Thus, it is hard to generalize approaches across patients, and what one learns from treating one patient may not be helpful in treating a different patient.

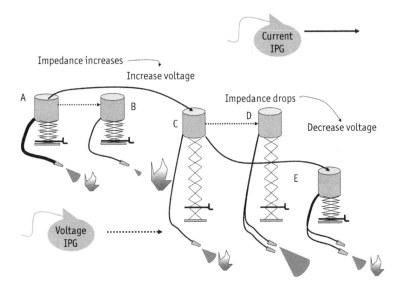

Figure 2.9: Schematic representation of the difference between constant voltage and constant current stimulation. Consider the situation in A compared to B where the two hydrostatic (voltages) are the same. Because A has a wider hose, there is less resistance and more water is delivered than in B, where the narrower hose has greater resistance. A patient may be in a situation like A where DBS is being delivered with relatively little impedance and the patient is having a beneficial effect. If there is an increase in the impedance, but the voltage is kept the same, as would be the case in constant voltage stimulation, now the patient is having a lesser electrical charge injected into the nervous system and consequently has less benefit. The constant current IPG would sense the loss of electrical current, B, and increase the voltage, C, to provide the same therapeutic electrical current. Consider a patient who is doing well in a situation analogous to C, but there is a decrease in the impedance, resulting in an excessive electrical charge being injected into the nervous system (D) because the voltage has been kept constant. The constant current stimulator would sense the increased electrical current and consequently reduce the voltage in order to keep the current at the therapeutic level.

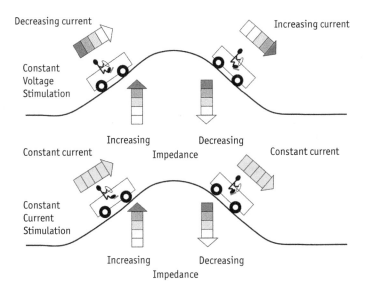

Figure 2.10: Analogy of constant voltage and constant current stimulation to cruise control in an automobile. The case of constant voltage like a driver keeping her foot at the same pressure when driving over a hill. When going uphill, analogous to increased electrical impedance, the automobile slows; and when going downhill, like decreased impedance, the automobile speeds up. In a car with cruise control, analogous to constant current stimulation, the gas pedal is depressed further automatically as the automobile proceeds uphill and then released as the automobile goes downhill.

NOTE REGARDING IMPEDANCES

With the proliferation of IPGs, and with each one using a different method for determining impedances, the programmer needs to be familiar with the nuances of each type of IPG he or she plans to use, particularly when using constant voltage IPGs. Changes in voltage, pulse width, and configuration of active contacts can affect the impedance, which in turn changes the amount of electrical current being injected into the brain. It is possible to exceed the accepted safety limits (*see Chapter 5—DBS Safety*).

As impedances depend on the frequency content of the stimulation, checks of the impedances with different frequencies in the same system will produce different results. Note that the frequency content of the stimulation train is not just the rate at which the DBS pulses are given. The waveform of each stimulation pulse also contributes to the frequency content (*see discussion of the Fourier Transform in Chapter 16—Oscillator Basics*). For checking electrode impedances for the electrical status of the devices (impedances measured at specific stimulation parameters and electrode configurations that are not specifically those used in providing therapy), the specifics of the stimulation frequency content are not as critical as the *therapeutic impedances* (the impedances based on the specific stimulation trains used to provide clinical effects). The electrode impedances are used primarily to test the structural and electrical integrity of the DBS systems. Most electrode impedances are tested with the manufacturer's default stimulation parameters. Some of these parameters may or may not be changed by the programmer. In some IPGs, the choice of voltage in the electrode impedance tests can affect the range of impedances that can be measured. For example, in one IPG, a voltage of 0.25 V allows specific impedance measures up to 4k ohms; 0.7 V up to 10k ohms; 1.5 V up to 20k ohms; and 3 V up to 40k ohms.

The dependence of impedance measures on the voltage for some constant voltage IPGs presents problems when assessing therapeutic impedances. For some IPGs, the voltage used therapeutically may not be sufficient to allow an accurate measure of the impedances. This could cause confusion regarding the structural and electrical integrity of the IPG. One way to check would be to measure the electrode impedances and note any discrepancies between the electrode and therapeutic impedances. For example, a patient can have very high therapeutic impedances, typically with a low stimulation voltage, suggesting an electrical discontinuity, such as a lead fracture, yet the electrode impedances are within normal operating limits. In that case, the therapeutic impedances could be checked with higher stimulation voltages. Also, the possibility of inaccurate therapeutic impedances potentially could affect ensuring the safety of the DBS if the therapeutic impedance underestimates the actual impedance, or could limit the efficacy if overestimating the actual impedance.

Some constant voltage IPGs often assume the impedance when assessing the safety of a particular electrode configuration and stimulation parameters. If the therapeutic impedance is significantly lower than the assumed impedance, the warning may not be issued when it should. If the therapeutic impedance is significantly higher, then a false warning may be given. Two newer IPGs have a two-tier safety warning. The first is based on assumed impedances. If the programmer continues with the planned electrode configuration and stimulation parameters, a second warning may be issued based on the measured impedances. The latter is more relevant for safe DBS. Consequently, it is not clear what the value of the first warning is, and its incorporation into the DBS programmer may be a legacy issue from prior IPGs. A problem might arise if the actual impedance is significantly higher than the assumed 500 ohms and the programmer does not elect to proceed but rather foregoes increases in DBS strength. Note, these problems are less likely to occur with constant-current IPGs.

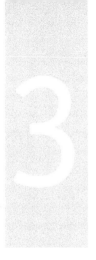

PRINCIPLES OF ELECTROPHYSIOLOGY

THERAPEUTIC MECHANISMS VERSUS DELIVERY OF THERAPY

While the nervous system is an electrical device and DBS works at the level of the electronics, in many ways post-operative DBS programming is prescribing electricity in much the same sense as prescribing medications (Table 3.1). The principles of pharmacokinetics and pharmacodynamics that guide the rational use of medications find parallels in DBS. Many drugs exert their effect by binding to ligand-gated channels, particularly channels that control the flow of electrical charges, in the form of ions across the cell membrane of the neuron in the soma. The binding of drugs to receptors can open the receptor in such a way as to approximate the normal opening by endogenous neurotransmitters; for example, as an agonist, or to block the channel from opening when endogenous neurotransmitters are released—in this case the drug is an antagonist. In the case of DBS, the electrical charges manipulated in the nervous system similarly affect neuronal membrane channels; however, these initially and primarily are voltage-gated ionic conductance channels, which are described in detail in this chapter (Table 3.1).

The pharmacological treatment of Parkinson's disease includes issues of dopamine action on striatal neurons and issues of how to get dopamine to the striatal neurons and not other neurons. Similarly, DBS includes issues of the effects of electricity on the neural elements responsible for its therapeutic effect, and issues of stimulating only the right neural elements. Thus, one principle of providing effective therapy is to differentiate between stimulation characteristics that relate to effective stimulation of the responsible neural elements, and the characteristics related to getting the electricity there. As described below, electrical current, pulse width, and frequency primarily relate to stimulating the neural elements effectively. Note, as will be discussed, that electrical current is more directly related to the effects of DBS and not voltage. Hence, *electrical current* rather than *voltage* will be the term used most frequently. As discussed in Chapter 2—Principles of DBS Electronics—electrical current can be derived from knowledge of voltage and impedance. Electrical current and the combination of active electrodes—for example, monopolar versus bipolar configurations—relate to getting the current to the right neural elements.

The therapeutic mechanisms of action of DBS are unknown. However, the general consensus is that DBS activates neural elements, whether axons or the termination of the axons in the presynaptic terminals. The activation results in the generation of an action potential, which is the basic unit of information in the brain (*see Supplemental essay, The Basic Unit of Information in the Brain, at http://www.greenvilleneuromodulationcenter.com/DBS_Programming_essays/*). Therefore, knowing the biophysics of neuronal action potential generation is important to understanding the therapeutic mechanism of action.

Table 3.1   Comparison of factors affecting the use of medications and DBS

Medications	DBS
Dose	Stimulation strength
Volume of distribution of drug—where does the drug go in the body, and how much is in each place?	Volume of the electrical field—Stimulation amplitude and electrode configuration
	Volume of tissue activation—Stimulation amplitude, pulse width, and electrode configuration
Time to peak dose effect—influences the dosing interval	Latency of clinical or adverse effect in order to assess effect and adjust
Selectivity of action—receptor specificity	Regional anatomy around the DBS electrical contacts
Agonist or antagonist actions at ligand-gated ionic conductance channels for many drugs	Action at voltage-gated ionic conductance channels

THE NEURON

By way of brief review, Figure 3.1 schematically demonstrates the architecture of an archetypical neuron. Derivative from the Cell Theory, the Neuron Doctrine holds that the neuron is the fundamental anatomical unit in the nervous system. Unfortunately, its place in the anatomy has been extrapolated to posit the neuron as the fundamental unit of function in the nervous system, which is not true (*see Supplemental essay, The Basic Unit of Information in the Brain, at http://www.greenvilleneuromodulationcenter.com/*

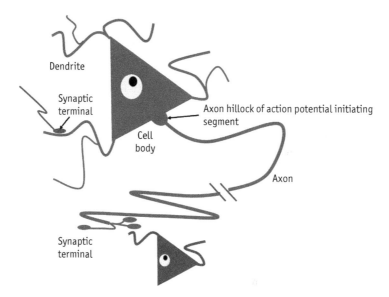

Figure 3.1: Schematic representation of the functional anatomy of an archetypical neuron. The input stage consists of the *cell body* and *dendrites*, together constituting the *soma*. These structures represent the input stage as they receive information from axon terminals from other neurons (presynaptic neurons). The information is encoded in the changes in the electrical potentials across the neuronal membrane in the soma consequent to action potentials' arriving at the presynaptic terminals. The changes in the electrical potentials across the neuronal membrane of the soma in the postsynaptic neuron consequent to inputs are integrated at the action-potential-initiating segment, which may be the axon hillock. Should the integrated inputs exceed some threshold (discussed later), an action potential is generated at the action-potential-initiating segment and relayed to the next neuron in the sequence.

DBS_Programming_essays/). The cell body of the neuron contains the metabolic machinery to maintain the life of the neuron. Exiting from the cell body are branchlike structures referred to as *dendrites*. The dendrites with the cell body comprise the *soma* of the neuron and can be conceptualized as the input stage of the neuron with respect to processing information. Exiting from the soma is the *axon*, which is the source, in most cases, of the output of the neuron. The transition between the soma and the axon is called the *axon hillock*.

The input and output regions of the neuron have very different electrophysiological properties, as will be discussed latter. Key to the output is a signal that can be transmitted over long distances in a reliable manner. For example, information related by the letter "*c*" entered at the beginning of the transmission must be the letter "*c*" at the end of the transmission. The axon is well structured to do so. The action potential represents a stereotypical pattern of changes in the electrical potential across the neuronal membrane of the axon. Because the action potential is stereotypical, the information is preserved. As will be discussed, the action potential is stereotypical because of positive and negative feedback mechanisms involved in the generation of the action potential.

The soma is very different from the action-potential-initiating segment and the axon. The soma is the location in the neuron where information is collected and integrated. Consequently, information must be encoded in such a way as to represent a wide range of information; and, most importantly, diverse information from varied inputs must be able to interact. This requires significant degrees of freedom (variability); for example, allowing the letters "*a*" and "*b*" in the input to combine to produce the letter "*c*" in the output. Action potentials are limited in the way they can represent information: the letter "*c*" that enters the axon must remain the letter "*c*" as it exits the axon.

At some point, there must be a transition from the inputs to the output in the neuron. In other words, input letters "*a*" and "*b*" must be combined into letter "*c*" at the beginning of the axon and be maintained as letter "*c*" at the end of the axon. This transition occurs at the action-potential-initiating segment, which typically, but not necessarily, is the axon hillock.

NEURONAL ELECTRONICS

Key to DBS's activating the neural elements is producing an action potential. The action potential is a particular change in the electrical potential across the neuronal membrane at the action-potential-initiating segment and in the axon. It is the action potential that conveys information among neurons, and it is the information in the action potential that is affected by DBS. The action potential is caused by flow of electrical charges across the neuronal cell membrane, which changes the voltage across the neuronal membrane that initiates a feedback-driven stereotypical electrical response. Moreover, the timing of the action potentials must be strictly controlled so as to properly encode information.

These events impose certain requirements on the neuron. First, there must be some force that will move the electrical charges. This is analogous to the electromotive force or voltage in an electrical battery. Second, this flow must be precisely controlled, and this is analogous to an electrical switch in an electrical circuit. Each neuron is like a battery in which there is a relatively positive pole and a relatively negative pole (Figure 3.2). Separating electrical charges creates the battery. Such separation gives rise to forces that can be put to work, such as driving electrical appliances or generating action potentials. In one instantiation of a battery, positive and negative ions in solution are randomly and evenly distributed; thus, there is no net electrical force (Figure 3.2). However, if the ions are separated by a semipermeable membrane, and the positive ions are moved to one side and the negative ions to the other side, the separation creates an electrostatic charge that could be capable of moving electrons through an electrical device (Figure 3.2).

Unlike in electrons in electrical appliances, the electrical charges are mediated in the nervous system by ions, such as the positive sodium (Na^+) and potassium (K^+) ions and negative chloride (Cl^-) ions, among others. The neuron pumps Na^+ ions outside its membrane, creating a greater number of positive ions outside the neuron than inside (Figure 3.3). There are two significant results from this. First, the inside of the neuron has negative voltage relative to the outside. This creates an electrostatic force that will drive Na^+ ions into the neuron. In addition, there is a chemical concentration gradient, with Na^+ in greater

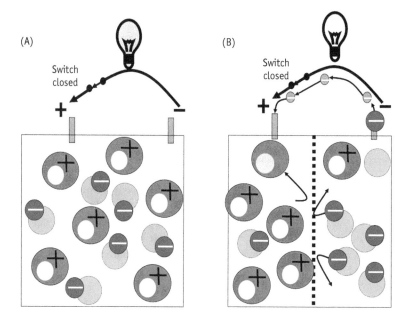

Figure 3.2: Schematic representation of one type of a battery consisting of a number of ions. Negative ions (light blue filled circles) have additional electrons (dark blue filled circles) relative to the number of protons in the atom, while positive ions (orange filled circles) have fewer electrons (represented by the hole in the orange filled circles) than protons. In A, the positively and negatively charged ions are randomly and evenly distributed in the solution. In B, the positive ions have been moved to the left side of the battery and are kept there by a semipermeable membrane (dotted vertical line), and similarly, the negative ions have been concentrated on the right side of the semipermeable membrane. As a consequence, the right side of the battery has a negative charge compared to the left side of the battery. This will cause an electrostatic force that could move electrons through the circuit, passing through the incandescent light to turn the light on. In A, even though the switch is closed and electrons could pass through, there is no electromotive force (voltage) to push the electrons through. In B, the negatively charged ion can give up its extra electron, which then moves through the circuit to reach the left side. There the extra electrons combine with the positively charged ion to fill the vacancy (gray filled circle within the larger orange circle) and thus make the atom neutral in its electrical charge.

concentration outside the neuron; thus, there is a chemical force that drives Na^+ ions into the neuron as well.

A similar situation attends K^+ ions, except that there is a relatively greater concentration of K^+ ions inside the neuron, which would drive K^+ ions out of the neuron (Figure 3.4). However, as there is a relatively greater number of positive charges outside the neuron than inside, there is an electrostatic force that would drive the K^+ ions into the neuron. Generally, the forces attendant on the chemical gradient are stronger than the electrostatic forces.

The chemical concentration gradients, and their subsequent electrostatic charges, are the consequence of an energy-requiring pump in the neuronal membrane. This pump pulls out of the neuron three Na^+ ions for every two K^+ ions that are pumped in. The net effect is to create a one-unit positive charge outside the neuron relative to the interior of the neuron. As the process is repeated, there is an increasingly negative charge in the interior of the neuron relative to outside the neuron.

It is important to note that a number of other ions are involved in maintaining or changing the electrical potential across the neuronal membrane. Calcium (Ca^{++}) and chloride (Cl^-) are particularly important. Generally, these ions do not play much of a role in action potentials at the axon; consequently, they are not directly affected by DBS. However, these ions are important in the soma of the neuron, and ultimately, the DBS effect is propagated to the soma.

Activating the neural element requires closing the circuit to allow electrons to flow through the membrane. Whereas electrons might flow through

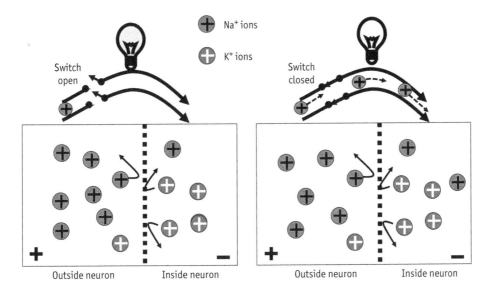

Figure 3.3: Schematic representation of the differences in Na$^+$ ion concentrations, with higher concentration outside the neuron than within. Furthermore, as there is a relatively greater number of positive ions outside the neuron, an electrostatic force is also created. Both of these forces would tend to drive Na$^+$ ions into the neuron. However, the neuronal membrane is not permeable to Na$^+$ ions, and there are special channels that open to allow the flow of Na$^+$ ions according to the chemical gradient and electrostatic forces. These special channels can be open or closed and thus control the flow of electrical charges just as a switch in a flashlight would do.

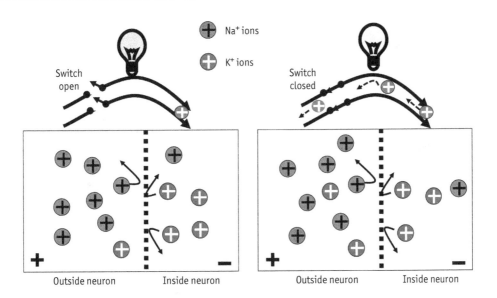

Figure 3.4: Schematic representation of the differences in K$^+$ ions concentrations, with higher concentration inside the neuron than without. This creates a chemical gradient that would drive K$^+$ ions out of the neuron. Furthermore, as there is a relatively greater number of positive ions outside the neuron, an electrostatic force is also created that would tend to drive K$^+$ ions from outside the neuron to the inside. However, the neuronal membrane is not permeable to K$^+$ ions, so special channels open to allow the flow of Na$^+$ ions according to the chemical gradient, which overcomes the electrostatic forces. These special channels can be open or closed and thus control the flow of electrical charges just like a switch in a flashlight would do.

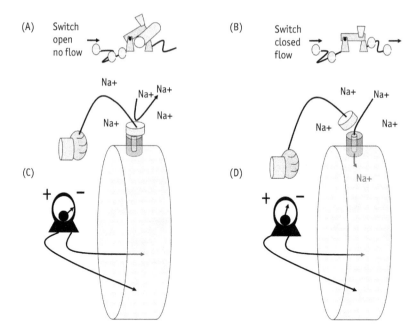

Figure 3.5: Schematic representation of the neuronal analogy to a switch in an electronic circuit. The switch in an electronic circuit allows electrical charges, typically in the form of electrons, to flow through the circuit to perform some function, such as turning on a light in a flashlight. In (A) the switch is held open by a bar that prevents the contacts of the switch from closing to make an electrical connection that allows the flow of electrons. In order for the electronic circuit to perform a function, the obstacle needs to be removed (B) so that the electrical contacts can mate and allow the flow of electrons. An analogous situation occurs in the resting neuron. The neuronal membrane does not allow Na$^+$ ions to pass through (C). Rather, there are channels in the neuronal membrane that, when open, allow Na$^+$ ions to pass through (D).

---

copper wire, electrically charged ions flow through neurons. Activating neural elements, such as axons, generates action potentials that are then conducted to neurons elsewhere in the brain. Turning on a light bulb (Figure 3.5) is analogous to generating an action potential. Furthermore, the sequence of "flashing lights" (action potentials) encodes information (or misinformation), just like Morse code. Neurons convey and process information by the sequence of action potentials they receive. When used to treat disease, DBS may be acting to control misinformation in the activities of the neurons affected by disease. Therefore, for DBS to work, it must close the circuit in the neural membrane to generate the action potential.

While the differences in the ion concentrations inside and outside provide the force for Na$^+$ to move into and K$^+$ ions to move out of the neuron, thereby producing an action potential, this process must be precisely controlled. The control mechanisms are determined by the voltage across the neuronal membrane, which is affected by the relative concentrations of ions on each side of the membrane. The control mechanisms are like valves, referred to as *ionic conductance channels*, which are closed at rest then opened to initiate an action potential. At rest, the neuronal membrane is steady at some negative voltage, typically −60 to −70 millivolts. If the neuronal membrane voltage becomes less negative (a process termed *depolarization*) to exceed a threshold, the valve opens to allow the flow of ions.

The switch in the neural membrane is created by protein units that in turn make up electrical channels that control the flow of ions, the electrical charge, across the membrane. The "switch" that activates neural elements is created when these channels open and allow ions to flow through the membrane. Generally, there are three types of switches, depending on the mechanism that opens the switch. Voltage-gated ionic conductance channels open, close, or change state in response to the electrical potential, voltage, across the neuronal membrane. DBS changes the electrical potential or voltage across the neuronal membrane,

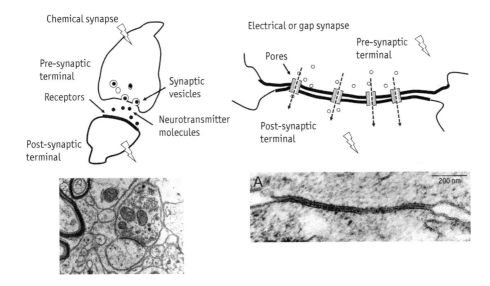

Figure 3.6: Examples of a chemical synapse that typically involves ligand-gated ionic conductance channels and an electrical or gap synapse or junction. In the chemical synapse, an action potential causes changes in the local neuronal membrane of the presynaptic neuron, which results in the release of neurotransmitters. These neurotransmitters diffuse across the synaptic cleft to bind to ligand-gated ionic conductance channels on the postsynaptic membrane to induce local changes in the neuronal membrane of the postsynaptic neuron. In the case of electrical or gap junctions or the synapse, there is physical continuity of the protoplasm of both the pre- and postsynaptic neurons that allows electrical charges to move through the gaps according to the electrostatic forces generated in the presynaptic neuron.

thereby affecting the voltage-gated ionic conductance channels.

The voltage-gated ionic conductance channels provide a unique dynamic because, as the voltage-gated ionic conductance channels open, the voltage across the neuronal membrane changes and thereby affects the very channels that caused the neuronal membrane voltage to change. This dynamic results in feedback mechanisms that can be positive and negative in effect. Indeed, it is these feedback mechanisms that determine the nature of the action potential.

Other types of ionic conductance channels open, close, or change state in response to the presence of a chemical neurotransmitter or neuromodulator typically released from the presynaptic terminals (Figure 3.6). These types of switches are called *ligand-gated ionic conductance channels*. As these channels typically are not affected by the neuronal membrane voltages, the consequence of their opening, closing, or changing state does not have a feedback dynamic. The ligand-gated ionic conductance channel receptor, n-methyl-d-aspartate (NMDA), is an exception where the neuronal membrane potential does affect the state of the receptor.

As the typical ligands are not influenced by subsequent changes in the electrical potential across the neuronal membrane, the NMDA receptor being an exception, there are few or no feedback mechanisms. Consequently, the changes in neuronal transmembrane voltages are passive and decay in amplitude as the changes in ions diffuse to adjacent areas, much like the ripples on a pool of water into which a stone has been dropped. This passive decay over space and time allows for important computational functions that will be discussed later. These types of switches typically are located over the soma, where a wider range of computational functions is implemented. These switches are not primarily affected by DBS.

The third type of switch is the *electronic* or *gap junction* in which there is physical continuity of the protoplasmic conductor between connecting neurons (Figure 3.6). Like most ligand-gated ionic conductance channels, these electrical or gap junctions are not affected by the neuronal transmembrane voltages and thus lack the feedback mechanisms of the voltage-gated ionic conductance channels.

VOLTAGE-GATED IONIC CONDUCTANCE CHANNELS AND ACTION POTENTIALS

What controls the switch is the *transmembrane voltage*, which is the difference between the positive charge outside the neural membrane and the negative charge inside the membrane. For many neurons, the relative difference between the positive and negative charges is roughly −70 microvolts. If this difference is reduced to some threshold—for example, to −60 microvolts—the channels open, allowing ions to flow across the membrane, just as electrons move through a completed circuit (Figure 3.7). Reducing the voltage difference is called *depolarization*. DBS works by depolarizing the neural membrane.

Once the neuronal membrane containing voltage-gated ionic conductance channels is depolarized (reduced electrical potential differences between the inside and outside of the neuron) above a threshold, a series of changes in ionic conductance channels ensues. First to change are the Na⁺ voltage-gated ionic conductance channels. These channels can exist in four states; open, closed, activated, and inactivated (Figure 3.7). The channel consists of a number of protein subunits that are in close proximity at neuronal transmembrane voltages below a threshold and thus block the flow of Na⁺ ions. Once the neuronal membrane has been depolarized sufficiently, the protein subunits change their structure to allow the flow of Na⁺ ions from outside to inside the neuron if the Na⁺ voltage-gated ionic conductance channels are in the activated state.

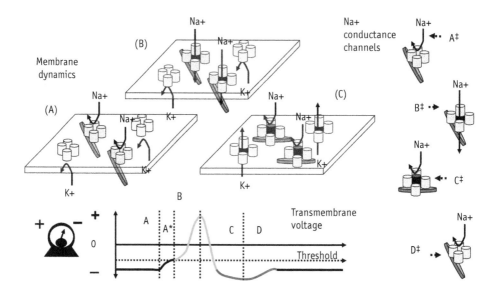

Figure 3.7: Schematic representation of the chain of changes in voltage-gated ionic conductance channels in the generation of an action potential. Initially, the neuron is in a resting state in which the electrical potential across the neuronal membrane has the voltage inside the neuron more negative than outside the neuron, typically approximately −70 mv (A). At this stage, the Na⁺ and K⁺ voltage-gated ionic conductance channels are in their closed state (A⁺). If the local neuronal transmembrane potential is made more positive (*depolarized*) (A*), for example up to −55 mv, then the Na⁺ voltage-gated ionic conductance channels open (B and B⁺) and Na⁺ ions enter the neuron. The inflow of Na⁺ ions causes further depolarization of the local neuronal membrane potential. The influx of Na⁺ ions can continue, even to the point of reversing the neuronal transmembrane electrical potential where the local voltage inside the neuron becomes positive relative to outside the neuron (B). Once a certain degree of depolarization occurs, the K⁺ voltage-gated ionic conductance channels open and allow an efflux of K⁺ ions due to the chemical concentration gradient (C). Also, the Na⁺ voltage-gated ionic conductance channels become inactivated (C⁺). With the inactivated Na⁺ and the open K⁺ voltage-gated ionic conductance channels, the neuronal membrane potential becomes more negative (*hyperpolarizing*) (C). Indeed, the neuronal membrane potential interior may be more negative than during rest, at which point the neuron is said to be hyperpolarized. During this phase, the K⁺ voltage-gated ionic conductance channels are closed, and the Na⁺ voltage-gated ionic conductance channels are activated and closed (D⁺).

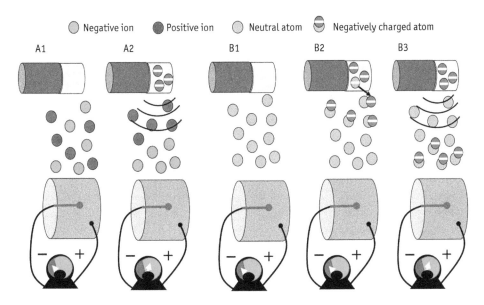

Figure 3.8: Schematic representation of the process of depolarizing a neuron in order to generate an action potential. The process involves moving negative charges in higher concentrations onto the surface of the neuron, which reduces the net positive charges outside the neuron. The reduced positive charges over the local neuronal membrane reduce, or depolarize, the neuronal transmembrane electrical potential to generate action potentials, as described in Figure 3.7. Figure A1 shows the situation where there is no electrical charge on the DBS electrode. As can be seen, there are equal numbers of positive and negative ions in the vicinity of the neuron axon (gray cylinder), and the electrical potential across the neuronal membrane is the resting voltage. When an electrical charge is applied to the DBS electrode, an electrostatic force is created that drives the negative ions towards the neuron such that there is a net reduction in the positive charges outside the neuron, and the neuronal membrane becomes depolarized (A2). In this case, the stimulation is due to capacitance between the electrode and the brain interface. Another mechanism may relate to converting neutral (uncharged atoms) when no electrical charge is on the DBS electrode (B1) to ions with electrical charges. As electrons are deposited onto the DBS electrode contact, some electrons bind to the neutral atoms (B2) to become negative ions. Subsequently, the newly created negative ions move towards the neuronal membrane, and as described in A1, the neuronal membrane becomes depolarized.

The inward flow of Na^+ ions through the now open and activated Na^+ voltage-gated ionic conductance channel causes a further depolarization that in turn opens other activated Na^+ voltage-gated ionic conductance channels, thereby generating a positive feedback-amplifying response. This response continues even as the local membrane potential moves from relatively negative voltage to positive, though briefly. At a certain neuronal transmembrane potential, the open Na^+ voltage-gated ionic conductance channels are inactivated and block any further flow of Na^+ ions (Figure 3.7).

Once the neuronal membrane has been sufficiently depolarized, the K^+ voltage-gated ionic conductance channels open, and K^+ ions begin to move outward according to the forces generated by the chemical concentration gradient (Figure 3.7). The result is a reversal of the depolarization, and the neuronal

membrane now becomes more negative, even to the level of being more negative than the voltage when the neuron is at rest, a state termed *hyperpolarization*. At a certain neuronal transmembrane potential, the K^+ voltage-gated ionic conductance channels are closed. The hyperpolarizing effects of the open K^+ voltage-gated ionic conductance channels are necessary to quickly reverse and stop the action potential, as Na^+/K^+ pump mechanisms would take too long. The hyperpolarized state also is important to activate those Na^+ voltage-gated ionic conductance channels that were inactivated. Until those channels are activated, no action potentials can be produced, and the neuron is said to be in its *absolute refractory period*.

Depolarization to activate the desired neural elements requires delivering an electrical charge into the fluid outside the neural membrane (Figure 3.8). Thus, the outside of the neural membrane is less positive, and the difference between the outside and inside is relatively less negative; that is, the neural membrane is depolarized. Once the membrane is depolarized sufficiently to some threshold, the channels open (analogous to the switch closing), and current flows through the membrane, producing an action potential.

DOWNSTREAM SECONDARY ISSUES

The effects of DBS-induced depolarization in the axon produce an all-or-none response because of the threshold to the initiation of positive and negative feedback mechanisms. These mechanisms play a less prominent role in the soma of the neuron. Rather, depolarization produces on the soma tend to dissipate over time and space on the neuronal membrane unless there is a convergence that is supra-threshold at the action-potential-initiating segment. However,

this temporal and spatial dissipation provides considerable opportunity for computation.

Typically, when an action potential arrives at the presynaptic terminal, there is a release of a neurotransmitter that then combines with ligand-gated ionic conductance channels on the postsynaptic membrane that open to allow the flow of specific ions across the neuronal membrane. Depending on the specific ions involved, the flow can produce depolarization or hyperpolarization of the local neuronal membrane.

The depolarizations or hyperpolarizations then spread out over the neuronal membrane, and the amplitudes of the changes in the electrical potentials across the neuronal membrane diminish over time. This provides an opportunity for a subsequent possynaptic potential to interact with residual changes from the prior event. For example, if there is a second action potential producing a post-synaptic

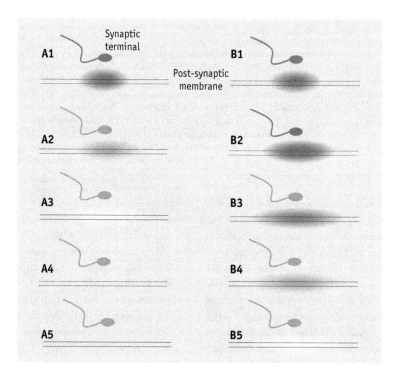

Figure 3.9: Schematic representation of temporal summation on the soma. In A, the arrival of an action potential in the presynaptic terminal induces change in the local neuronal postsynaptic membrane (A1), which dissipates over time (A2–A4). However, if there is a second action potential inducing a postsynaptic potential change (B2) following the prior event (B1), then the potentials will add. If the both changes in membrane potential are of the same polarity (depolarization or hyperpolarization), the result will be a change of greater amplitude (B2), which will persist over a longer time period (B2–B5). If the polarities are different, then the result will be a reduced amplitude.

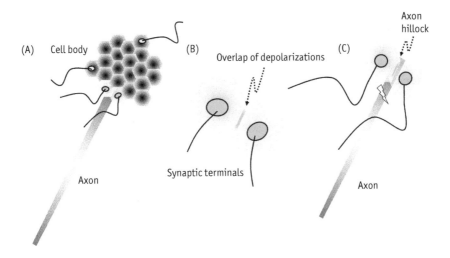

Figure 3.10: Schematic representation of spatial summation on the soma. In this case, each piece of neuronal membrane associated with a presynaptic terminal is represented as a mosaic (A). There are two postsynaptic depolarizations induced by presynaptic action potentials terminating on contiguous postsynaptic regions of the postsynaptic neuron. The initial depolarization is greatest just under the synaptic terminal and dissipates outwardly. Each of the individual postsynaptic potentials is insufficient to generate an action potential (B). However, the individual depolarizations overlap and combine in the overlap region to produce an action potential (C), indicated by the lightning bolt.

depolarization just before the prior depolarization fades, these potentials would sum to increase the effect of the second depolarization (Figure 3.9), a process called *temporal summation*. Similarly, two adjacent postsynaptic depolarizations can combine, and if the sum at the action-potential-initiating segment is above the threshold, an action potential can be produced (Figure 3.10), a process called *spatial summation*.

The primary effect of DBS is to produce action potentials in the axons, as these have the lowest threshold for activation (*see Chapter 6—Nervous System Responses to DBS*). However, these action potentials are conducted orthodromically to arrive at the synaptic terminals on downstream neurons to produce a postsynaptic event (Figure 3.11). Also, the action potential is propagated antidromically, and if the axon has a collateral, the antidromic potential then moves into the collateral branch, becoming an orthodromically conducted action potential. Thus, the indirect postsynaptic events can invoke both temporal and spatial summation as potential mechanisms of action.

The downstream secondary effects, such as postsynaptic changes in the neurons' transmembrane potentials, can affect spatial and temporal summation in the downstream neurons. For temporal summation,

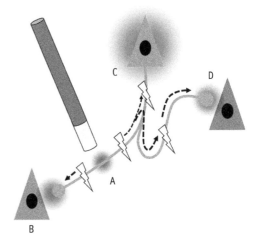

Figure 3.11: Schematic representations of the primary and secondary effects of DBS. DBS produces an action potential in the axon near the DBS contact (A). The action potential is conducted orthodromically to neuron B to produce a postsynaptic change in the local neuronal transmembrane electrical potential. The action potential also is conducted antidromically to neuron C, from which the axon originated. The axon activated may have an axon collateral or branch, which goes to neuron D. The antidromic action potential arrives at the branch point antidromically but then is conducted further in an orthodromic direction to neuron D and produces a postsynaptic change in the electrical potential across the local membrane of neuron D.

the DBS pulses must be given frequently enough so the effects of the prior pulse have not dissipated before the second pulse generates the subsequent change in the neurons' transmembrane electrical potentials. The minimum frequency to effect temporal summation depends on the time course of the ligand-gated ionic conductance channels. For some, such as the NMDA receptor, the time course may be up to 50 ms, in which case a DBS frequency of just over 20 pps may be sufficient to generate temporal summation.

The DBS pulse may affect spatial summation because the volume of tissue activation is very large compared to the packing density of axons in the vicinity of the DBS cathode (active negative electrical contact). Thus, it is likely that many axons are activated, and these may converge on the same neuron, thereby producing spatial summation. Both temporal and spatial summation may contribute to the physiological effects of DBS (*see Chapter 6—Nervous System Responses to DBS*).

CONTROLLING THE FLOW OF ELECTRICAL CHARGES

Chapter 3, Principles of Electrophysiology, described the mechanisms by which an electrostatic field generated by a DBS pulse leads to the generation of action potentials in axons by virtue of voltage-gated ionic conductance channels. The key to effective DBS treatment lies in generating action potentials in structures that lead to clinical benefit, while avoiding structures whose stimulation leads to adverse effects. Thus, the critical issue will be the precise control of electrical charges flowing from the active negative (cathode) DBS electrode contacts that determine the volume, shape, distribution, and intensity of the electrical fields generated by the DBS pules.

Chapter 2, Principles of DBS Electronics, discussed the electricity and electronic issues related to generating the electrostatic field. Following from Ohm's Law, the intensity of the electrical field is determined by the voltage applied to the active contacts, as well as the resistivity, particularly measured in impedance, of the tissue between the negative contact (cathode) and the positive contact (anode). However, following from principles outlined in Chapter 3, there are additional factors that determine whether action potentials are generated within axons located in the *volume of the electrical field*. These include pulse width, the direction of the lines of electrical force, and frequency-related resonance, as action potentials are propagated in a reentrant manner through closed loops within the basal ganglia-thalamic-cortical system with respect to movement disorders, though the same principles apply to other functional systems (*see Chapter 6—Nervous System Responses to DBS*). Thus, the *volume of tissue activation*, meaning the volume of tissue containing axons in which action potentials have been induced, is not the same as the *volume of the electrical field*. This chapter discusses how the factors that influence the volume of the electrical field and the volume of tissue activation can be controlled to produce clinical benefit and avoid adverse effects.

ORIENTATION OF THE LINES OF ELECTRICAL FORCE

For depolarization to work, electrical charges must be delivered to the neuron so as to affect the electrical potential across the neuronal membrane to affect voltage-gated ionic conductance channels. Thus, the orientation of the field of electrical charges to the neuronal membrane is critically important. Electrical charges flow from the negative contact to the positive contact. Neuronal membranes perpendicular to the lines of electrical charges coming from the negative contact will receive electrical charges that will affect the electrical potentials across the neuronal membrane, particularly to depolarize the neuronal membrane enough to generate an action potential (Figure 4.1, Neuron A). The negative electrostatic charge "pushes" negative charges onto the outer surface of the neuron, which will result in a

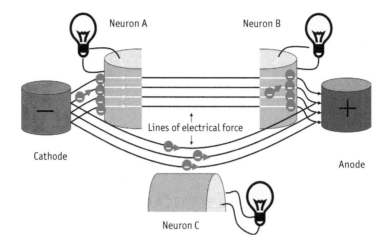

Figure 4.1: The importance of the orientation of the neuronal membrane relative to the lines of electrical force coming from the negative contact. The electrostatic field generated by the negative contact (*cathode*) will deposit negative charges onto the outer surface of the neuronal element (neuron A). The result will be a depolarization of the neuronal membrane of neuron A and, if sufficient, will generate an action potential. The same lines of electrical force will "push" negative charges onto the inner surface of neuron B, which will not depolarize the neuronal membrane, and no action potential will be generated in that portion of neuron B. Neurons whose membrane surfaces are oriented parallel to the lines of electrical force (C) will not respond to the electrical force entering the neuron, will not be depolarized, and will not generate an action potential.

depolarization of the neuronal membrane. Neurons near the positive contact will not have negative electrical charges deposited on the outer surface, will not be depolarized, and thus, are not activated (Figure 4.1, Neuron B). Likewise, neurons whose membranes are oriented parallel to the lines of electrical forces that move electrical charges will not receive the electrical charges and, consequently, will not be activated (Neuron C; Figure 4.1).

Although the orientation of the lines of electrical forces relative to the neuronal membrane (most often the axon) is important, it is difficult to know the exact orientation. Hypothetical examples are shown in Figures 4.2, 4.3 and 4.4. In Figure 4.2, the axon is predominantly oriented parallel to the lines of electrical force and hence is parallel to the flow of electrical charges, so those parts of the axon would not be excited. However, as shown in figure 4.3, the axon has a small S-shaped curve. On this small curve, the neuronal membrane is perpendicular to the lines of electrical force, so electrical charges may accumulate and may lead to depolarization of the neuronal membrane, initiating an action potential that will be conducted through the remainder of the axon. This variability of the axon's orientation limits the value of computational models of DBS, which assume

a smooth and regular orientation. For example, if the axon in Figure 4.2 is straight and not curved, it will not be activated. It is far more likely that axons have irregular shapes; consequently, the precise orientation of the axon in the electrical field cannot be predicted. Nevertheless, the orientation of the neuronal elements to the electrical field is important, as evidenced by the fact that reversing the polarity in bipolar stimulation can have a marked and different clinical effect.

A similar hypothetical situation is shown in Figure 4.4, but for the end of the axon that forms the synaptic terminal. Again, this difference in the orientation of the neuronal element could give rise to an action potential, especially because axonal terminals have the lowest excitation thresholds.

ORTHODROMIC AND ANTIDROMIC CONDUCTION OF ACTION POTENTIALS

Figure 4.4 shows the action potential going in both directions. The action potential moving toward the synapse is traveling orthodromically, which is usually the case in biological systems. The action potential moving in the opposite direction, toward the neuronal

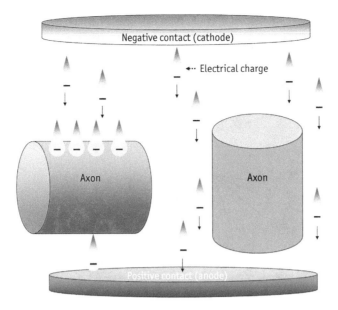

Figure 4.2: Hypothetical illustration of the importance of the orientation of the neuronal membrane to the lines of electrical force from the negative contact. Negatively charged ions move from the cathode to the anode. When the neuronal membrane is perpendicular to the flow of ions along the lines of electrical force, the negative charges can be thought of as accumulating on the surface of the axon (A). When enough negative charges accumulate, the resultant depolarization exceeds some threshold, and the axon responds with an action potential. When the axon (B) is parallel to the flow of the negative charges, negative charges will not accumulate on the neuronal membrane. The negative charges will continue to flow past the neuronal membrane. Consequently, an electrical charge will not accumulate, the axon will not depolarize, and no action potential is created.

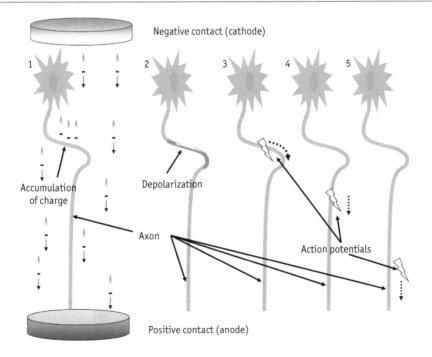

Figure 4.3: A hypothetical example of how an irregularity in the shape of an axon in the electrical field may result in an unanticipated excitation of the axon. In this example, the axon is generally parallel to the lines of electrical force and to the flow of electrical charges. Such an orientation would not be expected to result in an action potential. However, the axon with the S-shaped curve has a small portion that is oriented relatively perpendicular to the lines of electrical force. Consequently, negative charges can accumulate on this small region, and the membrane can be depolarized; if the depolarization is sufficient, it may result in an action potential that is conducted through the remainder of the axon.

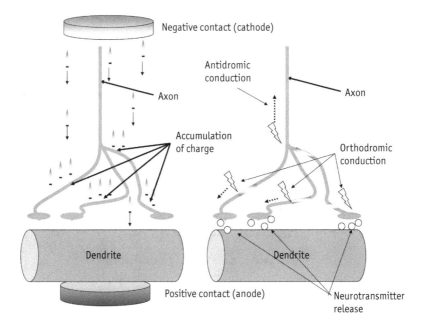

Figure 4.4: A hypothetical example of how changes in the orientation of an axon branching at the synaptic terminal can give rise to excitation of the axon, even though the majority of the axon is parallel to the lines of electrical force and the flow of the electrical charge. Even when the axon is oriented parallel to the lines of electrical force, the axon terminal branches may be relatively perpendicular to the lines of electrical force and become charged. This charge may result in an orthodromic conduction of action potentials to the synaptic terminals, either exciting or inhibiting the postsynaptic neuronal element, in this case a dendrite. At the same time, the action potential initiated in the axon branches is conducted antidromically to excite its associated neuron, which was the origin of the axon terminals being excited.

cell body or soma from which the axon originated, is traveling antidromically. Although not the usual circumstance, antidromic activation should have important physiological effects and may mediate much of the therapeutic mechanisms of DBS (*see Chapter 6—Nervous System Responses to DBS*). Figures 4.5 and 4.6 show the evidence of antidromic activations in neurons of the Vop thalamus and motor cortex. In these cases, DBS of the STN or GPi becomes synonymous with direct activation of the thalamus and motor cortex. The physiological implications are represented in Figure 4.7.

There is a tendency to only consider the effects of DBS at the local target site. However, in every relevant study, the effects of the DBS pulse are propagated widely throughout the network (Figure 4.7). Furthermore, the propagated pulse returns to the original site of the DBS pulse to resonate with subsequent DBS pulses (*see Chapter 6—Nervous System Responses to DBS*). Perhaps in the future

these resonance effects will be leveraged for more optimal DBS.

AXON DIAMETER

Neurons differ in how much electrical charge deposited by DBS is required to produce an action potential. Large-diameter axons require less electrical charge than small-diameter axons. DBS programming can exploit these differences. For example, the desired DBS therapeutic effect may require activating large-diameter axons, whereas activating medium-diameter axons causes unwanted side effects. DBS can be adjusted to activate only the larger-diameter axons without activating the medium-diameter axons. This differential response is accomplished as follows: Larger-diameter axons have a larger surface area, which means that more negative electrical charges can accumulate on the surface of the axon. This increased

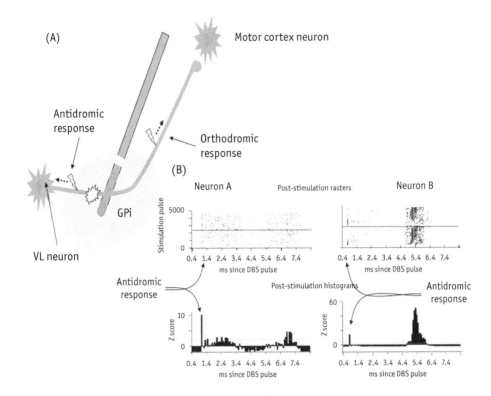

Figure 4.5: The consequences of initiating an action potential in axons passing near the DBS target. In this case, research has shown that DBS in the vicinity of the GPi activates axons from the Vop thalamus, causing antidromic activation of the thalamic neurons (Montgomery 2006) as shown in (A). Evidence for antidromic activation of two Vop neurons is shown in B. The top figures in B are post-stimulus rasters that show the discharge of the neurons in the 8 ms or so after each DBS pulse, which occurs at time 0. Each row represents the neuronal response to the DBS pulse, and each dot represents the discharge of the neuron. The responses in the rasters are then organized and summed in columns for increments of time to construct the histograms that show the average response over time after the DBS pulse.

The very short latency (about 1 ms) is highly consistent with an antidromic response (for further evidence of the antidromic response, see Montgomery 2006). The action potential generated in the axon of the thalamic neuron passing the near the GPi could be expected to result in an orthodromically conducted action potential, in addition to the antidromically conducted action potential. This orthodromically conducted action potential could then monosynaptically activate the motor-cortical (and other cortical) neurons, as shown in A.

All thalamic neurons recorded in this study show a reduction of reduced activity about 3.5 ms after the GPi DBS pulse (delivered at a high frequency), which is consistent with DBS activating the output axons of the GPi and not inhibiting the segment, as some current theories of DBS hold. Also striking for these two neurons and other thalamic neurons is the remarkable and robust increase in thalamic neuronal activity after the DBS-induced GPi inhibition. This post-hyperpolarization rebound activity is seen in both neurons. Neuron B displays two components of increased activity, including a very large later increase that is thought to reflect reentrant activity from the cortical neuron that was monosynaptically activated by action potentials generated in the thalamic neuronal axons passing near the DBS. The robust post-hyperpolarization rebound of increased excitability of the Vop neurons calls into question the basis for most current theories of basal ganglia physiology and pathophysiology (see Montgomery 2006).

charge results in a greater depolarization of the neuron and, therefore, a greater probability of generating an action potential. Thus, controlling the current flow within a volume of tissue allows control of how many and which axons will be activated. For an extensive view of electrophysiological responses to stimulation, see Ranck (Ranck 1975).

ELECTRODE CONFIGURATIONS

The volume, shape, and distribution of the electrical field created by the electrical current/voltage is very important. It is important to note that the volume of the electrical field generated by a DBS pulse is not the same as the volume of tissue activation. The electrical

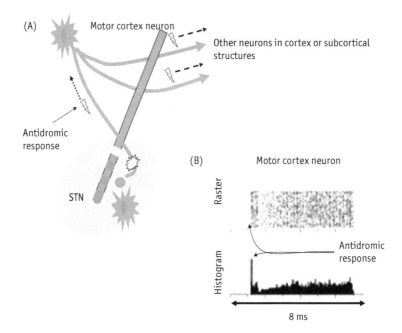

Figure 4.6: An example of the consequences of initiating an action potential in axons passing near the DBS target. In this case, research has shown that DBS in the vicinity of the STN antidromically activates axons from the cortex, which synapses in the STN (Montgomery and Gale 2008), as shown in A. The evidence for a motor-cortical neuron is shown in B. The top figure in B is the post-stimulus rasters that reveal the neuronal discharges of the neurons about 8 ms after each DBS pulse, which occurs at time 0. Each row represents the neuronal response to the DBS pulse, and each dot represents the discharge of the neuron. The responses in the rasters are then organized and summed in columns for increments of time to construct the histograms that show the average response over time after the DBS pulse. The very short latency (about 1 ms) is highly regular, as evidenced by the tall and narrow response at about 1 ms, which is consistent with an antidromic response. The action potential generated in the axon terminal of the motor-cortical neuron could be conducted antidromically towards the cortex. This action potential would then pass orthodromically down the collateral axons of the same neuron to the synapses on other neurons, either in the cortex, to other subcortical structures, or both. Thus, the effects of DBS in the vicinity of the STN are rapidly conducted widely throughout the brain, contrary to many theories of DBS that focus exclusively on local DBS effects (see Montgomery and Gale 2008).

---

fields are the spatial distributions of the current or flow of electrical charges. The volume, shape, and gradient or intensity of the electrical field can be greatly affected by the tissue resistivity and the configuration of active electrical contacts. "The volume of tissue activation" refers to the neural elements excited, such as generation of action potentials in axons within the volume of the electrical field. For example, a volume of the electrical field in which mostly large-diameter axons are contained will have a greater volume of tissue activation than the same volume of the electrical field containing only small-diameter axons. These principles can be exploited to provide DBS management of symptoms. Four electrical contacts on the typical DBS lead provide a large number of combinations of active contacts and, therefore, a large number of different fields of electrical current.

Generally, the combinations of active electrical charges can be divided into *monopolar* or *multipolar*, which are defined as the number and nature of active contacts within the DBS target. *Monopolar* refers to only negative contacts (cathodes) within the stimulated structure. The positive contact (anode) in the monopolar stimulation may be the IPG itself, which is typically placed under the skin over the chest. From an electrical standpoint, the positive contact on the pulse generator is an "infinite" distance from the negative contact in the brain; hence the stimulation of the brain can be considered as coming from a single electrical contact. *Multipolar* configurations have more than one active contact within the stimulated structure, and these necessarily include both negative and positive contacts. A bipolar configuration could have a single negative and a single positive contact

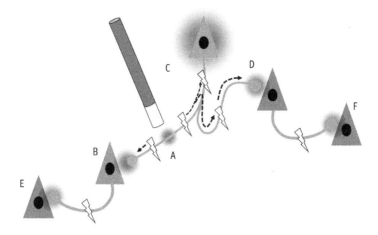

Figure 4.7: Schematic representation of how the effects of a DBS pulse can propagate widely beyond the local site of the DBS contact. The most likely effect of the DBS pulse is to generate action potentials in axons in the vicinity of the DBS active negative contact (cathode), as shown in A. The action potential can be propagated orthodromically to the next neuron in the chain of neurons that make up the network (B). At the same time, the action potential is conducted antidromically to the soma of the neuron from which the axon arose (C). If the axon has a collateral, the antidromic action potential can become an orthodromic potential at the branch point and go on to excite the next neuron in the chain of neurons that make up the network (D). If the temporal and spatial summations associated with the DBS pulse trains are sufficient, there may be propagation of action potentials further down the chain of neurons (E and F).

in the DBS target. The allowable combinations of negative and positive contacts may vary by manufacturer, and the reader is referred to the manufacturer's information.

The volume, intensity, shape, and distribution of the electrical current field are strongly influenced by the spatial relation between the negative and positive contacts and the nature of the brain tissue between them. With constant voltage IPGs, the volume and intensity of the electrical fields also depend on the impedance of the tissue between the negative and positive contacts. For both monopolar and multipolar configurations, the current flow is greatest next to the contacts and diminishes as the neural element is further away from the negative contact. However, in a monopolar configuration (Equation 4.1), the current flow falls off as the distance from the negative contact increases:

$$Electrical\ charge_{monopolar} \propto 1\,/\,r \qquad \textbf{Eq. 4.1}$$

where r is the distance of the neural element from the negative contact. Thus, doubling the distance from the contact halves the electrical current. However, for a bipolar configuration (Equation 4.2), electrical current is reduced by the square of the distance to the active contact, but is increased by the square of the distance between the negative and positive contacts:

$$Electrical\ charge_{bipolar} \propto d^2\,/\,r^2 \qquad \textbf{Eq. 4.2}$$

While the fact that the electrical charge increases with the distance between the anode and cathode (d) is counterintuitive, this fact has implications for the choice of DBS leads based on the spacing between electrodes. In order to maximize the intensity of the electrical field to ensure efficacy, one would want a DBS lead with widely separated contacts. On the other hand, wider spaced contacts make it more difficult to fine-tune the distribution of the electrical field in the long axis of the DBS lead that might be needed to minimize side effects. Of the two current available DBS leads, I prefer the lead with the wider spacing.

Often it is helpful to think of electrical fields as lines of electrical force that radiate out from the negative contact (Figure 4.8). In monopolar configurations, the lines of electrical force radiate outwards in all directions. In bipolar configurations, the lines of electrical force radiate out from the negative contact but are attracted to the positive contact. Thus, in

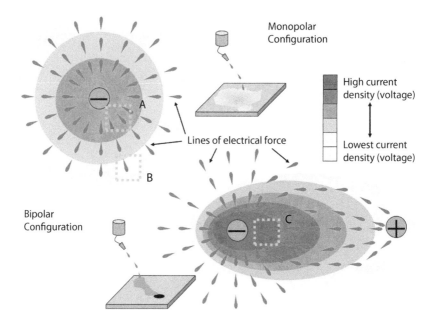

Monopolar
Configuration

High current
density (voltage)

Lowest current
density (voltage)

Lines of electrical force

Bipolar
Configuration

Figure 4.8: The *electrical field* can be pictured as lines of electrical forces emanating from the negative contact. In the case of monopolar stimulation (A), the lines of electrical force radiate out in all directions (B). In bipolar configurations (C), the lines of electrical force radiate from the negative contact but are attracted to or pulled in by the positive contact. Thus, the shape and spatial distributions of the electrical fields are different. The strength of the electrical field in any spatial location can be inferred from the lines of electrical forces traversing that volume (shown here as a box). In the case of monopolar stimulation, the intensity of the electric field is greater near the negative contact and rapidly diminishes as the box moves out. Figure C shows the hypothetical case of a wide bipolar configuration where there is a large distance between the cathode (negative) and anode (positive) contacts. Note that, as drawn, the intensities of the electric fields produced by widely separated negative and positive contacts (bipolar, figure C) are different that in monopolar (figure B). One could visualize this as the closer positive contact producing a greater attraction for the lines of electrical force emanating from the negative contact, thus bringing the lines of electrical force closer to the line connecting the negative and positive contacts.

bipolar configurations, the lines of electrical force are bent inwards.

One could represent the strength of the electrical fields by counting the number of lines of electrical force per unit volume (Figure 4.8). Thus, a box placed near the negative contact will have many more lines of electrical force than a box placed at a distance from the negative contact. In bipolar stimulation, the positive contact placed at a greater distance allows for more lines of electrical force at greater distances from a line connecting the negative and positive contacts compared to a closer positive contact. Thus, the intensity of the electrical fields a given distance from the negative contact will be less when the negative and positive contacts are adjacent

(narrow bipolar) than when they are separated (wide bipolar).

The equations indicate that the shapes of the electrical fields are different and depend on the configuration of the active electrodes. A hypothetical example is shown in Figure 4.9, which plots the relative intensities of the electrical fields as a function of distance from the negative contact and for the electrode configuration with one unit of electrical current/voltage (for example 1 milliamp or 1 volt). Consider the circumstance of a narrow bipolar stimulation where adjacent contacts are used, compared to when the negative and positive contacts are separated by one unused contact. For the same electrical current/voltage, the intensity of narrow bipolar stimulation is less than the wide

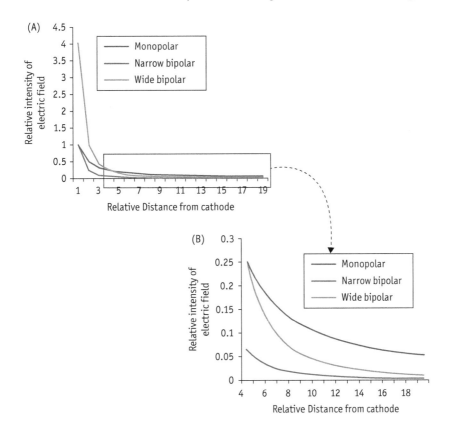

Figure 4.9: Hypothetical example of how the intensity of the electrical field decreases at increasing distances from the negative contact for monopolar, narrow bipolar (1 unit of separation between cathode and anode), and wide bipolar (2 units of separation) stimulation. The wide bipolar configuration provides the highest intensities near the negative contact (A), but the intensity falls off rapidly, such that at 4 units of distance, the intensity of the wide bipolar configuration is less than that of the monopolar configuration (the box in A is expanded in B). The narrow bipolar configuration produces the electrical field with the smallest volume and the least intensity.

bipolar configuration. The intensity of the electrical field falls off rapidly with bipolar stimulation. The intensity of monopolar stimulation closer to the negative contact is less, but it does not decrease as rapidly as the distance from the negative contact increases.

The effects of electrode configuration on electrical current are illustrated in Figure 4.8. The electrical charge from the negative contact flows to the positive contact. Imagine the flow of electrical charge as water flowing between the spigot (the negative contact) and the drain (the positive contact). For monopolar stimulation, the drain effectively is very far away. A different number of drains (positive anodes) in different configurations and relatively close to the spigot (the negative cathode) are analogous to multipolar stimulation. A bipolar

configuration is one in which there is a single spigot (a negative contact or cathode) and a single drain (a positive contact or anode) that are relatively close together.

An analogy of monopolar stimulation would be water flowing onto a table without a drain. The water would spread in all directions. The water would cover a large area but not to a great depth. The consequence would be activating larger-diameter axons at a large distance from the negative contact. However, the current would not be very high and would create a smaller charge density or electrical intensity (Figure 4.8). In a bipolar configuration, a drain would attract and focus the water, covering a smaller area but to a greater depth, which corresponds to a greater electrical charge density.

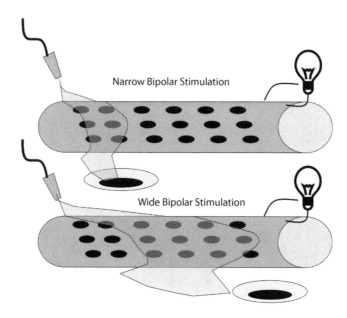

Figure 4.10: Heuristic device to remember the effects of wide versus narrow bipolar electrode configurations. With narrow bipolar, the anode (drain) is close to the cathode (spigot) so that most of the electrical current (water) flows into the anode (drain) with relatively less current (water) to activate neurons compared to the wide bipolar electrode configuration.

The analogy of flowing water to the flow of electrical current also helps illustrate why wide bipolar stimulation generates more intense, and therefore more effective, activation of axons (Figure 4.10). Water and electrical charges will be attracted to the drain, and electrical charges going down the drain rather than through the neuronal membrane will reduce the effects of electrical charge on the neuronal membrane necessary to activate the axon. When the drain or positive contact is near the spout or negative contact, such as in a narrow bipolar configuration, more water or electrical charge will go into the drain or positive contact than can get onto the neuronal membrane. When the drain or positive contact is further from the spout or negative contact, as it is in a wide bipolar configuration, more electrical charge will be applied to the neuronal membrane to activate the axon.

CURRENT INTENSITY IN MONOPOLAR AND BIPOLAR ELECTRODE CONFIGURATIONS

As described above, the strength of the electrical field diminishes as the distance from the negative contact increases. However, the strength falls off more rapidly

in bipolar stimulation than in monopolar stimulation. For example, the strength of the electrical field created by monopolar stimulation is reduced by one-half at a distance 1 mm from the negative contact, but that created by bipolar stimulation is reduced by one-quarter at a distance 1 mm from the negative contact. However, the strength of the electrical field created by bipolar configurations increases by the square of the distance between contacts. Thus, wide bipolar configurations generate a more intense electrical field close to the negative contact than do narrow bipolar configurations. Narrow bipolar configurations will generate a stronger electrical field than will monopolar stimulation. The monopolar stimulation will create a larger but less intense electrical field.

The differences in shape, size, and intensities generated by the different electrode configurations can be exploited to maximize the efficacy and minimize side effects of DBS. For example, monopolar stimulation of electrodes too close to the internal capsule, medial lemniscus, optic tract, or oculomotor fibers increases the chance of the electrical charge's reaching and activating axons in these structures, causing adverse effects.

Suppose that the therapeutic effect depends on the number of activated large axons (Figure 4.11A). In this case, monopolar stimulation at a current/voltage low enough not to stimulate axons in the internal capsule activates only two axons in the STN or GPi. Increasing the current/voltage increases both the size and the intensity of the electrical field (Figure 4.11B), increasing the number of axons activated in the STN or GPi to three, thereby increasing efficacy. However, higher-current/voltage monopolar stimulation would activate axons in the internal capsule, producing unwanted muscle contractions. In this case, changing to a wide bipolar configuration (Figure 4.11C) activates more axons (three) in the STN or GPi,

increasing efficacy but without activating the axons in the internal capsule that cause muscle contractions.

Why not use wide bipolar stimulation all the time? Consider the example where the electrode is not too close to the internal capsule (Figure 4.11D). Monopolar stimulation would activate more (four) axons in the STN or GPi, rather than only the three axons activated by the wide bipolar configuration.

Another example where the electrode configurations can be set to conform the volume of the electrical field to the regional anatomy is shown in Figure 4.12. In this hypothetical case, the DBS lead is placed too

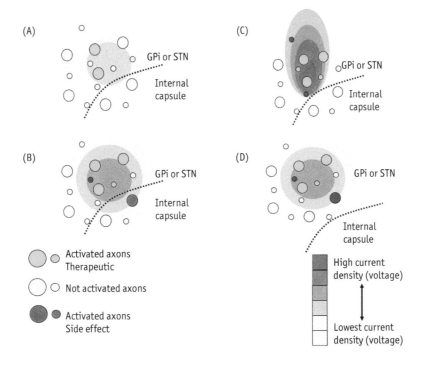

Figure 4.11: The differential effects of monopolar and bipolar stimulation. Here, effectiveness is determined by the number of axons activated within the STN or GPi, and side effects are caused by activation of axons in the internal capsule. Examples A, B, C, and D show the DBS electrode too close to the internal capsule. Stimulation spreading to the internal capsule would result in unwanted muscle contractions. Lower-current/voltage monopolar stimulation would not activate axons in the internal capsule but would be less effective because it activates only two representative axons (A). Increasing the current/voltage would increase the spread and intensity of the electrical field, thereby increasing effectiveness by activating three axons in the STN or GPi (B). However, this increase also activates the internal capsule, causing muscle contractions. Switching to a wide bipolar configuration creates a smaller but more intense electrical field. Consequently, no axons are activated within the internal capsule and, therefore, there are no side effects (C). In addition, effectiveness is greater because three representative axons are activated in the STN or GPi. However, wide bipolar stimulation is not always the most effective. For example, when the cathode (negative) contact in the DBS lead is further away from the internal capsule, monopolar stimulation activates more axons, in this case four representative axons in the STN or GPi, without activating axons in the internal capsule, thereby avoiding the side effect of muscle contractions (C). Figure D shows the effects of using the smaller current/voltage as shown in A, but with a longer pulse width, which results in more axons in the target being activated but no axons in the internal capsule being activated. However, a wider pulse width will increase the rate at which electrical charge is removed from the battery.

deep (ventrally) where the volume of the electrical field encroaches on the optic tract. Stimulation through the most ventral lead in a monopolar configuration leads to *phosphenes*. Similarly, the DBS lead is too posterior such that the volume of the electrical field spills over onto the posterior limb of the internal capsule. One could raise the negative contact (cathode) upward to the ventral contact, for example. The volume of the electrical field does not affect the optic tract. However, because the long axis of the DBS lead is running parallel to the posterior limb of the internal capsule, even raising the monopolar electrical field up the DBS lead will not escape stimulation of the posterior limb of the internal capsule, risking intolerable tonic muscle contractions that could limit DBS therapy. Alternatively, one could stimulate in a wide bipolar configuration that would narrow the volume of the electrical field to avoid both the optic tract and the posterior limb of the internal capsule.

The key concept is that the volume, shape, and intensity of the electrical fields can be tailored to the patient's unique anatomy relative to the location of the DBS electrodes. Controlling the size, shape, and intensity of the electrical fields allows you to maximize benefit and minimize side effects. Figures 4.13, 4.14, and 4.15, show various monopolar and bipolar configurations. By carefully selecting electrode configurations, currents/voltages, and pulse widths, you can control which regions of the anatomy surrounding the DBS negative contact are excited. Conceptually, this situation is no different than selecting a particular formulation of levodopa, such as immediate-release or controlled—or extended-release carbidopa-levodopa for Parkinson's disease. Different doses of levodopa in the carbidopa-levodopa preparation are analogous to the current/voltage used in DBS. Similarly, the use of multipolar configurations to constrain the size and shape of the electrical fields to control the regions affected is analogous to the adjunctive use of carbidopa to restrict the actions of levodopa to the brain, rather than to involve the rest of the body. Another useful analogy is the use of dopamine agonists with varying degrees of specificity to the D_1 and D_2 receptors, which is conceptually similar to the use

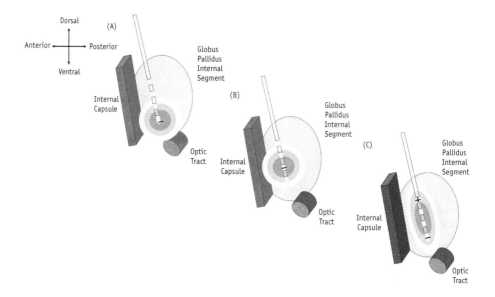

Figure 4.12: Schematic representation of a situation where the DBS lead is placed too deep (ventrally) and posteriorly in the GPi. Monopolar stimulation through the most ventral contact stimulates the optic tract, producing phosphenes, and the posterior limb of the internal capsule, producing tonic muscle contraction (A). Raising the volume of the electrical field dorsally, such as by monopolar stimulation through the ventral contact, avoids stimulation of the optic tract but continues to stimulate the posterior limb of the internal capsule (B). However, wide bipolar stimulation narrows and shortens the volume of the electrical field, thus avoiding both the optic track and the posterior limb of the internal capsule, and still stimulating sufficient GPi to provide clinical benefit.

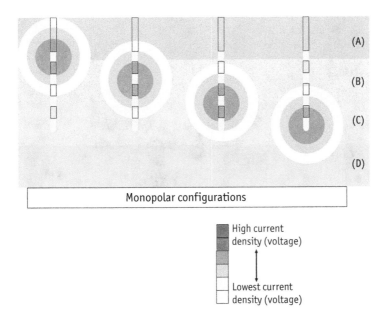

Figure 4.13: Schematic examples of relative distributions of electrical fields generated by various configurations of monopolar stimulation in the vertical direction (long axis of the DBS lead).

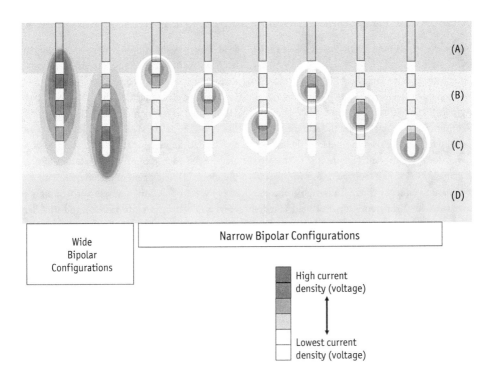

Figure 4.14: Schematic examples of relative distributions of electrical fields generated by various configurations of bipolar stimulation in the vertical direction (long axis of the DBS lead).

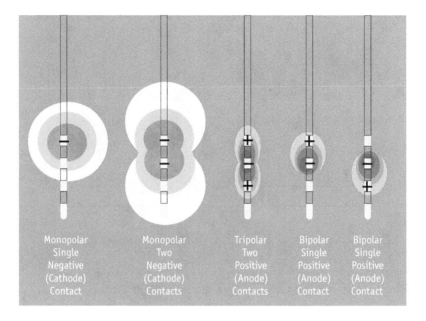

| Monopolar Single Negative (Cathode) Contact | Monopolar Two Negative (Cathode) Contacts | Tripolar Two Positive (Anode) Contacts | Bipolar Single Positive (Anode) Contact | Bipolar Single Positive (Anode) Contact |

Figure 4.15: The variety of electrical fields that can be created by multiple active contacts. Some situations may require unusual electrode configurations. For example, where greater therapeutic efficacy is needed, multiple active negative contacts can be used to generate larger electrical fields, as long as the electrical current does not spread to structures where axon activation is undesirable. The tripolar configuration can greatly restrict the horizontal spread of the electrical field to prevent side effects.

of pulse widths and currents/voltages to select axons of different sizes.

Two commercially available IPGs provide for nearly simultaneous delivery to two stimulus trains (called *groups*). The two trains have the same frequency but are offset (*phase delay*) so that the stimulus pulse in one group follows the stimulus pulse of the second group and does not overlap (Figure 4.16). The two groups can vary in current/voltage, pulse width, and polarity, but not frequency (rate). Thus each group can be associated with a different electrical field (Figure 4.16). Theoretically, the two groups could give an effective electrical field that is some combination of the two (Figure 4.16). This could be an advantage in shaping the electrical field for greater efficacy and fewer adverse effects. For example, the stimulation through the most ventral lead produces the greatest efficacy but greater adverse effects. In this case, the electrical field generated around the most ventral contact would have to be small. Stimulation through a more dorsal contact could be effective, but less so than stimulation through the most ventral contact, but it is also associated with fewer adverse effects and thus could have a larger electrical

field. It is possible that a synergistic combination of both fields could further increase the efficacy without increasing the adverse effects.

It is not clear that the phase delays between the DBS pulses of each group are such that the effects of the two groups are synergistic, resulting in an effective field, or rather that the effects are just those associated with each group. Hypothetically, if neither of the electrical fields generated independently by each set of electrode configurations and stimulus parameters is effective, and if the interleaved stimulation by both sets are not synergistic, then there may not be any value in combining them. Although the time of the phase delay is likely to be quite small (depending on the DBS frequency, with the delay between the two interleaved pulses equal to one-half of the time between two successive pulses of one group), it is unclear whether it is short enough to allow a synergistic effect. For example, DBS at 100 pps may not be effective, whereas DBS at 130 pps may be. Thus, the time difference in the inter-stimulus interval between the 100 pps and 130 pps DBS is approximately 2.3 ms, and this is enough to make a therapeutic difference.

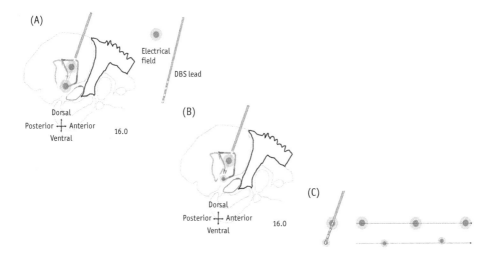

Figure 4.16: Schematic representation of DBS lead that is too posterior in the ventral intermediate nucleus of the thalamus. In this case, stimulation through the most ventral contact produced intolerable paresthesias because of the proximity to Vc posteriorly. Stimulation through the most dorsal contact did not produce paresthesias; however, alone it did not provide sufficient relief of tremor (A). One option is to apply a smaller stimulation current through the most ventral contact so as to reduce the volume of tissue activation that would affect Vc, in addition to a higher stimulation current through the most dorsal contact (B). Thus, while each active negative contact (cathode) alone fails to provide sufficient clinical benefit, the combination has a synergistic effect that is sufficient. In one commercially available system, the two different negative contacts (cathodes) operate as two independent pulse trains with the same frequency but different stimulation currents. The two pulse trains are combined into an interleaved single pulse train where each set of pulses alternates. Note that the pulse in one contact is delivered halfway between a pair of pulses in the other contact. Thus, the phase delay is 50% of the interval between pulses on one contact. The delay will vary based on the overall frequency of DBS. Note: in some commercially available systems, the maximum DBS frequency is less than when no interleaved stimulation is used and may not be optimal.

There also is the concern that the electrical fields generated by each group could overlap. This could cause a potentially dangerous additive charge density, particularly at long pulse widths. Consequently, the manufacturer limits the frequency to 125 pps. The rationale for limiting the maximum frequency in the interleaved mode to 125 pps is unclear. It is not clear how effective such limitations will be, in that clinical studies demonstrate many patients requiring higher DBS frequencies (rates). Furthermore, neurons in the overlapping area theoretically could be subject to DBS at twice the frequency (rate) as neurons in the non-overlapping area. At the time of publication of this monograph, there was insufficient evidence known to the author regarding the potential additive effect of the two different groups; whether the effects would be any different than either group given alone and what advantages this would have clinically.

The discussions above evidence the value of being able to sculpt the electrical field, and in large part this ability is related to the physical structure of the electrodes and the ability to deliver varying electrical currents to the electrodes. Currently, commercially available DBS leads use a linear array of electrodes that wrap around the full circumference of the lead shaft. While having these electrodes at different lengths along the long axis of the lead allows one to move the electrical field up and down the shaft of the lead, this arrangement does not allow directing the electrical field in a restricted direction in the plane orthogonal to the long axis of the DBS electrode array. In other words, controlling the electrical field in front, back, medial, or lateral to the DBS lead is problematic. A segmented electrode that was only a part of the circumference would allow for better directional specificity (*see Supplementary essay—The Ideal DBS System, at http://www.greenvilleneuromodulationcenter. com/DBS_Programming_essays/).

Monopolar and bipolar stimulations are the most commonly used. However, in other circumstances,

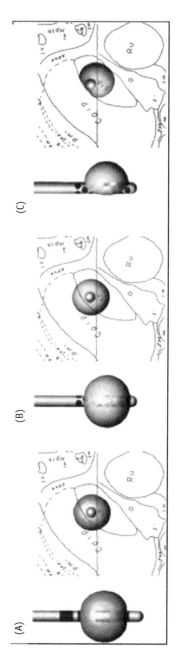

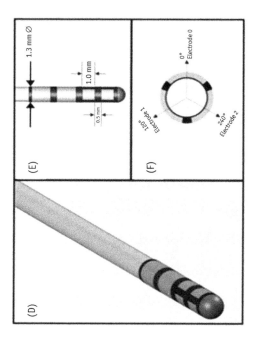

Figure 4.17: Schematic representations of two types of segmented DBS leads whose use in human studies have been reported: A–C (Contarino et al. 2014) and D–F (Pollo et al. 2014). Figure A shows a typical, currently available, unsegmented DBS lead. Figures B and C show another lead that consists solely of segments that lack any continuous circumferential contact. As shown in B, however, the active negative contacts (cathodes) may be configured to approximate a continuous circumferential contact. Figures D, E, and F show a DBS lead whose two upper circumferential contacts are unsegmented and whose bottom two circumferential contacts are segmented.

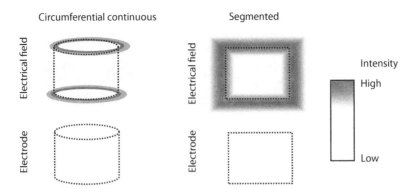

Figure 4.18: Schematic representation of "edge effects" where the stimulation intensity is greater at the edges of the electrical contact. As can be seen, the number of edges in the cylindrical, circumferentially continuous contact is less than that of the segmented contact and consequently may have fewer "edge effects." These edge effects may complicate the selection of active contacts. One must take into consideration that it is the edge of the segmented contact that will determine the response and not the center of the contact. Further, the edge effects that are greater with segmented DBS leads could add when multiple segmented contacts are active, raising safety concerns.

multiple negative contacts or tripolar configurations are needed because of their unique shapes and spatial orientations (Figure 4.15). The principles determining the shape, size, orientation, and intensities for these configurations are the same principles as described above for monopolar and bipolar configurations (Equation 4.3). For example, for tripolar configurations, the intensity of the electrical field falls off as the cube (power of 3) of the distance from the negative contact, as described below.

$$Electrical\,charge_{bipolar} \propto d^2 / r^3 \qquad \text{Eq. 4.3}$$

SEGMENTED DBS LEADS

It is anticipated that soon new types of DBS lead architectures will become commercially available. The currently available DBS leads have electrical contacts that are continuous around the circumference of the long axis of the DBS lead—like a ring. New DBS leads may divide the continuous contact into segments of smaller contacts (Figure 4.17). The availability of segmented DBS leads will be a boon to patients. While the current DBS leads allows for control of the spatial distribution along the long axis of the DBS lead, there is no selectivity in the plane orthogonal to the long axis of the DBS lead. For patients in whom the DBS lead is too close to a structure whose stimulation

produces adverse effects, finding electrode configurations, stimulation parameters, and pulse trains that produce sufficient benefit without intolerable adverse effects often is difficult and may even be unattainable. The ability to focus the electrical field away from the structure that when stimulated produces adverse effects may make all the difference between a successful outcome and failure.

A potential concern with segmented DBS leads is the possibility of "edge effects" on the stimulus intensity (Kim et al. 1990) (Figure 4.18). The intensities at the edges of an electrical contact are greater than over the center of the electrical contact. The concern is that the segmented DBS contacts could increase the "edge effects," with the potential of exceeding the safety limits on the stimulation current at the edges.

The consequence will be a tremendous increase in the electrode configurations that will be available and potentially overwhelming for the programmer. The hope is that automated assistive DBS programming devices or algorithms will be available to offload some of the complexity from the DBS programmer. However, the development of such automated assisted DBS programming systems is very problematic (*see Supplemental essay—Automated Assisted DBS Programming* at http://www.greenvilleneuromodulationcenter.com/DBS_Programming_essays/). Nonetheless, the principles outlined in this chapter still apply, and the programmer's sound knowledge and understanding should make the use of segmented DBS leads efficacious.

Once segmented DBS leads are available, there is a compelling argument to use them. Even if in the majority of instances, the circumferentially continuous contacts, such as those currently available, are sufficient, one cannot know ahead of time whether a particular patient is going to be in the majority for whom the continuous circumferential contacts would be sufficient, or in the minority in which successful DBS critically depends on the segmented lead. The position of only using the segmented lead in the circumstance of a failed DBS lead due to continuous circumferential contacts would mean subjecting the patient to an entire additional DBS lead-implantation surgery with its attendant risks and costs.

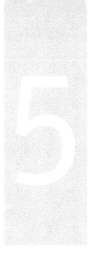

DBS SAFETY

THE RANGE OF SAFETY CONCERNS

DBS is not just about passing electrical current charges into the brain; rather, DBS is integrated into a complex ecological system that involves not only electricity but medications, biologics, rehabilitation, and a range of human issues including ethics, psychology, sociology--indeed, the full gamut of human activities. Furthermore, these human activities of concern include not only the patient and the patient's family members, caregivers, and friends, but also physicians and healthcare professionals (Montgomery 2015b). Space and time limit the excursion here into these issues. The focus necessarily falls on issues directly related to DBS.

INJURY SECONDARY TO ELECTRICITY

Excessive electrical charges can damage tissue. The safety limit typically is defined as the *charge density*, which is the amount of electrical charge delivered, divided by the surface area of the electrical contact. The generally accepted safety limit is 30 $\mu C/cm^2/$phase. *Microcoulombs* are the number of units of electrical charge administered into the brain, and *cm^2* is to the surface area of the active electrical contacts. *Phase* refers to the negative (cathodal) and positive (anodal) phases of an individual DBS pulse (Figure 5.1). The phase is the part of the DBS pulse associated with one polarity of electrical current. The negative (cathodal) phase is associated with negative electrical charges flowing out of the electrical contact. A positive (anodal) phase is associated with negative electrical charges flowing into the contact. The negative (cathodal) and positive (anodal) phases of the individual DBS pulse should not be confused with the negative (cathode) and positive (anode) electrical contacts (see below). The difference in the neurophysiological (and hence clinical) effect between the negative and positive contacts is that the height of the negative (cathodal) current at the negative contact in the first phase is sufficient to activate axons, whereas that during the second (anodal) phase at the positive contact it is not.

The *electrical charge density* is the total charge per pulse divided by the surface area of the active DBS contact. The *total charge* is the current times the pulse width. The *current* is the voltage divided by the impedance. Thus, a 10-volt DBS pulse through a contact with 1000 ohms of resistance for a pulse width of 90 μs delivered through a DBS contact that is 1.5 mm (0.015 cm) in length and 1.2 mm (0.012 cm) in diameter results in a charge density of 1.86 microcoulombs/$cm^2/$phase, where the phase is the pulse width in seconds.

For current commercially available IPGs, the two phases of the DBS pulse differ in the height and duration of electrical current/voltage (see Figure 5.1). Programmers should consult the manufacturer

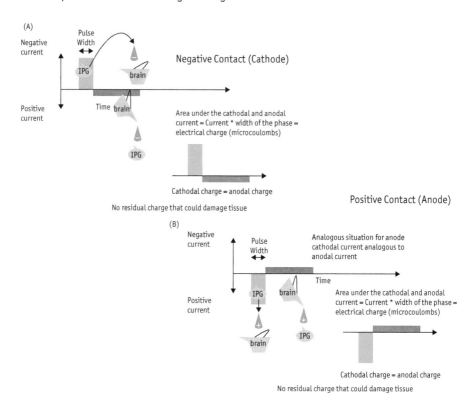

Figure 5.1: Waveforms of individual DBS pulses illustrating the distinction between a negative (cathode) contact and negative (cathodal) current or phase, and the similar distinction between a positive contact and positive (anodal) current or phases of electrical current administered into the brain with each DBS pulse. The distinction is important. Note that both contacts that are designated the cathode (negative) and anode (positive) contacts pass both negative and positive electrical current. The naming convention of the contacts is based on the initial phase or component of the stimulus waveform. A shows the situation for a cathode (negative) contact where negative current is going from the IPG into the brain during the first phase. During the second phase, negative current is going from the brain back into the IPG. Alternatively, considered from the standpoint of the brain, this is a positive current going into the brain counterbalancing the initial or first phase of the DBS pulse. B shows the configuration where the contact is an anode (positive) contact because the first phase of the DBS pulse can be considered a relatively positive current. The second phase would be an negative current. Note that this is the circumstance of B with the commercial IPGs available at the time of publication—this arrangement requires a bipolar configuration, as the IPG cannot act as a cathode (negative) contact nor can it act as an anode (positive) contact if one of the DBS lead contact(s) acts as an anode (positive) contact. Also note, the area under each phase is the same. The initial phase, either cathodal (negative) or anodal (positive) contacts, has a higher electrical current but a briefer duration than the following phase with reversed current. However, the same amount of electrical charge administered during the first phase is returned during the second phase.

regarding the specific IPG used. In some IPGs, the initial phase is higher, meaning that a greater intensity of electrical current/voltage is applied, but for a briefer period than in the second phase. However, the area under the curve for each phase of the individual DBS pulse is the same. This equality means that the total amount of charge administered during the first phase by the negative (cathodal) current is taken back in by the second positive (anodal) phase. An imbalance in the area under the curve, representing a

surplus of electrical charge on the neural membrane, can damage brain tissue. Some IPGs available at the time of publication are capable of cycling mode stimulation wherein the DBS stimulation train is turned on for a defined period of time and then turned off for a defined period of time. For some IPGs, cycling mode stimulation could cause a charge imbalance that could be sufficient to cause brain injury. You should check with the manufacturer regarding cycling mode stimulation.

Tissue can be damaged through *electrolysis*, in which water molecules are broken down into hydrogen and oxygen gas bubbles. Fortunately, this process is reversible, so that when the current reverses between the first and second phases of each DBS pulse, the hydrogen and oxygen bubbles recombine to form water. However, if bubbles accumulate, they can tear and damage tissue. Residual electrical charges resulting from charge imbalances, as described above, can result in marked bubble formation and possibly tissue damage.

Another way that DBS can damage the brain is by the heat generated when electrical current is passed through the brain. Passing electrical current through a conductor with resistance (or impedance in the case of DBS), generates heat. The more electrical current that passes through the impedance of brain tissue, the higher the risk of overheating and tissue damage. Factors related to the risk of heat damage include increases in voltage, pulse width, and the rate that pulses are delivered (DBS frequency).

The safety of electrical stimulation is directly related to the electrical current density, which is determined by the amount of administered electrical charge and the surface area of the cathode. For the same voltage, as provided by constant voltage IPGs, multiple cathodes reduce impedance, increasing the current that is administered into the tissue. Counterbalancing the decrease in the impedance is the greater surface area offered by multiple cathodes, which decreases current density. However, this decrease is non-linear, so that halving the impedance does not counterbalance doubling the surface area. Also, all contacts and the IPG case can act as either cathodes or anodes. Thus, a contact designated as the "anode" in one electrode configuration during programming becomes a "cathode" during the second DBS phase.

When the IPG case is the anode in the electrode configuration, its large surface area is likely to more than compensate for any reduction in therapeutic impedance. However, the same is not true for the DBS lead anode in bipolar electrode configurations. The larger electrical charge administered from multiple cathodes during the first phase becomes the cathodal current administered into the brain through the anode during the second phase. If there are fewer designated anodes than cathodes, the current densities at the designated anodes can be higher than anticipated. For example, consider the electrode configuration where there are two cathodes (negative contacts) and a single anode

(positive contact) that is on the DBS lead rather than the IPG case. During the first and second phases of the DBS pulse, current will be flowing out of and then into two cathodes. The electrical charge delivered at the two cathodes (negative contacts) will be diluted by the doubling of the surface area because two contacts are used. However, that same amount of current that flows out of and then into the two cathodes (negative contacts) must flow in and then out of the single contact, and the charge density at the anode (positive contact) will be twice that at the two cathodes (negative contacts). This could be a serious problem if the using the multiple cathodes (negative contacts) significantly reduced the impedance. In the situation where the IPG case is used as the anode (positive contact), the large surface area would greatly reduce the charge densities.

Many IPGs may have built-in safety warnings. Some commercially available IPGs make assumptions about the impedance of the electrode configurations when calculating the electrical current to be administered into the brain. Some IPGs assume that the impedance is 500 ohms. *If the actual impedance is less than 500 ohms, harmful stimulation may occur before the warning is given.* If the impedance is substantially higher than 500 ohms, the warning may be expected but false, and you may decide not to use parameters that would benefit the patient. *You should review the appropriate manufacturer manuals for the IPG you are using.*

Some IPGs allow the patient or caregiver to change certain DBS stimulation variables, such as voltage. However, these IPGs may not warn the patient or caregiver if the safe stimulation level is exceeded when the patient or caregiver modifies the stimulation parameters. Usually the professional programming device will provide a warning when the limits of the allowable patient or caregiver-controllable parameters are programmed. However, this is based on assumed impedances that may or may not be accurate (see preceding discussion). Consequently, you should always determine the upper limit of the stimulation variable that the patient can use safely, and limit the patient's ability to exceed those limits. Review the appropriate operation and safety manuals of the systems you use, and when in doubt, consult the manufacturer.

MEDICAL COMPLICATIONS

DBS acts in synergy with other treatments, such as medications. Indeed, much of the post-operative care involves establishing an optimal synergy, which requires expert knowledge not only of DBS but of the other treatments as well. Ethical concerns arise when persons assume responsibility for post-operative DBS management who do not have a reasonable understanding of the other therapies.

Synergies between DBS and other treatments, particularly medications, have both a positive and negative side. For example, for patients with Parkinson's disease and a history or risk of dyskinesia, STN DBS can exacerbate the dyskinesia. Fortunately, reduction of medications with optimal DBS can reduce the dyskinesias. However, the reduction in medication renders the patient more dependent on the DBS for control of symptoms. Should there be a sudden uncontrolled failure of the DBS system, the patient may experience a sudden and potentially severe worsening of their symptoms. In the case of patients with Parkinson's disease who are at risk for a neuroleptic malignant-like syndrome with sudden discontinuation of dopaminergic medications, there have been concerns regarding possible neuroleptic malignant-like syndromes associated with sudden discontinuation of DBS.

ADVERSE EFFECTS RELATED TO ACTIVATION OF NEURAL NETWORKS

The neurophysiological effects of DBS relate to the generation of action potentials in axons in the vicinity of the active negative contacts (cathodes). Note, in many cases axons just passing by the active negative DBS contact (cathode) with no specific neurophysiological relationship to the intended DBS target may be activated. That is why it is a mistake to talk about DBS of a specific target such as the STN. Rather, the more appropriate description is DBS "in the vicinity of" the DBS target, such as the STN. Discrimination among axons in which action potentials are generated within the volume of the electrical field depends on factors such as pulse width, stimulation intensity, the direction of lines of electrical force, and frequency affecting reentry resonance. Thus, there are potential safety issues based on a prior knowledge of the physiology and pathophysiology of the DBS target and its surrounding regional anatomy, but there also are safety issues with unintended activations. Many are

relatively easy to associate with DBS; some are not. Of particular concern are psychological and psychiatric complications that make take considerable time to manifest and more time to be recognized.

It is critical not to dismiss any complaint of an adverse effect out of hand or because these complaints have not been encountered in prior experience. There is still much about DBS that is unknown or unclear. These complaints should be investigated with an open mind by those responsible for the patient's post-operative care. While it is clear that rapid decline of post-mortem human studies (autopsies) has led to the concern that "we are burying our mistakes," another way to bury them is to ignore them. It is important to note that the term "mistake" is not pejorative, nor an accusation of malfeasance, but it does imply a responsibility to learn from DBS complications so as to avoid them in the future.

THE POTENTIAL PSYCHOSOCIAL CONSEQUENCES OF DBS

After years of disability and dependence, patients experiencing the often dramatic and relatively rapid improvements in their neurological disabilities may become distressed (Schüpbach, Gargiulo et al. 2006). Such distress is related not only to the mood changes that can accompany successful DBS treatment, but also to their effect on the personal relationships between patient and family. The psychological and sociological adaptations to the patient's disease may suddenly become maladaptive when the patient has greater functioning and perhaps independence. In my experience, this phenomenon is not unique to patients with neurological disorders who have been treated with DBS. It also occurs in patients treated with levodopa and, indeed, in many instances in which chronic dependence is suddenly relieved by effective therapy.

These psychosocial stresses are difficult to predict but, fortunately, are not frequent. However, they can be catastrophic, so you need to anticipate them and monitor the patient closely. Often, establishing a rapport and familiarity with the patient and caregivers through frequent and unhurried contact over time can help you detect these stresses early.

6

NERVOUS SYSTEM RESPONSES TO DBS

The technology related to DBS has advanced considerably. DBS implanted pulse generators (IPGs) have greatly increased their capabilities, providing opportunities for different combinations of DBS pulses and stimulation trains. On-demand or closed-loop DBS pulse generators may soon be available. Yet therein lies a dilemma. An increase in technical capabilities increases the degrees of freedom, or number of controlling variables, for therapeutic stimulation. In other words, the various types of DBS that may be possible will increase exponentially, leading to a bewildering and potentially befuddling number of possibilities to consider. For example, the modest recent advances in DBS technology employing constant current and partitioning stimulation of multiple electrical contacts have not translated to any change in typical practice in order to take advantage of the technology.

A growing need to reduce the range of DBS options to a manageable number makes itself felt in the face of the growing range of options and functionality. The range of options presently on hand makes it unlikely that any effective and efficient DBS programming algorithm will rest purely on empirical observation. In other words, randomized controlled trials (RCTs) of every possible combination of electrode configurations, stimulation parameters, and pulse trains is infeasible. The best hope for effective and efficient stimulation lies with an understanding of DBS's therapeutic mechanisms of action on which to base any such algorithm. There do exist algorithmic approaches that lend themselves to a type of automation, but these are primarily anatomical. As such, they lie some distance from the meaningful controlling variable: physiology. This latter issue will be taken up in the *Supplemental essay, Automated Assisted DBS Programming at http://www.greenvilleneuromodulationcenter.com/DBS_Programming_essays/.*

KNOWLEDGE OF NERVOUS SYSTEM RESPONSES VERSUS KNOWLEDGE OF THERAPEUTIC MECHANISMS

A growing body of remarkable research has demonstrated a range of neuronal responses to DBS. Yet though the catalogue of nervous system responses has increased, there has resulted no increased insight into those responses productive of DBS's therapeutic effect, which would thus recommend themselves as targets for greatest clinical benefit. This situation owes in part to some confusion about the nature of nervous system responses and how to investigate them. And it perhaps owes in larger part to confusion about what the therapeutic effects ought to be. In other words, the state of knowledge is currently such that it remains entirely unknown what it is that DBS is supposed to correct at the neuronal level. This confusion is addressed in Chapter 8, Pathophysiological Mechanisms.

This chapter catalogues the various responses of neuronal elements to a DBS pulse. The basics

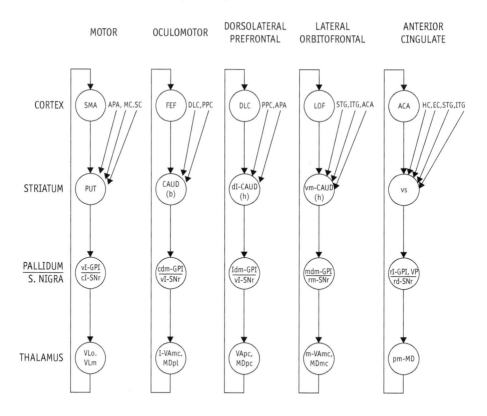

Figure 6.1: Parallel organization of the five basal ganglia–thalamocortical circuits. Each circuit engages specific regions of the cerebral cortex: striatum, pallidum, substantia nigra, and thalamus. *Abbreviations* are as follows: ACA: anterior cingulate area; APA: arcuate premotor area; CAUD: caudate, (b) body (h) head; DLC: dorsolateral prefrontal cortex; EC: entorhinal cortex; FEF: frontal eye fields; GPi: internal segment of globus pallidus; HC: hippocampal cortex; ITG: inferior temporal gyrus; LOF: lateral orbitofrontal cortex; MC: motor cortex; MDpl: medialis dorsalis pars paralamellaris; MDmc: medialis dorsalis pars magnocellularis; MDpc: medialis dorsalis pars parvocellularis; PPC: posterior parietal cortex; PUT: putamen; SC: somatosensory cortex; SNr: substantia nigra pars reticulata; STG: superior temporal gyrus; V Amc: ventralis anterior pars magnocellularis; Vapc: ventralis anterior pars parvocellularis; VLm: ventralis lateralis pars medialis; VLo: ventralis lateralis pars oralis; VP: ventral pallidum; VS: ventral striatum; cl-: caudolateral; cdm-: caudal dorsomedial; dl-: dorsolateral; l-: lateral; ldm-: lateral dorsomedial; m-: medial; mdm-: medial dorsomedial; pm: postero-medial; rd-: rostrodorsal; rl-: rostrolateral; rm-: rostromedial; vm-: ventromedial; vl-: ventrolateral.
Verbatim from Alexander et al. 1986, page 364.

of neuronal electroneurophysiology and electrical stimulation are reviewed in Chapter 2, Principles of DBS Electronics, and Chapter 3, Principles of Electrophysiology, which focus primarily on generation of action potentials in axons of neurons and action-potential-initiating segments of neuronal cell bodies located in the vicinity of a DBS electrode.

Chapter 7, DBS Effects on Motor Control, discusses the effects of DBS on motor control, particularly in movement disorders. And it does so in light of the realization that the range of future clinical applications for DBS is likely to extend beyond the treatment

of movement disorders. Nonetheless, a detailed discussion of the effects of DBS on motor control is valuable because it stands as a metaphor for investigations of indications beyond movement disorders. One reason for optimism is that by considering the anatomy through which DBS-generated action potentials percolate, one may arrive at an understanding of DBS effects on motor control of patients with Parkinson's disease and other movement disorders (Figure 6.1). There is remarkable similarity among different functional domains served by the same anatomical architecture. Anatomical architecture probably influences to some degree nervous system responses to DBS, thus also influencing potential therapeutic mechanisms.

The responses of neuronal elements is probably due to the introduction of negative (cathodal) rather than positive (anodal) electrical charges (current) to a neuronal element's membrane electrical (*see Chapter 3—Principles of Electrophysiology*). This is demonstrated in an isolated neuron preparation (Ranck 1975). Furthermore, experience in postoperative programming has shown this author that the majority of effects—adverse effects related to unintended stimulation of structures in the vicinity of DBS, for example—directly relate to the higher-voltage cathode or negative stimulation, typically in the first phase of the DBS pulse. This is evidenced by the fact that reversal of bipolar stimulation's polarity creates quite different behavioral effects. In the case of DBS, having as the negative contact (cathode) the ventral-most contact closest to the medial lemniscus in the vicinity of the STN and the dorsal-most contact as the positive contact (anode) in bipolar stimulation may produce paresthesias. Yet, when the polarity is reversed, the ventral-most contact becoming the positive contact (anode) and the dorsal-most contact the negative contact (cathode), paresthesias may not result. Clearly, passing negative (cathodal) current through the ventral-most contact does not produce the same effect as does passing same electrical charges as positive (anodal) current.

EFFECTS MEDIATED BY VOLTAGE-GATED IONIC CONDUCTANCE CHANNELS IN THE NEURONAL MEMBRANE

Introduction of electrical charges in the vicinity of various neuronal elements changes the membrane electrical potential (*see Chapter 3—Principles of Electrophysiology*). These changes in turn affect conductance of electrical charges in the form of ions through the neuronal membrane. Thus, the distribution of voltage-gated ionic conductance channels is likely to have a large effect on the neuronal responses to the DBS pulse. If, for the sake of discussion, one assumes that the primary effect of DBS on ensembles and networks of neurons is mediated by action potential generation, then those voltage-gated ionic conductance channels that lead

to depolarization sufficient for generating an action potential probably play a large role in DBS. Thus, distribution of such channels over the entire surface of a neuron, including the axon, plays a determining role in the neurons' response. What is important, then, is distribution of voltage-gated depolarizing ionic conductance channels combined with the biophysical properties that are based on the geometry of the neuronal elements as well as the presence or absence of myelin.

Major voltage-gated depolarizing ionic conductance channels include the sodium (Na^+) channels. These are usually localized in an axon, particularly at an action-potential-initiating segment and at the internodes of Ranvier in myelinated axons. DBS negative (cathodal) stimulation is thus likely to affect Na^+ voltage-gated ionic conductance channels, which, when they produce sufficient depolarization, leads to action potential generation.

Of the other voltage-gated depolarizing ionic conductance channels, some are located on the dendrites, a fact which suggests that a DBS pulse may affect dendrites. For example, calcium (Ca^{++}) spikes, which are analogous to an action potential, may be generated in dendrites. Also, the N-methyl-D-aspartate (NMDA) ligand-mediating ionic conductance channel has at least three states: (1) at rest and closed to positive ion conductance; (2) an open state that allows passage of ions; and (3) a state of greater conductivity that owes to the removal of a magnesium (Mg^{++}) ion from a receptor's interior. The transition to a state of greater conductivity provides for a regenerative process quite similar to the kind seen in the generation of Na^+ and potassium (K^+) mediated action potentials in an action-potential-initiating segment and axon (Larkum et al. 2009).

The role played by dendritic spikes is not clear. In the case of NMDA-associated spikes, individual spikes do not propagate for any great distance. For this reason, their potential for summing to produce an output action potential at the action-potential-initiating segment may be limited. Though this may be true for initiating dendritic spikes under normal conditions, DBS is not a normal condition. As the electrical fields generated by DBS and utilized to produce a physiological affect are orders of magnitude larger than the typical dendrites', it is likely that many dendritic spikes may be initiated simultaneously. This could result in sufficient depolarization at the action-potential-initiating segment and, consequently, an increase in output action potentials.

The neuronal elements that have the lowest threshold to negative (cathodal) current to generate an action potential are, in order: axon terminals, axon hillock or action-potential-initiating segment, axon nodes of Ranvier in myelinated axons, unmyelinated axons, and cell bodies and dendrites (together constituting the soma).

POST-HYPERPOLARIZATION REBOUND EXCITATION, DEPOLARIZATION BLOCKADE, AND NEUROTRANSMITTER EXHAUSTION

Hyperpolarization of the neuronal membrane, such as that which results from positive (anodal) current injection, may lead to an initial reduction in the probability of action potential generation. However, the same hyperpolarizing membrane potential may be followed by a rebound as an increased probability of generating action potentials. Following termination of the hyperpolarizing current, Na^+ ionic conductance channels are activated. Thus, when a hyperpolarization ends, a neuronal membrane responds with depolarization, the event of which may be sufficient for the generation of action potentials. This phenomenon is referred to as *post-hyperpolarization rebound excitation*. (The other term for it, "post-inhibitory rebound excitation," is inaccurate.) It also important to note that post-hyperpolarization rebound need not be related directly to a DBS pulse. Rather, it may be related to excitation of an axon terminal by a DBS pulse that releases a hyperpolarizing neurotransmitter. The latter, though it may initially decrease the probability of action potentials, is followed by a rebound increase in action potential generation.

In a case report, neurons of the Vop, which receives afferents from the GPi, were recorded during DBS in the vicinity of the GPi (Montgomery 2006). Figure 6.2 shows the results of an analysis of a representative neuron. Evident is a very short latency (less than 1 ms) highly consistent (narrow peak) response. This probably represents antidromic action potentials owing to excitation of axons from the Vop that project to the cortex. After a span of approximately 3.5 ms, there occurs a reduction in action potentials recorded from the thalamic neurons. This event is consistent

with afferents from the GPi, the activation of which liberates gamma amino butyric acid (GABA), thereby causing a hyperpolarization of the thalamic neurons that lasts approximately 3.5 ms. This is followed by a rebound in the form of increased generation of action potentials. For many neurons, a rebound increase in action potentials results in a net increase of thalamic neuron discharges.

In recordings of non-human primate neuronal response to DBS-like stimulation of the STN, antidromic activation was observed in the cortex and GPe neurons (Figure 6.3) (Montgomery and Gale 2008). In humans, recordings for STN neurons demonstrate antidromic responses to DBS in the vicinity of the contralateral STN. Also, recordings of electroencephalographic activity evoked by stimulation pulses with DBS in the vicinity of the STN demonstrate very short latency responses, which are consistent with antidromic activation (Walker et al. 2011). Other studies of electroencephalographic activities evoked by paired-pulse DBS in the vicinity of the STN demonstrate very short refractory periods, which are indicative of axonal activations and therefore consistent with antidromic activations (Baker et al. 2002).

Some have argued that DBS suppresses neuronal activity by creating a depolarization blockade of Na^+ voltage-gated ionic conductance channels. However, most studies have shown that action potentials increase rather than decrease. Yet there persists nonetheless the claim that prolonged depolarization results in inactivation of Na^+ voltage-gated ionic conductance channels (*see Chapter 3, Principles of Electrophysiology*). However, the time course of reactivation of Na^+ voltage-gated ionic conductance channels, as evidenced by the refractory period, is on the order of 1–3 ms. Thus, any period between successive DBS pulses that runs longer than a few milliseconds provides ample opportunity for reversing the effects of subthreshold depolarization.

Some have argued that high-frequency DBS produces repetitive firing of neurons of such intensity that neurotransmitters become depleted. This author was unable to find any direct empirical demonstration of this concept. The claim rests on the presumption that the neuron discharges at a high rate in response to the frequency DBS. Recordings of STN neurons made during DBS in the vicinity of the contralateral STN, however, demonstrate that approximately only 10% of the DBS pulses are associated with an

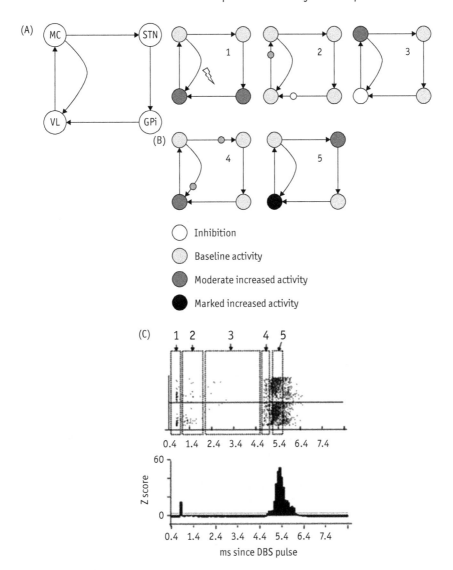

Figure 6.2: Some Vop neurons (designated VL in the figure) demonstrate a remarkable post-hyperpolarization (post-inhibitory) rebound increased excitability (C). A potential mechanism is schematically represented (B). A nested two oscillator system is shown (A). The first oscillator is the disynaptic feedback loop between the motor cortex (MC) and Vop or basal ganglia relay nucleus of the thalamus. The second loop consists of the MC to the STN, GPi, Vop, and motor cortex once again. Each numbered step (B) shows the subsequent activations, which begin with the synchronized activation of Vop and GPi neurons in step 1. The activity in Vop is then transmitted to MC, and activity in GPi is transmitted to Vop in step 2. This results in excitation of MC and inhibition of VL in step 3. MC activity is then transmitted back to Vop and is followed by a post-inhibitory rebound increased activity in Vop in step 4. The excitation from MC in step 4 combines with the post-inhibitory rebound increased excitability in Vop to produce a marked increase in activity, as shown in step 5.
Modified from Montgomery 2006, page 2698.

antidromic response. Thus, the effective stimulation rate of high-frequency DBS is far lower and, as such, is unlikely to deplete neurotransmitters. Additionally, because low-frequency DBS can be as effective as high (*see Chapter 10—Approaches to Programming*), it is unlikely that neurotransmitter depletion occurs or that neurotransmitter depletion is a therapeutic mechanism of action.

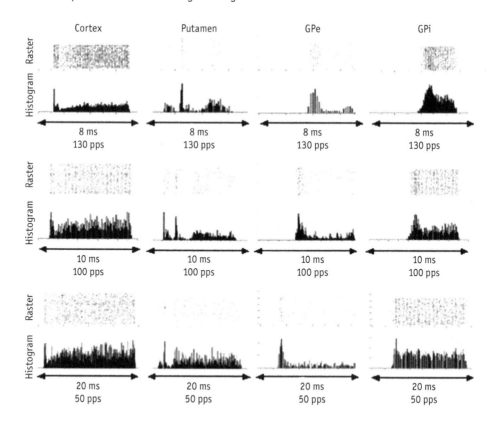

Figure 6.3: Representative post-stimulus rasters and histograms of neuronal activity recorded from the cortex, putamen, GPe, and GPi. The top portion of each figure is a raster of neuronal activity. Each dot represents the time of an extracellular action potential. Each row represents a segment of neuronal activity between each stimulation pulse. Division of the time into bins and summation across rows result in a histogram that appears in the lower portion of each figure. For stimulation at 130 pulses per second (pps), the time of the rasters and histograms is 8 ms; for 100 pps, it is 10 ms; and for 50 pps, it is 20 ms. Observable is a pattern of response in the first 8 ms, which, when compression of the time scale is accounted for, is the same regardless of the stimulation frequency.

From Montgomery and Gale, 2008, page 396.

DISSOCIATION OF EFFECTS ON ACTION-POTENTIAL-INITIATING SEGMENT, DENDRITES, AND CELL BODIES

There prevails a belief that DBS of a specific structure affects only the neurons of that structure. As will be discussed, this is not the case: Evidence demonstrates widespread propagation of the effects of a DBS pulse (Figure 6.3). For this reason, this discussion refrains from presenting DBS as being related to a specific target, such as the STN. Rather, it discusses DBS as being in the vicinity of a target.

The tendency to view DBS solely according to its effects on neurons at or near its target follows from the Neuron Doctrine, in which the neuron is posited as the nervous system's fundamental unit of function. In this sense, the Neuron Doctrine is probably incorrect. (The reasons for this are discussed in *Chapter 8—Pathophysiological Mechanisms.*) Yet it is clear that there may be a dissociation of DBS effects on cell bodies and dendrites compared to the action-potential-initiating segment. Observations of neuronal discharges in a DBS target made by use of extracellular recordings depend on the back-propagation of an action potential generated from an action-potential-initiating segment into the dendritic field where it may be recorded. Action potentials in axons, such as those that exit the target nucleus, are usually quite difficult to record. For example, either depolarization of synaptic terminals in a target structure releases hyperpolarizing neu-rotransmitters, or stimulation induces hyperpo-larization in the cell bodies. In either case, such hyperpolarization prevents an action potential from back-propagating into cell bodies and dendrites, resulting in no recordings of action potentials in neurons of a DBS target. At the same time, action potentials are, unobserved, generated in axons and then influence downstream neurons. This dissoci-ation between effects on dendrites and cell bodies as different as those on action-potential-initiating segments has been demonstrated electroneuro-physiologically (Coombs et al. 1957, Llinas et al. 1964, Steriade et al. 1974) and has been provided a robust explanation utilizing computational model-ing (McIntyre and Grill 1999).

NETWORK EFFECTS OF DBS

Another consequence of the Neuron Doctrine is that it directs focus to DBS's effects on a DBS tar-get's neurons. However, DBS's effects are propagated throughout networks that span multiple anatomical structures. The problem is that, if an investigator stud-ies only neurons in a DBS target structure, s/he will see changes correlated with DBS but not see more extensively propagated effects. S/he is then likely to presume that the effects s/he observed do indeed represent the therapeutic mechanism of action of DBS. This presumption instances the logical Fallacy of Confirming the Consequence," which is expressed in the following form: If "*a implies b*" is true, and if *b* is true, then *a* must be true. This is fallacious because *b* may be true for reasons other than *a*. In the present example, *a* is DBS of the STN and *b* is improvement in Parkinsonism: The investigator does see improvement in the subject's Parkinsonism and concludes that it is the result of DBS of the STN.

The foregoing fallacy is a major problem with the use of DBS to conduct physiological and behavioral studies. A great many investigators claim to have gained insight into the physiology or functions of the STN, for example, by using DBS in the vicinity of the STN. Because those studies cannot be interpreted, they are of little use.

It has been clearly demonstrated that DBS in the vicinity of the STN causes antidromic activations in a number of structures (Figure 6.3). Antidromic

activations may lead to orthodromic propagation to a site at which the original action potential was gen-erated (Figure 6.4). A summary of some of the local effects of generation of action potentials in axons in the vicinity of the DBS-induced electrical field is shown in Figure 6.4, which is a schematic representa-tion of the way in which an antidromic action potential may be propagated. Shown are local—in the physio-logical rather than anatomical sense—responses. By "local" is meant physiological interaction via axonal connections rather than neurons that belong to the same anatomical structure. For example, applica-tion of the schematic to a neuron (E in Figure 6.4) in the GPi reveals that the orthodromically propa-gated action potential quite probably affects the Vop (C in Figure 6.4) rather than another neuron in the GPi, because the latter contains few physiologically active interconnections between neurons of the GPi, as evidenced by a lack of cross-correlations in dis-charge activities recorded simultaneously in groups of GPi neurons. Consequently, the neuron in the Vop is physiologically closer to the GPi neuron than it is to another GPi neuron. An example of this effect is observed in the reduction of neuronal activities of neurons in the Vop in response to DBS in the vicinity of the GPi, shown in Figure 6.2.

Consider the situation of DBS in the vicinity of the STN. In this case, the antidromic action potential is generated in the axons of neurons in the cortex (E in Figure 6.4) that project to the STN neurons (neurons receiving input from C in Figure 6.4). The antidromi-cally conducted action potentials (B in Figure 6.4) invade the soma of the cortical neuron. Evidence for this effect is shown in Figure 6.3, the recorded action potentials of which are derived from action potentials that have invaded the soma. (It is quite difficult to record action potentials in axons.) The antidromically conducted action potentials may reach a branch point and then orthodromically travel (D in Figure 6.4) to a point at which they monosynaptically activate the neuron that is the target of the axon collateral. In this case, it is a striatal neuron, as shown by the response with a latency of approximately 4 ms in Figure 6.3.

Importantly, there is reason to believe that the DBS effect continues through multiple synapses. Shown in Figure 6.3 are later increases in neuronal activities approximately 6 ms to 8 ms after the DBS pulse. These are consistent with a disynaptic orthodromic propa-gation. It is important to note also that an antidromic

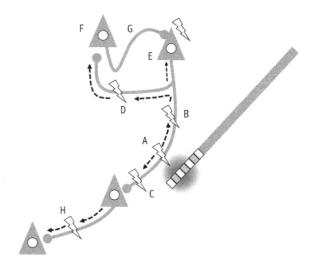

Figure 6.4: Schematic representation of antidromic action potential propagation. Local responses (in the physiological rather than the anatomical sense; see text). In A, the electrical field generated by the DBS electrode excites an action potential in the axon near the electrode. The action potential is propagated antidromically (B) to the neuron from which the axon originated and travels orthodromically (C) to the neuron receiving the axon's synapses. Antidromically traveling action potentials may encounter a branch point to an axon collateral. If this happens, the antidromic action potential is carried orthodromically (D) to another neuron (F), which in turn may send an action potential to other neurons or to the neuron (G) that originates the axon in which the antidromic action potential was initiated. Neuron C, which receives the influences of action potentials generated in the axon at A, may propagate that effect to the next neuron (H). The antidromic action potential may also invade the originating neuron (E), back-propagating into the soma and dendrites to effect information processing in that neuron.

action potential probably invades the soma of a neuron that originates an antidromically activated axon. The action potential back-propagated into the soma can have a profound effect on the status of electrical potentials across a neuronal membrane in the soma and thus affect the immediate processing of information therein. Finally, antidromic activations may occur in axons that have nothing to do with the various neuronal elements proper to the DBS target nucleus. An electrical field generated by a DBS pulse does not discriminate among axons activated by means other than biophysical properties, such as their diameter or the state of being myelinated. For example, DBS in the vicinity of the STN generates axonal action potentials in neurons in the contralateral STN. Ashby and colleagues provide evidence, based on electromyographic recordings, that DBS in that vicinity causes activation of corticospinal fibers (Ashby and Rothwell 2000), and it is believed that these fibers do not synapse onto neurons of the STN or striatum.

Figure 6.2 depicts a possible disynaptic propagation. There occurs an increase in activity of a Vop neuron to DBS in the vicinity of the GPi less than 1 ms after the DBS pulse. This activity is consistent with antidromic activation and is followed by a return to normal discharging until approximately 3 ms after the DBS pulse, during which neuronal activity decreases until approximately 5 ms, consistent with hyperpolarization of the thalamic neurons consequent to action potentials' arriving at the synaptic thermals of axons exiting the GPi. After 5 ms, there occurs a net increase in neuronal activity, which is consistent with post-hyperpolarization rebound excitation, followed by a remarkable increase in neuronal activity. On close inspection of the raster, it is observed that with continued DBS comes a gradual falloff in the antidromic response and a progressive increase in the late increased activity occurring at 5 ms. This correlation suggests that increased activity coming late after the DBS pulse prevents the antidromic response. This tendency probably owes to an orthodromically induced action potential, possibly from feedback activation from the cortex that collides with the antidromic action potential to prevent it from invading the dendrites and cell body and producing a detectable spike.

The above-mentioned feedback mechanism suggests the presence of a reentrant disynaptic oscillator that consists of thalamic and cortical neurons. The progressive accumulation of the late response suggests a positive resonance between a DBS pulse train, whose periodic pulses are equivalent to an oscillator—a discrete oscillator, to be exact, whose nature is discussed in detail in Chapter 18, Discrete Oscillators—and a reentrant oscillator, which consists of a disynaptic circuit between thalamic and cortical neurons. Also discussed below is the potential for resonance interactions between the DBS, which functions an oscillator, and oscillators that consist of polysynaptic reentrant circuits in the basal ganglia–thalamic-cortical system.

CRITICALLY IMPORTANT CAVEATS CONCERNING INTERPRETATION OF NERVOUS SYSTEM RESPONSES TO DBS

DBS is not normal. An exaggerated example serves to illustrate this observation. Application of DBS in the service of coming to understand nervous system function is similar to inference of nervous system mechanisms arriving from observation of lightning bolts as they strike a subject's head. Lightning strikes to an individual's head are indiscriminant, simultaneously affecting millions of neurons, as well as such other structures as glia. Information processed in the nervous system depends on differences and distinctions the site and moment of action potential generation. Information is encoded in activated axons that occupy a physiological pathway. If all are activated, or if none are, the information encoded is greatly reduced. Similarly, information is encoded in the pattern of action potentials. When an individual hums, she conveys far less information than when she speaks. Intonations and inflections produced during speech convey information. The degrees of freedom and thus range of information conveyed are greatly reduced when an individual produces sustained sound at a single pitch.

Though DBS is different from a lightning bolt, the difference is perhaps quantitative rather than qualitative. A DBS pulse is no more discriminatory than would be a tiny lightning bolt striking a specific region of the nervous system. Indeed, the combination of nonspecific means of excitation with the precision of genetic control of susceptibility to nonspecific means of excitation represents the great hope of optogenetics.

Fortunately, there is produced no simultaneous action potential in every axon in the vicinity of a DBS pulse, because the latter is quite inefficient. Indeed, if it were the opposite, it would probably worsen, rather than improve, motor function, because it would overwrite important information conveyed in spatially and temporally encoded action potentials. Indeed, this possibility probably explains why, at higher stimulation currents and voltages, motor function observably worsens.

Many reasons exist to explain why a DBS pulse is inefficient. Indeed, only on the order of 10% of DBS pulses result in an action potential, the low incidence owing to such factors as the size and geometry of an axon, and whether it is myelinated or not (*see Chapter 3—Principles of Electrophysiology*). Any generated action potential's propagation is also inefficient. Conduction through a branch point, for example, depends on the relative diameters of the parent—an axon segment that precedes a branch point—and daughters: axon segments that follow a branch point. If daughters are smaller than a parent segment, the antidromic action potential is less likely to propagate from the former to the latter.

Despite the inefficiencies of a DBS pulse, it is highly unlikely that DBS replicates normal nervous system function. One must exercise great caution, therefore—indeed, far more than is currently applied—if one attempts to gain understanding of normal nervous system functions by way of responses to DBS. Yet, in at least one way (if there are not in fact several ways), DBS helps us restore normal information processing. As such, it lends itself to an understanding of nervous system function. This process may be DBS-induced stochastic resonance, which is discussed in Chapter 8, Pathophysiological Mechanisms. Also, DBS may be used as a negative experimental method by purposefully disrupting normal function, much in the same way as transcranial magnetic stimulation that disrupts normal nervous system functioning to produce observable changes attributable to the region of nervous system disrupted.

One might notice that, thus far, there has been no discussion of local field potentials as indicators of nervous system responses to DBS. This lack owes to the fact that, as indicators, they are quite poor. As such, they likelier to obscure rather than illuminate the nature of nervous system responses. In fact, local field potentials are more likely artifacts that stem from the methods of recording of local field potentials. This is not to say that local field potentials are never any help in developing automated methods for adjusting electrode configurations, stimulation parameters, and pulse trains. They may be helpful in the same way as is the Venereal Disease Research Laboratory (VDRL) test of a patient's blood against an extract of beef heart for the presence of an antibody. A test for syphilis infection, it has been in use since 1906.

A local field potential represents the summed changes in electrical potentials across many dendritic trees and over many neurons. Under ideal circumstances, the special resolution of local field potentials is on the order of millimeters, which is vastly greater than that of most dendritic fields. Also, selection of areas of the nervous system sampled by local field potential recordings is relatively indiscriminant. An analogy is that local field potentials are to action potentials what a crowd at a sporting event is to an individual fan's voice. Someone listening in cannot understand any one fan's words when they are spoken amid the general din. One may be speaking about a recent call by the referee, and another about politics or some other subject completely unrelated to the action on the field. The best a listener may gather is what may be considered an average of those conversations and others, which would probably not be terribly intelligible. This is not to say that someone listening cannot learn from the sounds of the crowd that something has happened—that a point had been scored, say, or a player for the home team has been fouled in an egregious way. It is to say that there is nothing in the roar of the crowd itself that enables the listener to know exactly what has happened.

Though a local field potential lacks spatial resolution, it has relatively high temporal resolution, which is limited only by the electrical characteristics of a recording device, such as the filters used. Temporal information in the neuronal elements involved in production of a local field potential, however, does not reflect the information in those elements any more than does the average. By analogy, a size 9 pair of shoes for adult males do not provide any information about the shoe size of a given individual. Information

contained in neuronal elements is irretrievably lost in the very act of recording a local field potential.

A local field potential is misleading if one makes the mistake of ascribing meaning to it. Illustrative of this fact is the average value of 10, which can be achieved by component values of 5, 5, 5, 15, 15, and 15. Nowhere in the sample may be found the value 10, despite the fact that it is the average. The problem is that, if given only the average value of 10, as would be the case in the average voltages of the local field potential, one cannot know whether the sample that results in the average of 10 is 5, 5, 5, 15, 15; 15, 10, 10, 10, 10, 10, and 10; or 10 10, 11, 12, 9, and 8. The problem becomes deeper because the component values of the local field potentials are positive and negative. Consequently, the average, such as might occur when recording local field potentials, may be −5, −5, −5, 5, 5, and 5. The average being zero, it would be a mistake to assume that there are no component values.

Signals in the dendrites are analog signals that vary in frequency of content over time. Integration of these time-varying analog signals results in positive and negative resonance, of which beat interactions are an example. The signal actually recorded in local field potentials partially depends on the difference between the frequencies in the component signals. Thus, summing a 100 Hz and a 120 Hz signal gives a beat signal of roughly 20 Hz. The same is true of a 20 Hz and a 40 Hz signal; it also is true of a potentially infinite number of pairs of signals whose frequency only differs by 20 Hz. The mistake, then, is inferring from a 20 Hz signal recorded in a local field potential that there actually is a 20 Hz signal in the nervous system's electrical activity.

These concerns are relevant to one theory of the pathophysiology of Parkinson's disease, which posits that excess nervous system activity in the high beta (approximately 20 Hz), as recorded in local field potentials, is causal to motoric effects of Parkinsonism. This is not to say that an increased amount (power) of a high beta frequency is not in the local field potential recording in patients with Parkinson's disease. It is to say only that one cannot interpret from the local field potential that there exists, in an ontological sense, a high beta frequency oscillator rather than a set of gamma or even higher frequency oscillators whose difference is in the high beta frequency range. However, as will be demonstrated latter, there is independent evidence of a high beta oscillator, at least in the electrical potentials across the neuronal membranes of some STN neurons. High beta frequencies in local field potential recordings in patients with Parkinson's disease are analogous to the presence of an antibody in an extract of beef heart, which predicts a possible infection with the syphilis organism. Indeed, as is discussed in *Supplemental essay, Automated Assisted DBS Programming at http:// www.greenvilleneuromodulationcenter.com/DBS_ Programming_essays/*, the presence of power in the high beta frequencies has been explored as a biomarker for closed loop DBS.

REENTRY PROPAGATIONS AND RESONANCE

The above discussion suggests that it is likely that the effects of each DBS pulse are propagated downstream through links of pre- and postsynaptic neurons in an open or closed loop feed-forward mechanism, initiated by both anti- and orthodromic action potentials generated in the axon in the vicinity of the DBS. This was demonstrated in the above-mentioned case of neuronal responses to DBS-like stimulation in the vicinity of the STN, as shown in Figure 6.3. It is also possible that the chain of neurons closes back to form a feedback reentrant loop, as shown in Figure 6.2.

In a study of non-human primates that made use of paired-pulse DBS-like stimulation, the responses of neurons to pairs of pulses with different inter-pulse intervals were recorded (Montgomery and Gale 2008). In this study, pairs of DBS-like pulses were applied in the vicinity of the STN in non-human primates. Recordings of the action potentials of neurons in a number of targets were made. The time between pulses—the inter-pulse interval—varied. The concept explored is represented schematically in Figure 6.5. The hypothesis is that the initial pulse of the pair initiates an action potential whose effects propagate through a closed loop reentrant pathway. If the second pulse is delivered at the moment at which effects of the first pulse return to the site of stimulation, the effects on the subsequent neurons would be additive, owing to resonance. The inter-pulse intervals that resulted in the additive effect indicate the time required for effects of the initial pulse to traverse the closed loop. As such, it is also a measure of the frequency of the oscillator, which consists of the closed loop.

An example of the analysis of a representative neuron appears in Figure 6.6. Each row represents the effects of a specific inter-pulse interval DBS. The colored tic mark indicates a response that is at least two standard deviations above the neuronal activity recorded prior to DBS. The colors indicate the z-score of the change in neuronal activities. Also, the colored tic mark indicates the time following the second of the paired pulses at which the response occurred. Observable in the bottom row, which corresponds to an inter-pulse interval of 1 ms, is a maximum response that occurs approximately 3.8 ms after the second pulse. Because the pulses were separated by only 1 ms, it is likely that the effects of the second pulse temporally summed with the effects of the first pulse on the same neuronal element (*see Chapter 3—Principles of Electrophysiology*). Interestingly, there again occurred increased action potentials in the recorded neuron at approximately 7.6 ms and approximately 15.2 ms, which are first and third harmonics of the first response at 3.8 ms. Because these harmonics occurred between pairs of DBS pulses, they cannot be ascribed to the direct effect of the DBS pulse. They suggest, rather, an oscillation ongoing between sets of DBS pulse pairs. Furthermore, these latencies suggest the presence of an underlying oscillator of approximately 263 Hz.

Interestingly, the modeling of the neuronal electrical potentials by Hodgkin and Huxley predicted oscillations in the neuronal membrane potential. Subsequently demonstrated biologically, it revealed that, in dampened oscillation, there occurred slight displacements from a normal resting electrical potential resulting in oscillations whose periods were on the order of 7–8 ms (Hodgkin and Huxley 1952), which may explain the occurrence of a second peak at approximately 7.6 ms, which in turn may explain the occurrence of a peak at approximately 15.2 ms.

Several increases in neuronal activities are observable at different inter-pulse intervals. These occur at different latencies and do not follow from an early response, as was observed with the 1 ms inter-pulse interval. These responses thus appear not to be the result of dampened oscillations consequent to a neuronal membrane's inherent dynamics. The different inter-pulse intervals with significant increases in neuronal activities include 4 ms, 5 ms, 7 ms, and 8 ms, and they correspond to reentrant frequencies of 250 Hz, 200 Hz, 143 Hz, and 125 Hz. These frequencies

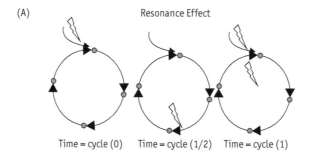

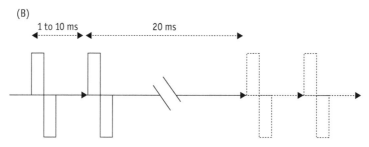

Figure 6.5: The top figure (A) is a schematic representation of the resonance effect. The first stimulation (conditioning pulse) causes an excitation to traverse the closed loop. If the second stimulation (test pulse) is delivered precisely at the moment at which the excitation effect from the first or conditioning pulse returns to the original site, temporal summation on the neuronal cell membrane will amplify the response. The bottom figure (B) schematically represents the paired-pulse stimulus trains. The inter-stimulus interval represents a specific frequency (1/interval). This study examined the frequencies represented by the intervals from 1–10 ms (1000 Hz–100 Hz) at 1-ms increments.

fall within the range of normal neuronal spike trains of many neurons within the basal ganglia–thalamic-cortical system.

Figure 6.7 shows the effects of varying the inter-pulse interval on the neuronal responses in the cortex, putamen, and GPi neurons to DBS-like paired pulses delivered in the vicinity of the STN in a non-human primate. The DBS pulse train was randomized to produce different inter-pulse intervals with an overall rate of 130 pps. The data were segregated according to the inter-pulse intervals between successive DBS pulses, unless the next pair of pulses occurred for fewer than 7.5 ms. According to this analysis, the first pulse of the pair is regard as a conditioning pulse that affects the

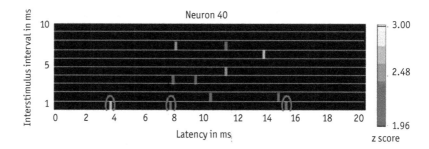

Figure 6.6: Results of paired-pulse experiments for a neuron recorded in the motor cortex of a non-human primate. Each row represents the changes in the probability of a neuronal discharge from baseline for each inter-stimulus interval of paired-pulse stimuli. Colored bars represent z-score changes of greater than 1.96 compared to baseline. The horizontal axis represents the latency of the resonance effect following the second or test pulse of the pair.

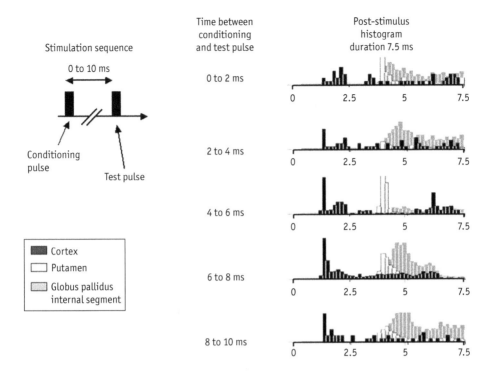

Figure 6.7: Activities of a single neuron in the cortex, putamen, and GPi following delivery of a second pair of DBS-like pulses in the vicinity of the STN. The DBS pulse train was randomized to produce different inter-pulse intervals whose overall rate was 130 pps. The data were segregated according to the inter-pulse intervals between successive DBS pulses unless the next pair of pulses occurred for fewer than 7.5 ms. According to this analysis, the first pulse of the pair is regard as a conditioning pulse that affects the response to the second or test pulse. The conditioning pulse was delivered at different moments other than those during which a test stimulus pulse was delivered. A conditioning stimulus pulse preceded each test stimulus pulse at different intervals. The post-test stimulus pulse histograms, which were constructed as described, were not normalized to the pre-stimulus activity.

From Montgomery 2004a, page 407.

response to the second or test pulse. The conditioning pulse was delivered at different moments other than those during which a test stimulus pulse was delivered. A conditioning stimulus pulse preceded each test stimulus pulse at different intervals. The post-test stimulus pulse histograms, which were constructed as described, were not normalized to the pre-stimulus activity (from Montgomery 2004a).

Observable in Figure 6.7 is a highly consistent, short-latency narrow peak in most of the responses to the DBS pulse delivered to the cortical neuron. This is consistent with antidromic activation. The responses are observably different for each neuron in the different structure, and each neuron's response differs according to the inter-pulse interval. Interestingly, the responses of the putamen and the responses of GPi neurons are reciprocal. Because the neurons of the

putamen use the hyperpolarizing neurotransmitter GABA, the increased activity in the putamen neuron results in monosynaptic hyperpolarization and reduced action potential generation in the neuron of the GPi. These observations suggest that the DBS response percolates through multiple synapses.

Another example of reentrant oscillatory activity initiated by a DBS pulse in the vicinity of the STN in a non-human primate appears in Figure 6.8. The figure shows rasters and histograms of action potentials, which are indicated by the dots in the raster, following each DBS pulse's delivery at its particular frequency at time 0. Each row of dots represents a response to a single DBS pulse. The number of dots in a column across a raster appears in the histogram beneath each raster. The lengths of the rasters and histograms represent the time period between DBS pulses. As is

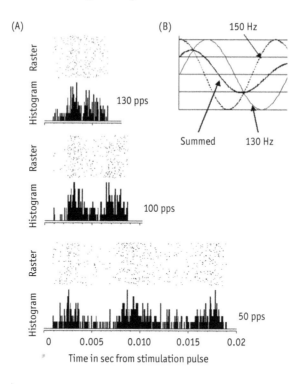

Figure 6.8: Figure A shows a post-stimulus raster and histogram of a cortical neuron recorded in a non-human primate with use of DBS-like stimulation delivered in the vicinity of the STN. The stimulus pulse occurred at time zero, and the raster and histogram show the periodic neuronal activities during the inter-stimulus pulse intervals. Each dot in the raster represents the onset of an action potential. Each row represents the responses to a single DBS pulse. The number of dots in columns across the raster appears in the histogram below each raster. The length of the raster and histogram represent the time interval between DBS pulses. In the raster and histogram associated with the 50 pps DBS, a recurring peak of increased neuronal activity is evident. The truncated appearance of the third peak suggests that the time period associated with the frequency of the reentrant oscillatory activity is not an integer multiple of the time interval between the DBS pulses. This suggests interaction between the oscillator generating the recurrent activity and the oscillator composed of the DBS spike train (B). This observation may be explained by an interaction between a 130 Hz DBS oscillator and a 150 Hz oscillator intrinsic to the neuron.

evident in Figure 6.8A, DBS at 130 pps produces a biphasic increase this cortical neuron's activity. At 100 pps DBS, two peaks occur in the interval between DBS pulses more separated than associated with DBS at 130 pps. At 50 pps three peaks occur in the 20 ms that elapse between DBS pulses. One interpretation is that DBS produces an oscillation in neuronal activities with a frequency of approximately 150 Hz. The responses at each DBS frequency represenst interactions between the underlying fundamental frequency and the DBS frequency (Figure 6.8B).

Interestingly, the third peak in the 50 pps DBS response appears truncated. These observations are consistent with a reentrant oscillatory increase in neuronal activities time-locked to the DBS pulse, and thus caused by it. As observed in the 50 pps DBS, the oscillatory reentrant activity is also truncated, suggesting that its period is not the same as the inter-pulse interval of the DBS train or the period of the DBS oscillator. The truncation of the third peak may be due to the interaction of two oscillators, represented in Figure 6.7B. The first is the 130 Hz DBS oscillator, and the second, an intrinsic oscillator at 150 Hz.

SYNCHRONIZATION AMONG NEURONS

It has been argued that DBS produces desynchronization of a neuronal ensemble's activities. This argument rests on the observation that experimentally induced Parkinsonism in non-human primates produces excessive synchronization (Heimer et al. 2006). Because DBS improves the symptoms of Parkinson's disease, it presumably also reverses the abnormalities thought to be causal of Parkinsonism. However, it is not likely that DBS reduces synchronization of neuronal activities in the basal ganglia–thalamic-cortical system. If DBS did cause desynchronization, it would be unlikely to produce evoked potentials in the electroencephalogram, for reasons that are discussed below. At the very least, any neurons that respond antidromically will be highly synchronized. One study estimated that approximately 10% of neurons in the GPi and externa were antidromically driven (Zimnik et al. 2015, McCairn et al. 2009). Recordings of action potentials of neurons throughout the basal ganglia–thalamic-cortical system in the non-human primate in response to DBS-like pulses, however, demonstrate remarkable synchronization beyond that which is associated with antidromic activation.

From a study of two naïve non-human primates, post-stimulus intensity histograms showed the statistically significant changes in neuron activities in the somatosensory and motor cortex in one animal

each (Figure 6.9). Each row represents an individual neuron, and the color indicates the change in neuronal activity expressed as z-score changes from pre-stimulation time periods. Observably remarkable synchronization occurs across the large majority of neurons.

One study that examined the effects of DBS-like stimulation in the vicinity of the GPi in non-human primates on motor cortex neuronal activity demonstrated decreased synchronization (McCairn et al. 2015). However, the methods employed may have been too conservative to be able to detect the above-mentioned noisy synchronization. This has been demonstrated by computational modeling of a four-node oscillator whose outputs from node 1 to node 2 extend to node 3, which in turn extends to a fourth node that projects to node 1 (Figure 6.10). Each node consists of 1,000 integrate-and-fire neurons. Each neuron in one node connects to each node in a subsequent node. The probability of generation by a set of action potentials in a preceding node of an action potential in a neuron in the subsequent node was adjusted low enough to avoid saturation of oscillations while maintaining them. Figure 6.10 shows a set

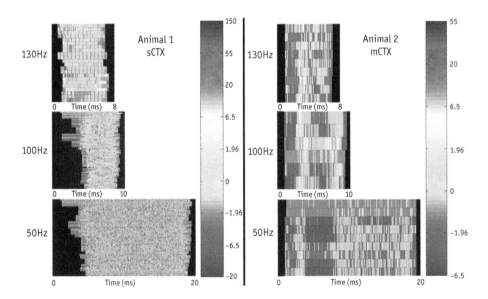

Figure 6.9: Intensity plots of peri-stimulus histograms showing the change in neuronal discharge rates of motor cortex (mCTX) and sensory cortex (sCTX) neurons following a DBS pulse delivered at time 0 for 130 Hz, 100 Hz, and 50 Hz in time bins of 0.0012 ms for animal 1. The x-axis for each plot is a neuron number, and the y-axis is time (ms). Each refers to color scales for each plot for statistical power. (It must be noted that the color scale is transformed by the natural log of the absolute value of the z-score.) The black area represents data loss owing to stimulus artifact.

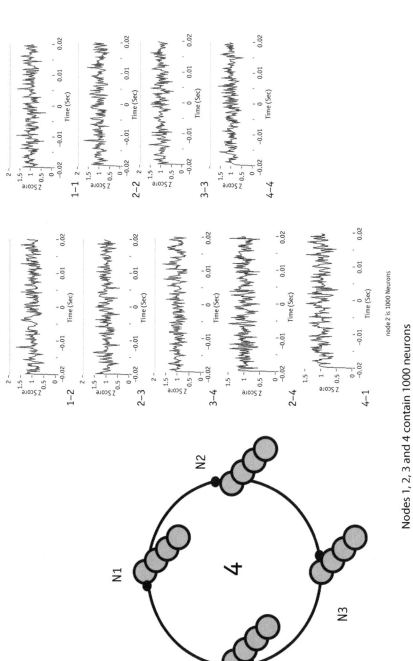

Figure 6.10: Cross-correlograms between representative pairs of neurons across and within nodes (see text). Despite the fact the model establishes a type of synchrony among neurons within and between nodes, the cross-correlation method was too conservative (insensitive) to detect the synchronization.

of cross-correlations between a representative pair of neurons across nodes and within nodes. The cross-correlogram shows the probability of one neuron's action potential's preceding or following an action potential in another, or index, neuron. A peak in the cross-correlograms indicates a physiological link between the two neurons. Notable is the fact that there is no demonstrable cross-correlation, though the modeling creates synchronized activities within nodes (noisy synchronization that will be explained in *Chapter 8—Pathophysiological Mechanisms*).

Even more notable is the fact that the cross-correlogram—as well as possibly measures of coherence—may not be able to detect synchronization despite the existence of a form of synchronization. This is shown in Figure 6.11, in which the same modeling as described above is changed in such a way that the number of neurons in node 2 is reduced to 200. This required an increase in the probability that a neuron in node 2 would respond to a neuron in node 1. Also, the effect of a neuron on a neuron in node 3 would be increased, because the convergence of inputs from neurons in node 2 has a higher probability of an action potential. Observable in Figure 6.11 is a high cross-correlation between a neuron in node 2 and a neuron in node 1 and 3. The cross-correlation between a neuron in node 3 and a neuron in node 4, however, is lower; that between a neuron in node 4 and a neuron in node, is lower still.

Other studies that recorded neuronal activities in non-human primates in response to DBS-like stimulation in the vicinity of the GPe in non-human primates do not specifically address the issue of synchronization (Vitek et al. 2012). Yet post-stimulus histograms of neuronal activities during the inter-pulse interval pooled over 50 neurons, from nearly as many neurons recorded, demonstrated definite structure, which probably would not be the case were the DBS pulse results in desynchronization.

A study of the flexor carpi ulnaris muscle response to M-waves—orthodromic action potentials generated in a peripheral nerve by electrical stimulation of the ulnar nerve—provided insight, at the level of the alpha lower motor neuron if nowhere else, into the issue synchronization (Aldewereld et al. 2012). Figure 6.12 illustrates the experiment's rationale. The basis for the experiment is that external electrical stimulation applied to a motor nerve axon in the refractory period that follows a spontaneous action potential does not excite the axon and thus meets with no response from a muscle. The result is a smaller electromyographic M-wave response, recordable from the skin surface over the muscle, which is inversely proportional to the number of motor neuron axons in the refractory period. If a large number of axons had just a moment before experienced simultaneous spontaneous action potentials—which implies greater synchronization of action potentials generated in an alpha lower motor neuron—they all would simultaneously experience a synchronized refractory period. Stimulation applied externally during this period would elicit a small M-wave response from the muscle. A few milliseconds following the refractory period, the externally applied electrical stimulation activates all the axons involved to produce a much larger M-wave response. Were the timing of spontaneous action potentials in an axon of the motor nerve completely desynchronized, the magnitude's M-wave response would follow a normal or Gaussian probability distribution. Were there to occur a higher degree of synchronization, the distribution of M-wave responses would be wider (greater variance) and skewed toward smaller M-wave responses.

The results appear in Figure 6.13. The distribution of the M-wave amplitudes for normal controls has an approximately normal or Gaussian distribution. The distribution for subjects with Parkinson's disease in an off-medication, off-DBS condition skews towards small-amplitude M-waves, suggesting increased synchronization of action potentials generated by the alpha lower motor neurons. Interestingly, therapeutic DBS in the vicinity of the STN further skewed the distribution of M-wave magnitudes to smaller amplitudes, which indicates even greater synchronization of action potentials generated by the alpha lower motor neuron. It is reasonable to expect that the increased synchronization of alpha lower motor neurons reflects increased synchronization, consequent to DBS, of efferent neurons in the motor cortex.

The evidence demonstrates that DBS synchronizes neuronal activities, albeit in a unique manner. The unique synchronization owes to the fact that a DBS pulse is quite inefficient in generating action potentials. Evidence shows that only some 10% of DBS pulses result in an antidromic action potential. It is well known that synaptic inputs are very inefficient in generating action potentials. Thus, feed-forward orthodromic activations are probably also

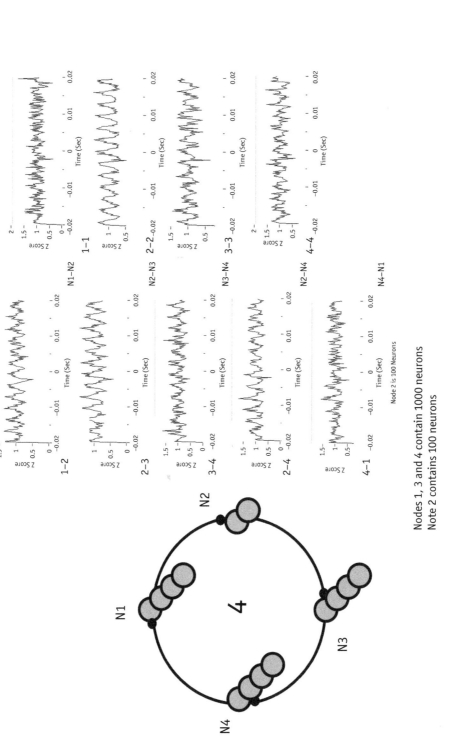

Figure 6.11: Cross-correlograms between representative pairs of neurons across and within nodes (see text), as they appear in Figure 6.10. The number of neurons in node 2 decreased from 1,000 to 100. Increased cross-correlations between neurons in node 2 and neurons within node 2 clearly indicate synchronization within the neural oscillators.

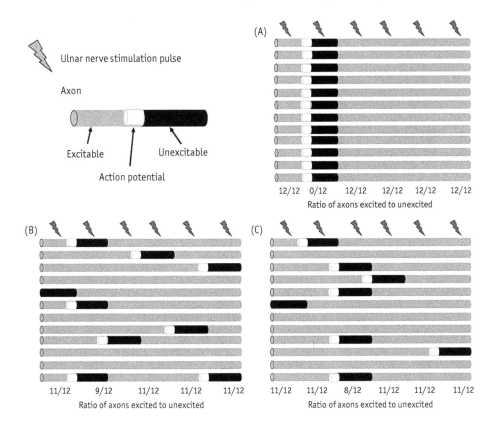

Figure 6.12: Schematic representation of a possible effect of synchronization of spontaneous action potentials in the ulnar nerve with sustained flexor force on the magnitude of an M-wave in response to supramaximal stimulation of the ulnar nerve. Action potentials are spontaneously generated in the nerve with sustained flexor force exerted by the subject. Shown is an axon that is excitable immediately prior to a spontaneous action potential and not excitable in the refractory period that follows the latter. In A, synchronization is maximal such that an ulnar nerve stimulation during the excitable period will elicit action potentials in all axons and result in a maximal M-wave. The size of the M-wave is given by the ratio of axons actually excited to the total number of potentially excitable axons. However, should ulnar nerve stimulation occur during the synchronized refractory period, no action potentials will be initiated, and the M-wave will be zero. In B, the spontaneous action potentials are asynchronous, and the refractory periods are consequently asynchronous. Any ulnar nerve stimulation sees roughly the same average number of excitable axons. This results in homogenous M-wave magnitudes. In C, an intermediate degree of synchronization results in a wider range of axons activated and a consequently wider range of M-wave amplitudes, including an increase in the number of small axonal activations and smaller M-wave amplitudes compared to B.

inefficient—an estimated 10% or lower. The synchronization may be described as "noisy synchronization" (Figure 6.14). The consequence is that the synchronization is a probability of discharging a great many neurons at a specific latency to the DBS pulse. The probability is likely to be no more than approximately 10%.

Synchronized probability, as it is presented in the forgoing discussion, may be important for physiological reasons, because the same phenomenon is observed in a group of neurons that participate in a behavior. Figure 6.15 shows the timing of action potentials in five neurons recorded simultaneously in the STN of a person saying "*la la la la la.*" The figure shows a raster of the neuronal activities, each symbol therein representing the time of onset of an action potential for each of the five neurons. The neurons observably synchronize their activity with the speaking of each *la* and with each other. Yet no individual neuron generates action potentials in each repetition of the task. Thus, there is a higher probability of each neuron's generating an action potential with speaking of the syllables. Nonetheless, the probability is much less than one.

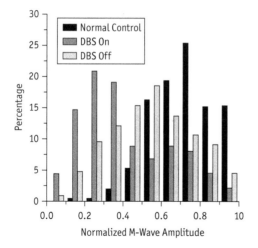

Figure 6.13: Interval histogram of the normalized area under the M-wave for each trial combined within subjects (normal and PD) and conditions (subjects with Parkinson's disease who are in off-DBS and on-DBS conditions).

Noisy synchronization may be an important mechanism of the therapeutic DBS response in the manner of stochastic resonance. This phenomenon bespeaks the counterintuitive notion that to improve the signal-to-noise ratio—the degree to which information contained in a signal can be distinguished from the accompanying noise—one must add more noise to the activities (Figure 6.16).

The relative lack of efficiency of the DBS pulse in driving action potentials in axons in the vicinity of the electrical field generated by the DBS pulse may explain the U-shaped response of progressive improvement with increasing stimulation intensity, and then a progressive worsening. The U-shaped response occurs when increasing the strength of DBS initially improves motor function and then worsens it. The strength of DBS can be increased by increasing the frequency in pulses per second, or increasing current/voltage. The U-shaped response related to different DBS frequencies has been addressed in Chapter 9, Approaches to Programming. The U-shaped response related to increased DBS stimulation current is addressed below.

The U-shaped response has at least three practical implications (Figure 16.17). First, you should increase the voltage in small increments, on the order of 0.5 mA (or 0.5 volts). Second, it is important to begin

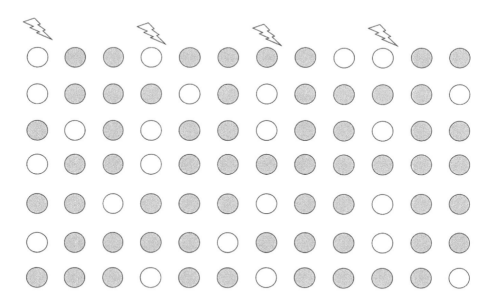

Figure 6.14: Schematic representation of the concept of noisy synchronization effected by DBS. Each row corresponds to a neuron whose activities are shown over multiple times, each time corresponding to a column. The lightning bolts illustrate delivery of a DBS pulse. Each DBS pulse observably produces a greater probability of a neuronal response at the time locked to the DBS pulse than it does at other times. However, each DBS pulse does not produce a guaranteed response in a neuron. Rather, whether a neuron responds to a specific DBS pulse is a probabilistic function and may be considered a "noisy" (probabilistic) synchronization.

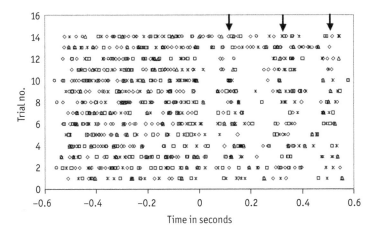

Figure 6.15: Raster of time of onset of action potentials for five neurons, each represented by a different symbol, recorded simultaneously at a single site in the STN as a patient with Parkinson's disease says "*la la la la la*." The first three *la*'s are associated with changes marked by the arrows. Each row represents a different trial. Though each neuron's participation is inconsistent, the aggregate activity is highly consistent with the behavior.

From Montgomery 2004a, page 413.

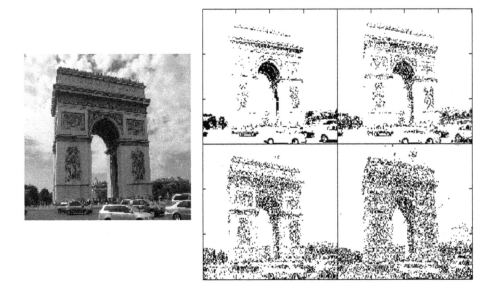

Figure 6.16: The above 256-grayscale-level images of the Arc de Triomphe result when the original is modified by the addition of noise and the performance of a nonlinear threshold operation. Each panel shows a different level of noise variance: a standard deviation of 10 grayscale levels in the top left, 50 levels in the top right, 100 in the bottom left, and 150 in the bottom right. Different panels enable the best detection of various features. The bas reliefs on the pillars are best seen in the top right, for instance, and the full outline of the Arc is best seen in the bottom left. The appearance of features also changes as the size of the image changes—the result of averaging of the image. This may be observed by viewing the image at different distances.

Verbatim from https://en.wikipedia.org/wiki/Stochastic_resonance_(sensory_neurobiology), and "ArcFull2" by Jamesvoltage—Own work. Licensed under Public Domain via Commons—https://commons.wikimedia.org/wiki/File:ArcFull2.png#/media/File:ArcFull2.png.

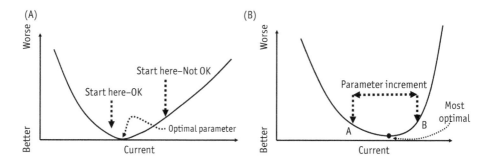

Figure 6.17: Implications of the U-shaped response to increasing DBS stimulation current. The U-shaped response demonstrates continued improvement with increasing stimulation current until a specific point is reached. Thereafter, there is a progressive worsening of the response. A shows the effect if the starting stimulation current is too high, and the programming begins beyond the optimal parameter. B shows the effect of starting at the appropriate stimulation current but taking too large an increment in the stimulation current, bypassing the optimal parameter.

with lower stimulation current/voltages. Increasing the strength in larger increments or by beginning with higher currents/voltages increases the risk of missing the U-shaped response, and you might miss the optimal parameters.

The U-shaped response has important implications for the therapeutic mechanisms of action of DBS. The worsening of symptoms with DBS in patients with Parkinson's disease may be specific to the region of the GPi being stimulated. In fact, some authors have suggested that DBS of the dorsal GPi is pro-kinetic (improving movement), whereas stimulation of the ventral GPi is anti-kinetic (worsening movement). One alternative explanation is that the worsening of symptoms is caused by the stimulation current spreading to the internal capsule, which is more likely with stimulation of the ventral GPi. Recent studies show that DBS of the STN can worsen Parkinsonian symptoms, but without spread of excessive electrical current to the internal capsule (Montgomery and Sillay 2008). This raises doubt about a pro-kinetic dorsal GPi and an anti-kinetic ventral GPi DBS.

Theories that posit suppressed neuronal activity as a mechanism of action are hard-pressed to explain why further suppression, such as that caused by increasing stimulation, would cause the recurrence or worsening of Parkinsonian symptoms. This difficulty is a problem, whether the suppression was cause by presynaptic release of inhibitory neurotransmitters, depolarization blockage, exhaustion of presynaptic excitatory neurotransmitters, or increased accumulation of adenosine (Bekar, Libionka et al. 2008).

The Systems Oscillator Theory (*see Chapter 8—Pathophysiological Mechanisms*), which conceives of the basal ganglia–thalamic-cortical system as a set of nested and interconnected, polysynaptic reentrant oscillators (Montgomery 2004a), can explain this paradoxical response. Collections of neurons in the anatomical structures represent nodes in the oscillators. Neurons within each node do not fire with every cycle of oscillatory activity, but they fire probabilistically, such that the average discharge frequency of an individual neuron is less than the frequency of the oscillator. Thus, the neurons operate within a specific range of probability of firing that is influenced by overall excitability.

DBS activates the output of neurons in the stimulated target, as well as afferent axon terminals and axons in passage. DBS is highly inefficient, with less than 10% of DBS pulses resulting in a neuronal response (Montgomery 2006). Consequently, increasing the strength of DBS may increase the excitability at a specific carrier frequency. This frequency in turn resonates with and amplifies the signal generated in the basal ganglia–thalamic-cortical system and improves function, just as an AM radio becomes tuned to the broadcast frequency. However, if the DBS stimulation–induced excitability of the neurons becomes too great, the signal deteriorates. In a sense, the signal "saturates" the structures interfering with the modulation of the neuronal spike train necessary to encode information. This concept has been verified in computational simulations (Montgomery and Sillay 2008).

Figure 6.18 shows a hypothetical example. The rasters consists of five neurons. At each cycle of the oscillation, some or none of the neurons discharge. In the normal condition, the number of neurons discharging at each point in time gradually increases and decreases. This process is represented in the histogram, which is the sum of neurons discharging in each column, representing each cycle of the oscillator. This would be analogous to the proper modulation of neuronal activity over time to drive behaviors. Next, consider the circumstance of a disease that reduces the probability of a neuron's discharging with each cycle of the oscillator. The histogram reflects a degraded signal that is very dissimilar to the normal pattern. Now consider the circumstance where there is a weak input signal, analogous to a relatively inefficient DBS but associated with optimal clinical response, at the same frequency as the normal variations represented in the histogram of the normal condition. This input increases the probability of a neuron's discharging with each cycle. The new histogram is more like the normal histogram. If the input signal is too strong, analogous to DBS stimulation parameters on the upward slope of the U-shaped curve, then the probability of a neuron's discharging is too high, and the rasters and histogram "saturate." The resulting signal is less like the normal condition compared to the condition of a weak input signal. Thus, the input of a weak signal improves the neuronal activity, thereby improving symptoms over the disease condition. The input of the strong signal degrades the neuronal activity, and the symptoms worsen, resulting in a U-shaped curve.

INTERACTIONS BETWEEN DBS PULSES IN INTRINSIC NEURONAL MECHANISMS

As stated above, a DBS pulse is highly inefficient when it comes to producing an antidromic action potential. The question naturally arises: Why is this so? Is this a purely stochastic process, or is there some underlying determining mechanism, such as the specific dynamics in the neuronal membrane potentials or ionic conductances? If the antidromic action potential represents the backfiring into the neuronal cell body and dendrites of an action potential arising in the axon, does the probability of an antidromic action potential depend on some condition within the neuronal cell body and dendrites? If

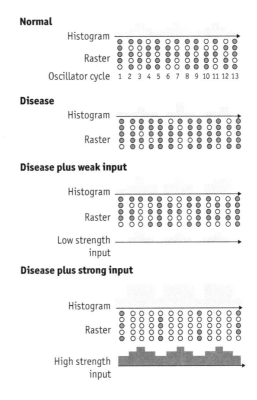

Figure 6.18: Hypothetical illustration of a possible mechanism underlying the U-shaped response to DBS. Each part of the figure contains a raster and a histogram. The raster represents the five neurons, some of which discharge during each cycle. A gray circle indicates no discharge, and a yellow circle indicates a neuronal discharge. The histogram represents the total number of neurons discharging in each cycle of the oscillator. Assume that a sinusoidally varying normal signal gradually increases and then decreases the probability of the neuron's discharging. In disease, the probability of neurons' discharging is reduced, and consequently, the information in the neuronal discharges degrades over time. This degradation is reflected in the difference in the histograms between the normal and disease conditions. The degraded information results in the symptoms and signs of the disease. Next, assume a weak input, such as therapeutic DBS, that increases the neuronal discharge probability in a waxing and waning pattern at the same frequency of the inherent changes under the normal condition. In this case, the information represented in the histogram is more like the normal condition than it is during the disease condition. This case is associated with improved symptoms and signs. Next, assume that the input signal, such as high current/voltage DBS, greatly increases the probability of a neuronal discharge. Now, nearly all the neurons are discharging with each cycle, and the histogram "saturates" and loses information, in contrast to the normal histogram and the histogram of the disease state plus a weak input. This case is associated with a worsening of symptoms and signs, giving rise to a U-shaped response.

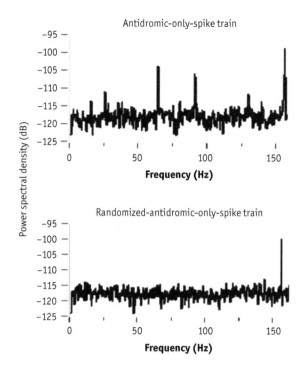

Figure 6.19: Representative power spectral density of a *antidromic-only spike train* and its *randomized antidromic-only spike train* counterpart for 160 pps DBS.

it does, then the probability of an antidromic action potential must reflect the conditions in the cell body and dendrites, which in turn must reflect the effects of synaptic inputs onto the neuron (Chomiak et al. 2007; Rosen 1981). This implies that the presence or absence of an antidromic action potential may reflect the status of the excitability of a neuronal cell body and dendrites over time.

Another analysis (Montgomery et al. 2012) used neuronal microelectrode recordings of the STN in subjects with Parkinson's disease (PD) that were made, in a manner described elsewhere, during DBS in the vicinity of the contralateral STN (Walker et al. 2011). Stimulation was at 160 pulses per second (pps) and 30 pps. Fifty-eight neurons were recorded from eight STN nuclei in eight subjects.

From the microelectrode recordings of STN neurons made during DBS in the vicinity of the contralateral STN, trains of antidromic action potentials were extracted for the purpose of constructing an antidromic-only spike train. Then the antidromic-only spike train was randomized. For a representative neuron, the power spectral density results for DBS at

160 pps appear in Figure 6.19 and in Figure 6.20 for 30 pps. The only peak in the power spectral densities in the randomized antidromic-only spike trains occurred at the DBS frequencies. In the antidromic-only spike train with DBS at 160 pps, peaks also were noted at 66 Hz and 92 Hz, the latter probability representing a beat interaction between the intrinsic oscillator at 66 Hz and the DBS frequency. In the 30 pps DBS condition, peaks were found at multiple frequencies. Subsequent analyses demonstrated two main intrinsic frequencies at 66 Hz and 26 Hz beyond the harmonics of these frequencies, the DBS frequencies, and beat interactions between the intrinsic frequencies and the DBS frequencies.

These observations suggest that at least two oscillators include neurons of the STN. It cannot be determined whether the source of these oscillations lies in mechanisms intrinsic to the neuron, which were mentioned in the above discussion of the Hodgkin and Huxley models of neurons' biophysical properties (Hodgkin and Huxley 1952), or in the fact that these neurons are embedded in polysynaptic reentrant oscillators.

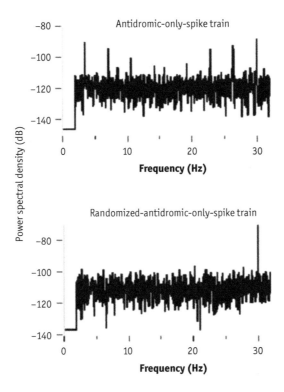

Figure 6.20: Representative power spectral density of a *antidromic-only spike train* and its *randomized antidromic-only spike train* counterpart for 30 pps DBS.

Importantly, these observations suggest that the DBS pulse train, which is considered an oscillator, interacts with neural oscillators intrinsic to the neurons of the basal ganglia–thalamic-cortical system. The degree to which the oscillator mechanisms in neurons are the result of the dynamics intrinsic to the neuronal membrane's biophysical properties and to the dynamics of activity—that is, information—percolating in a reentrant manner through the basal ganglia–thalamic-cortical systems remains to be determined.

EFFECTS ON BEHAVIORALLY RELATED INTRINSIC NEURONAL DYNAMICS

As discussed in Chapter 7, DBS Effects on Motor Control, the control of behaviors implemented by muscles requires the precise recruitment and de-recruitment of motor units. This orchestration of motor units takes place over time scales that,

depending on the behavior, range from milliseconds to many seconds. As motor units are driven by the alpha lower motor neuron, which are in turn driven by the basal ganglia–thalamic-cortical system as well as (among others such as the cerebellar systems) the dynamics of precise orchestration of neuronal activities occur throughout these motor systems. These precise changes are information that is encoded and processed within the nervous system. In Figure 6.21 an example appears of the activities of a striatal neuron (probably a tonically active cholinergic interneuron) in a non-human primate as it performs a wrist joint rotation in response to a visual commencement signal. The question thus arises: How does DBS affect these intrinsic information dynamics? Some have argued that DBS drives neuronal activities to "overwrite" the information, as it were, in what has been identified as "information ablation." If the information is faulty, then overwriting the misinformation could have a beneficial effect. Yet the inefficiencies of DBS in producing neuronal action potentials renders the notion of information ablation problematic.

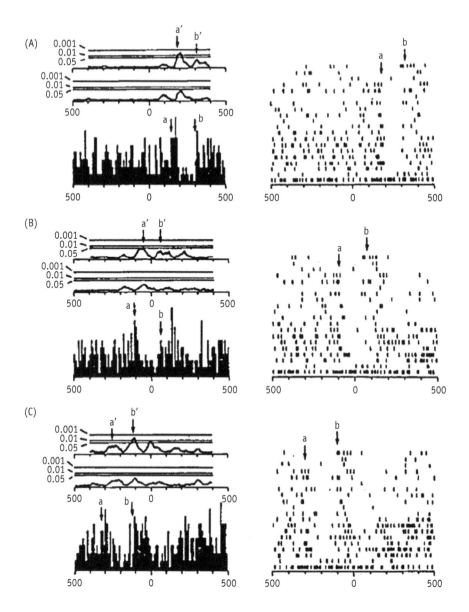

Figure 6.21: Three sets of representations of the same data set of a putamen neuron activity during the performance of a wrist flexion and extension task in a non-human primate. The data on the right represent peri-event rasters in which each row corresponds to a sequence of neuronal action potentials for each trial of the task. These rows are summed vertically from the histograms on the left. Over each summed histogram are two statistical measures that relate the change in neuronal activity between two adjacent sliding windows, and a lower measure that relates the activity of a sliding window to the baseline activity preceding the commencement signal. The associated graphs plot the *p* value of the statistical comparisons of the windows. There are two peaks in histograms "a" and "b." The top set of rasters and histograms is centered on the "go" signal. The middle set is centered on movement onset, whereas the bottom set is centered on reaching the target. The peak "a" is most consistently related to and follows the appearance of the "go" signal, whereas the peak "b" is most consistently related to and precedes the movement of reaching the target, as demonstrated by a maximum *p* value.

From Montgomery and Buchholz 1991, page 225.

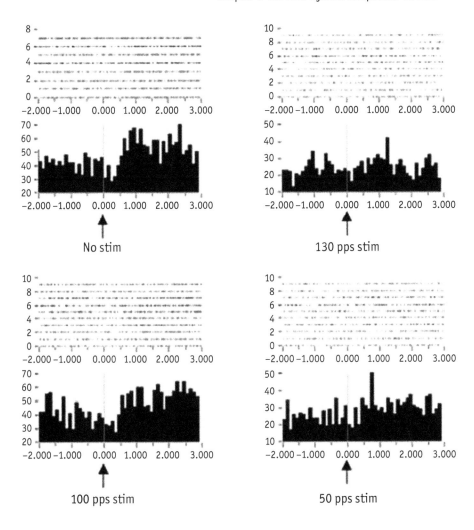

No stim

130 pps stim

100 pps stim

50 pps stim

Figure 6.22: Peri-event rasters and histogram showing a caudate nucleus neuron's activity before and after the onset of the commencement signal indicated by the up arrow. Each dot in the rasters represents a neuronal discharge, and each row represents a trial. Summing a column in the raster produces the histogram. With no stimulation, with 100 pps DBS and (to a lesser degree) with 50 pps DBS, there is an increase in neuronal discharge following the onset of the commencement signal. This dynamic modulation is lost with the 130 pps DBS. The post-stimulus histograms show the change in neuronal discharge probability following each stimulation pulse. The varying lengths of data represent different inter-stimulus intervals. There is very little difference in the early and intermediate responses to the stimulation pulse with the different DBS frequencies. Also, DBS drives neuronal activity even when the peri-event rasters and histograms demonstrate no modulation of neuronal activity with the behavior during stimulation at 130 pps.

From Montgomery and Gale 2007, page 398.

Recordings of neuronal activities made as non-human primates perform behaviors show a range of effects of DBS on the information or intrinsic dynamics. For the most part, the movement-related dynamics are preserved in neurons of the GPi during DBS-like stimulation in the vicinity of the STN in non-human primates (Zimnik et al. 2015). Other studies indicate that DBS markedly alters information in some neurons.

A second study involved recordings of neurons in multiple structures of the basal ganglia–thalamic-cortical system. Figure 6.22 shows activity in a non-human primate's caudate nucleus neuron related to the onset of an upper-extremity reaching task

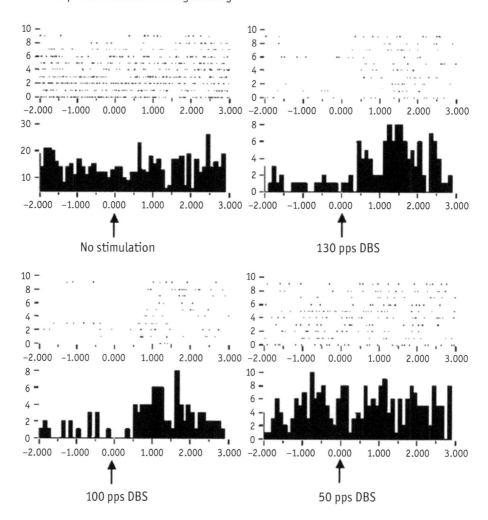

Figure 6.23: Peri-event rasters and histograms for a neuron recorded in the putamen of a non-human primate. There is no meaningful modulation of neuronal activity with behavior (appearance of the commencement signal at time zero is indicated by the up arrow) under the no-stimulation condition. However, consistent modulation occurs with 130 pps and (to a lesser extent) 100 pps DBS, suggesting that the DBS has enlisted the neuron into being meaningfully related to the behavior. This is consistent with, if not proof of, a resonance effect as described in the text (Gale, 2004). It bears noting that the baseline activity prior to the commencement signal is reduced.

From Montgomery and Gale 2007, page 401.

performed during DBS-like stimulation in the vicinity of the STN. There are observable dynamic modulations of neuronal activities related to the behavior under the no-DBS condition, and a significant reduction in modulation with increased DBS frequencies. For DBS frequencies that are typically therapeutic, normal dynamics were completely lost.

For another neuron recorded in the putamen, there was no modulation under the no-DBS condition (Figure 6.23). With increasing DBS frequency came progressively greater dynamic modulation of neuronal activities correlated with the behavior. Information encoded in the dynamic modulation probably did not inhere in the DBS pulse train; DBS interacted with intrinsic mechanisms to produce the modulation. The information may possibly have been the neuronal activities under the no-DBS condition, albeit with an inadequate signal-to-noise ratio. DBS, by a process of stochastic resonance, may have improved the signal-to-noise ratio to the point that information

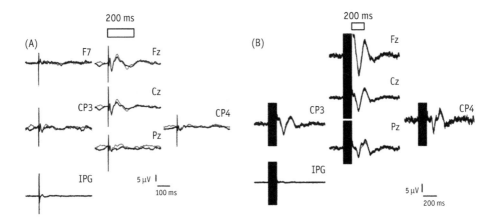

Figure 6.24: Electroencephalographic-evoked responses to DBS pulses in the vicinity of the left STN in a patient with Parkinson's disease. The left panel shows the responses to a single pulse delivered every 2 seconds, and the panel on the right shows the response to a 100 ms train of DBS at 130 pulses per second. The rectangle is 200 ms in duration, for comparison. The duration of the evoked potential is observably shorter than the train of pulses. Also, the evoked potential associated with a single pulse appears over frontal midline electrode (Fz), the central midline electrode (Cz), and the left-central parietal electrode (CP3). The evoked potential associated with the train of DBs pulses appears in the same locations as it did in the single pulse and the parietal midline electrode (Pz) and, at a longer latency, in the contralateral central parietal electrode (CP4). Modifed from Baker et al. 2002 page 974 and 978.

became manifest. (The topic of DBS and stochastic resonance is discussed in greater detail in *Chapter 8, Pathophysiological Mechanisms.*) The point to be made here is that stochastic resonance depends on frequency. Improved signal-to-noise ratio with high-frequency DBS suggests an interaction with an intrinsic mechanism or noise that operates at a similar frequency.

TEMPORAL EVOLUTION OF NERVOUS SYSTEM RESPONSES

Just as there is a tendency to focus on neuronal responses within the anatomical structure targeted by DBS, there is also a tendency to focus on responses to individual pulses. However, it is likely that the nervous system response to an individual pulses lasts for a relatively long period of time relative to the inter-pulse interval in a continuous DBS pulse train. A sequence of pulses may have an additive effect, resulting in nervous system responses that evolve over time. The variability in the latencies of the DBS effect raises questions about the temporal evolution of neuronal responses to DBS (Rizzone et al. 2001; Lopiano et al. 2003).

The nervous system response to an individual pulse may be different from the response to a sequence of pulses. This difference in effect may be seen in the electroencephalographic response evoked from DBS pulses. In Figure 6.24, the electroencephalographic-evoked response to individual DBS pulses and to a short series of DBS pulses in the vicinity of the STN is shown. The evoked potentials from the train of DBS pulses are observably longer in duration and distributed over a larger portion of the nervous system, particularly the contralateral central parietal area. The response to the train of DBS pulses on the contralateral central parietal area has a notably longer latency, suggesting that the effects of the DBS pulse take longer to reach the mechanisms underlying the evoked potential on the contralateral side.

The majority of studies examine nervous system responses to individual DBS pulses even when the pulses are delivered in a train of pulses. Such analyses depend critically on whether the response to each DBS pulse is the same during the entire course of the DBS train of pulses. One study examined that assumption, certain results of which are presented here. This preliminary study took advantage of recent demonstrations of both antidromic and orthodromic activation of neurons in the STN by use of DBS in the vicinity of the contralateral STN and elsewhere (Walker et al. 2011). In this case, cycling-mode DBS

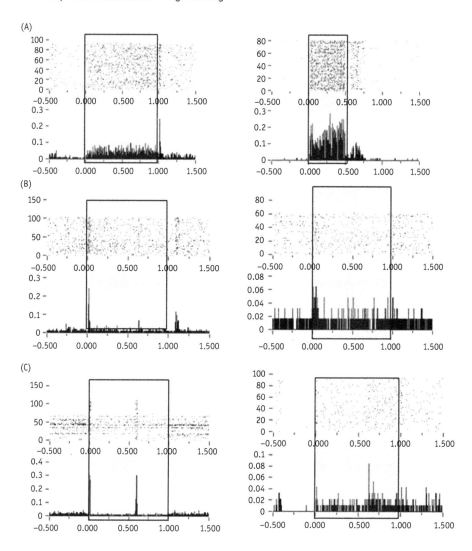

Figure 6.25: Representative examples of peri-event rasters and histograms centered on the onset of the DBS cycle. The top half of each figure displays rows of dots. Each dot represents the discharge of a neuron, and each row represents a single cycle of DBS. The bottom half of each figure is a histogram, which is constructed by collapsing the rows into columns. Time zero is the onset of the cycle of DBS. The box demarcates the onset and duration of the DBS cycle relative to the neuronal activities. Neuronal responses that followed the cycle are not interpretable, because the stimulation was not cleanly halted at the end of the cycle.

was used. Post-stimulus rasters and histograms may be constructed on the onset of the first DBS pulse, and the neuronal responses over the next 0.5–1 sec may be analyzed.

One hundred fifty-two neurons were recorded and analyzed. Twenty-nine neurons demonstrated a response to DBS in the vicinity of the contralateral STN. Three types of responses during the DBS cycle were found. The first was characterized by a progressive buildup, which was followed by sustained increased neuronal activity in six of the 29 responsive neurons (Figure 6.25, row A). The second type was an initial increase followed by return towards similar levels of activity between cycles (Figure 6.25, row B) in 19 of 29 responsive neurons. The third type demonstrated brief periods of increased activity within the DBS cycle (Figure 6.25, row C) in four of 29 responsive neurons.

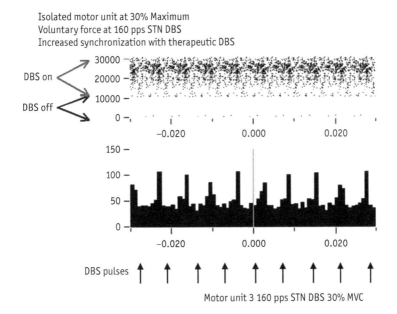

Isolated motor unit at 30% Maximum
Voluntary force at 160 pps STN DBS
Increased synchronization with therapeutic DBS

Figure 6.26: Raster and histogram of electrical activity generated by a motor unit (a combination of muscle fibers innervated by a single axon from an alpha lower motor neuron in the spinal cord as the subject creates a muscle force that is 30% of the subject's maximum force). The subject has a DBS electrode implanted in the vicinity of the STN, the activation of which stimulates at a rate of 160 pulses per second (pps). In the raster, each dot represents the electrical discharge of the motor unit. Each row represents the onset of a DBS pulse centered on the index pulse at time 0. The histogram counts the number of dots in columns across the rows in the raster to provide another view of the overall response. The length of the raster and histogram is longer than the time interval between DBS pulses for the purpose of providing a better sense of the change in responses. An observably significant change in the response of the motor unit occurs as the DBS continues.

These results mean that caution is needed, because reports of average changes in neuronal activities during DBS may not reflect the actual nature of the neuronal responses. Consequently, any explanation of DBS effects on larger-scale measures, such as averages of neuronal responses, local field potentials, and neurometabolic imaging during DBS, is quite difficult, because the actual neuronal responses may be quite non-stationary at the time scales used by these measures.

Another example of the evolution of the neuronal responses over time to sustained DBS appears in Figure 6.2. In this case, the response of a representative neuron in the Vop changes over the time course

of DBS in the vicinity of the GPi. Another example is shown in Figure 6.26, in which the electromyographic activity generated in a motor unit (the combination of muscle fibers innervated by the axon from a single alpha lower motor neuron in the spinal cord) changes during the course of DBS in the vicinity of the STN. One may reasonably extrapolate from this that the evolution of the motor unit activity reflects a parallel evolution of action potential generation in the alpha lower motor neuron in the spinal cord, which in turn reflects the evolution of neuronal activities in the basal ganglia–thalamic-cortical system with sustained DBS in the vicinity of the STN.

7

DBS EFFECTS ON MOTOR CONTROL

Use of DBS extends beyond what are typically referred to as *movement disorders*, for which issues of motor control are paramount; currently approved for treatment of refractory obsessive-compulsive disorder (OCD), DBS is expected to gain approval as a treatment for epilepsy, as well. Indeed, no neurological or psychiatric disorder ought to be excluded *a priori* from consideration as a potential indication for DBS. Post-operative management of DBS for these other disorders will benefit from a better understanding of the mechanisms of action. An understanding of the ways the brain responds to DBS (*see Chapter 6— Brain Responses to DBS*) related to motor control may therefore serve as an important metaphor for understanding the use of DBS for other conditions.

The relevance of an understanding of motor control to other neurological and psychiatric disorders is supported by commonalities in the circuitry of the basal ganglia–thalamic-cortical systems that underlie motor, limbic, and cognitive functions, which appear in Figure 7.1 (Alexander et al. 1986). Very roughly, commonalities in architecture suggest that these different domains, which range from movement, to emotions, to thinking, may share similar mechanisms that may prove highly relevant to attempts at improving with DBS disorders of movement, emotion, and thinking.

Even in the domain of movement disorders, there is plenty of room to improve DBS's clinical efficacy. For example, specific stimulation frequencies clearly help some motor behaviors and worsen others. High frequency stimulation in the vicinity of the STN can improve upper extremity function. Yet it often does so at the expense of worsening gait, postural control, speech, language, and swallowing. Even with respect to upper extremity function, some aspects, such as strength or force generation, are improved, and other aspects, such as the precise control of forces, are not. How these issues play out in determining the overall improvement in quality of life is difficult to know. Nonetheless, for the question to be answered, these issues must be considered and investigated.

ORCHESTRATION OF MOTOR UNIT ACTIVITIES

The motor manifestations of movement disorders, which are currently the major target of DBS therapy, are determined by the precise contraction of muscle fibers. This orchestration occurs among relatively small groups of muscle fibers and cannot be understood by analyses that are limited to the actions of whole muscles. A major controlling influence of the activities of these groups of muscle fibers is wielded by alpha lower motor neurons that reside in the spinal cord and brainstem and connect to and activate them. The group of muscle fibers innervated by a single alpha lower motor neuron is known as a *motor unit*. Discussion to follow will henceforth be couched in terms of motor units.

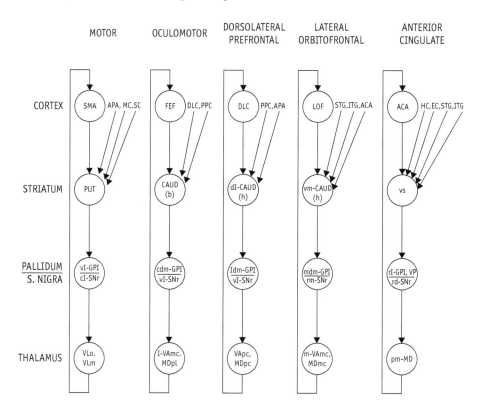

Figure 7.1: Parallel organization of the five basal ganglia–thalamocortical circuits. Each circuit engages specific regions of the cerebral cortex: striatum, pallidum, substantia nigra, and thalamus. *Abbreviations* are as follows: ACA: anterior cingulate area; APA: arcuate premotor area; CAUD: caudate, (b) body (h) head; DLC: dorsolateral prefrontal cortex; EC: entorhinal cortex; FEF: frontal eye fields; GPi: internal segment of globus pallidus; HC: hippocampal cortex; ITG: inferior temporal gyrus; LOF: lateral orbitofrontal cortex; MC: motor cortex; MDpl: medialis dorsalis pars paralamellaris; MDmc: medialis dorsalis pars magnocellularis; MDpc: medialis dorsalis pars parvocellularis; PPC: posterior parietal cortex; PUT: putamen; SC: somatosensory cortex; SMA: supplementary motor area; SNr: substantia nigra pars reticulata; STG: superior temporal gyrus; V Amc: ventralis anterior pars magnocellularis; Vapc: ventralis anterior pars parvocellularis; VLm: ventralis lateralis pars medialis; VLo: ventralis lateralis pars oralis; VP: ventral pallidum; VS: ventral striatum; cl-: caudolateral; cdm-: caudal dorsomedial; dl-: dorsolateral; l-: lateral; ldm-: lateral dorsomedial; m-: medial; mdm-: medial dorsomedial; pm-: postero-medial; rd-: rostrodorsal; rl-: rostrolateral; rm-: rostromedial; vm-: ventromedial; vl-: ventrolateral.
Verbatim from Alexander et al. 1986, page 364.

The orchestration of motor units is organized over multiple spatial and temporal scales or dimensions. Frequently, these different levels of organization are mistakenly described as "higher versus lower" or "complex versus simple." Connotations of such terms have inherent presuppositions that are invalid. As such, they may be the source of misleading inferences. The descriptors "high" and "low" often connote a hierarchical organization of components, which further leads to the inference that such components operate in a sequential manner. Such terms are used to describe the motor cortex as occupying a higher level than the alpha lower motor unit. But this is

mistaken, because it minimizes the roles of feedback and interaction with all levels of the nervous system and with the environment in shaping any activities in the motor cortex.

One level of orchestration of motor unit activities is the recruitment of motor units for generating a muscle force that rotates joints or pulls on other structures that are not mediated by joints, such as muscles that deform the skin for the purpose of creating facial expressions. In the 1950s it was discovered that there is a range of motor unit sizes, and they are determined by the number of muscle fibers innervated by a single alpha lower motor neuron. These range from a few to hundreds. Small motor units create small forces, and larger motor units generate larger forces. One level of control over the forces is thus generated by controlling the activation of motor units of different sizes. When a small force is required, small motor units are recruited (activated). As larger forces are required, the smaller motor units discharge more frequently, and larger motor units are recruited. This type of orchestration is called the *Henneman Size Principle*. Precise control of movement requires precise orchestration of the way in which motor units are recruited and de-recruited. If larger motor units are recruited first, the initial force will be relatively large and may thus be incapable of providing fine resolution of force control.

Since the 1950s it has been presumed that orchestration at the level of motor unit recruitment was a property of the alpha lower motor neurons and had little to do with other components of the motor system—the basal ganglia, for example. Small alpha lower motor neurons associated with small motor units were activated more easily than larger alpha lower motor neurons. The biophysical properties of the alpha lower motor neurons were thought sufficient for providing this level of precise control. Consequently, it was reasoned that the basal ganglia, whose physiology and pathophysiology underlie most movement disorders, played no role in motor unit recruitment and de-recruitment. No abnormalities of motor unit control owing to movement disorders, such as Parkinson's disease, at this level were considered. This notion may be largely responsible for the paucity of investigations of possible abnormalities at this level of motor control in Parkinson's disease and other movement disorders.

A study described below demonstrates that the Henneman Size Principle is abnormal in patients with Parkinson's disease, and that DBS in the vicinity of the STN helps restore the recruitment of motor units in way that is consistent with the principle (Huang et al. 2012). A representative example appears in Figure 7.2. Raw electromyographic (EMG) recordings obtained from intramuscular fine wire hook electrodes are shown. EMG spikes of different amplitudes are shown. As can be appreciated in the raw EMG under high frequency DBS, there is a progression, over time and increasing muscle force, of sequential activations of EMG spikes of larger amplitudes, providing a "stair-step" appearance consistent with the Henneman Size Principle. However, following an

overnight fast for anti-Parkinson medications and with the DBS turned off, the "stair-step" appearance is absent, with a more random pattern of EMG spikes of different amplitudes.

The raw EMG recordings in Figure 7.2 were analyses to extract the spike waveforms associated with individual motor units and the "size" of the motor unit calculated as the area under the curve of the EMG spike (Figure 7.2). Rasters are shown above the raw EMG. Each row in the rasters shows the time of each EMG spike associated with the isolated motor units. As can be seen under the high frequency DBS, larger motor units were recruited later (indicated by the red arrow). However, under the no medication and no DBS condition, all the motor units became active simultaneously without regard for motor unit size.

The force level at which each motor unit began to discharge for each DBS condition is shown in Figure 7.3 for a representative patient with Parkinson's disease who had also been receiving DBS at different frequencies. Linear regression lines were fitted for each DBS condition. As can be seen, only the high frequency DBS condition had a large positive slope consistent with the Henneman Size Principle. These findings suggest that this level of motor unit orchestration is abnormal in Parkinson's disease, which in turn suggests a role for the basal ganglia in determining motor unit recruitment order. As such, the latter shows promise as a therapeutic mechanism of DBS for Parkinson's disease, even if for no other movement disorders.

The issues that attend recruitment of motor units with increasing force also apply to the orchestrated reduction of motor unit activities known as *de-recruitment*. De-recruitment normally follows the opposite course of that which is identified in the Henneman Size Principle. Whether de-recruitment is also abnormal in such movement disorders as Parkinson's disease is unknown.

Other studies have demonstrated increased muscle force production with DBS in the vicinity of the STN and in the vicinity of the GPi (Sturman et al. 2010; Alberts et al. 2004). These observations also suggest that DBS has an effect on motor unit recruitment.

Another level of motor control relates to acceleration and deceleration of rotations about a joint. As the rotation around a joint goes from rest to some velocity, it accelerates. Because a joint cannot rotate indefinitely, it clearly must decelerate. In both cases,

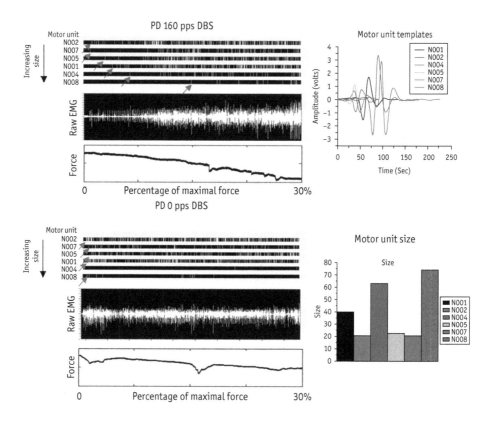

Figure 7.2: Representative example of raw, intramuscular electromyographic (EMG) activities in a subject with Parkinson's disease under conditions of 160 pps DBS (therapeutic) and 0 pps DBS. The raw EMG under 160 pps DBS has a stair-step appearance. Each step is associated with recruitment of a large motor unit. The same six motor units were identified under both conditions, and their waveforms and size are shown. The waveform associated with each motor unit is distinct and varies in size from its fellows. The size was determined by measuring the area under the curve. The time of occurrence of a motor unit discharge appears in the raster, with one row for each motor unit. The red arrow indicates onset of activities as the force generated progressively increases. Observable in the 160 pps DBS condition is an orderly recruitment (indicated by the red arrows): Consistent with the Henneman Size Principle, smaller units are recruited first, followed by progressively larger motor units. Under the 0 pps DBS condition, the orderly recruitment of motor units is lost, and the units are recruited nearly simultaneously. Large motor units are recruited early in the task and at small forces.

accelerations and decelerations require the application of force to overcome inertia. This follows from Newton's First Law of Motion, which holds that an object in motion or at rest tends to remain in motion or at rest unless acted upon by an outside force. Also, the forces required for overcoming inertia are directly related to the mass of an object, which in this case is the limb distal to the joint that is moved in the joint rotation. The mass of the hand, for example, affects accelerations and decelerations of rotations about the wrist.

In addition to inertia, joint rotations involve interactions with the elastic properties of muscles, tendons, and ligaments. These tissues may be considered as "springs" on each side of an axis of rotation of a joint. In joint rotation, the muscle being stretched by the rotation creates resistance to further rotation.

The potentially complicated effects of inertia may further complicate the orchestration of motor unit recruitment and de-recruitment. For example, a slow joint rotation invokes little resistance because of inertia. However, a quicker rotation requires greater force. Consider the act of a rapid hand rotation about the wrist that moves in the direction of extension and begins with flexion. The motor units in the wrist flexor muscles are initially recruited in order to overcome the elastic forces generated in the extensor muscles, because the wrist has flexed beyond the neutral

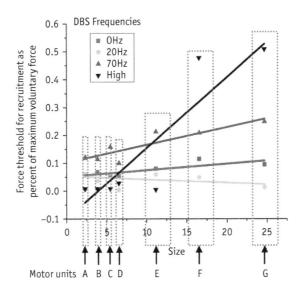

Figure 7.3: Relationship between percent of maximum force at which each of the seven motor units was recruited and the size of the motor units for different DBS conditions for a representative subject with Parkinson's disease. The seven motor units (A–G) are ordered according to motor-unit size: A is the smallest and G the largest. Each symbol and color represents the various DBS conditions. A flat or small slope indicates that the Henneman Size Principle did not hold under that DBS condition. An initially relatively flat slope that greatly increases with therapeutic (high) DBS frequency characterizes the untreated patient (0 Hz DBS), suggesting that motor unit recruitment has become normalized.

point (Figure 7.4). With the onset of extension joint rotation, motor units in the wrist flexor muscles are de-recruited. Then the motor units in the wrist extensor muscles are recruited to generate a force sufficient for accelerating the mass of the hand. If initial acceleration is unchecked, the hand often moves beyond the intended target. Consequently, motor units in the extensor muscles are de-recruited before the hand reaches the intended target in the extension position. This de-recruitment is followed by recruitment of motor units in the wrist flexor to decelerate the wrist joint rotation. Finally, motor units in the wrist extensors are recruited to bring the hand to the target position in extension, and these motor units continue their activity in order to maintain the hand in the extension position against the elastic forces of the stretched flexor muscles that would move the wrist to a neutral position.

There is considerable evidence that the above-mentioned orchestration of motor unit recruitment and de-recruitment is abnormal in Parkinson's disease. First, in normal subjects, de-recruitment of motor units in the muscle that oppose the intended joint rotation occurs prior to recruitment of motor units in the muscle that move the hand

in the intended direction. In the case illustrated in Figure 7.4, the motor units in the wrist flexor muscles are de-recruited (Figure 7.4.A) before the motor units in the wrist extensor muscles are recruited (Figure 7.4.D). In subjects with Parkinson's disease, however, motor unit activities in the muscles that oppose the intended joint rotation continue even as motor units are recruited in muscles that move the hand in the intended direction (Montgomery et al. 1991). This results in a co-contraction between the muscles that oppose the intended joint rotation and those that facilitate it. Also, it is known that the magnitude of the second motor unit recruitment—box E in Figure 7.4, for example—is less than normal, and the joint rotation often falls short of the intended target position. These features improve with DBS in the vicinity of the STN (Vaillancourt et al. 2004).

The above-mentioned issues for rotations about a single joint also apply to multi-segmented or multi-joint movements. Illustrative of this fact is the act of reaching for and grasping a cup. The movement involves simultaneous rotations about multiple joints, each of which has to account for the above-mentioned inertial and elastic forces. Interestingly, changes about each joint occur simultaneously, happening as if

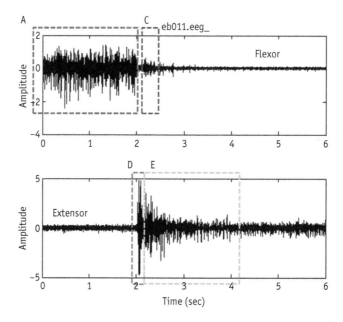

Figure 7.4: Example of the electrical activities generated by motor units in the wrist flexor and extensor muscles in a task that involves rapid wrist extension from a position in wrist flexion. Motor units of the wrist flexor muscles are initially active in holding the wrist in a flexed position in order to counter elastic forces generated by stretched extensor muscles (A). With the onset of wrist extension, motor units in the wrist extensor muscles are de-recruited, as is reflected by the paucity of electrical activity between the events marked by boxes A and C. In the same moment, motor units are recruited in the wrist extensor muscles (D). In order to prevent rapid acceleration in the extensor direction, which causes the hand to move beyond the intended target, there occurs a burst of motor unit activity in the flexor muscles (C) to decelerate the movement. This is followed by a recruitment of motor units in the wrist extensors to bring the hand to the intended position and maintain it in the extended position against the elastic forces that would move the hand more in the direction of flexion.

programmed as a single unit. The hand begins to form a shape that is consistent with that of the object to be grasped as proximal joint rotations carry it to that object. Patients with Parkinson's disease are abnormal in this coordination, which improves with DBS in the vicinity of the STN (Schettino et al. 2009).

Yet another level of orchestration—synergy in motor unit recruitment and de-recruitment of motor units—involves integration of intended movements with their base of support. When you move your arm from your side and extends it before yourself, for example, you shift your center of gravity. For you to maintain it over its base of support in order to avoid falling, motor units of the trunk and lower extremities must be recruited and de-recruited. Postural adjustment often begins prior to any shift in the center of gravity. This indicates that, rather than simply reacting to the shift, the necessary orchestration of motor units in the trunk and leg muscles anticipates it.

And yet another level of motor control occurs at the level of orchestration of a complex sequence of actions appropriate to specific contexts. This control may be impaired, despite an apparent absence of abnormalities at other levels of orchestration of motor unit recruitment and de-recruitment. Often referred to as *apraxias*, these abnormalities are observed in patients with Parkinson's disease (Villardita et al. 1982; Quencer et al. 2007). This observation has met some controversy. One problem with applying the term "apraxic" to describe patients with Parkinson's disease stems from the original definition of apraxias as disorders of movement that have no disorder of sensation attending them and no apparent abnormal components of the behavior. It would appear that, by definition, a diagnosis of apraxia could never be made in patients with Parkinson's disease, because, were it to be pressed, it would reveal itself to be mere sophistry. Most sophisticated observers recognize that there is an abnormality at this level of motor control that cannot be dismissed simply because other motor abnormalities are present as well (Swash 2007). How this level of motor control is affected by DBS is unknown.

ORCHESTRATION OF MOTOR UNIT RECRUITMENT AND DE-RECRUITMENT OVER DIFFERENT TIME SCALES

The above-mentioned levels of motor unit recruitment and de-recruitment described may also be conceptualized as operating at different time scales. For example, the first level —namely, onset of motor unit activity that increases in discharge frequency with increasing force and decreases in discharge frequency and de-recruits with decreasing force—operates over brief time intervals and thus, at high frequencies. For example, as shown in Figure 7.4, the timing between the recruitment, de-recruitment, and subsequent recruitment of motor units in the extensor muscles, and the de-recruitment, recruitment, and subsequent de-recruitment of motor units in the flexor muscles occurs over a hundred or so milliseconds.

The orchestrated recruitments and de-recruitments are organized on another time scale in what are called *envelopes of motor unit activity*. For example, recruitment–de-recruitment occurs in an envelope of time (Figure 7.4), which operates over a longer period than do the motor unit recruitment and de-recruitments. The successive envelopes of motor unit activities in various muscle groups in a complex multi-joint movement, such as reaching for a cup, are organized over a longer time scale, usually on the order of seconds. Also, during the course of a multi-joint movement, different muscles become involved. This argues for a spatial orchestration of motor unit recruitment and de-recruitment as well.

The different levels of orchestration of motor unit recruitment and de-recruitment are programmed simultaneously. When an individual reaches to grasp an object, motor units are recruited and de-recruited to shape his hand in conformity with it as motor units of the more proximal limb musculature carry his hand toward it. Also, at the same moment as his limb moves, motor units in the muscles of his trunk and lower extremities adjust in anticipation of changes in his center of gravity. The coordination of motor recruitments and de-recruitments in these complex synergies is affected by Parkinson's disease and appears to improve with DBS in the vicinity of the STN (Bleuse et al. 2011).

The question arises: How can DBS affect the different temporal time scales of orchestration of motor unit recruitment and de-recruitment? The latter may be regarded as having a counterpart in oscillator mechanisms whose period of frequencies corresponds to the time scales of motor unit orchestration. As is discussed in Chapter 6, Nervous System Responses to DBS, DBS may be regarded as an oscillator because of its repetitive and rhythmic discharge rates, which are introduced to oscillator activities in the basal ganglia–thalamic-cortical system. As such, a DBS oscillator may resonate positively (additive resonance) or negatively (destructive resonance) with neural oscillators. Resonance interactions depend on the frequencies of interacting oscillators. Thus, high frequency DBS may interact with some sets of oscillators, the therapeutic effect of which may explain improvements of motor control, at the appropriate time scale; but they may also disrupt oscillators at different time scales and thus interfere with the corresponding level of motor unit recruitment and de-recruitment.

A striking demonstration of the concept of complex interacting oscillators producing complex movements is seen in the medieval mechanical prayer monks. These automata were powered by a clockwork mechanism that consisted of interconnected gears and levers. They appeared to walk, turning approximately every 20 inches or so to turn their head, open and close their mouth, and direct their eyes at a crucifix carried in one hand as they beat their breast with the other (http://io9.com/5956937/this-450-year-old-clockwork-monk-is-fully-operational).

LESSONS TO BE LEARNED

The many discussions of DBS's mechanisms of action in the published literature pay scant attention to DBS's role in controlling the various manners of orchestration of motor unit recruitment and de-recruitment, despite the fundamental importance of motor unit orchestration. The silence may be due to the original presumption that the biophysics of the alpha lower motor neurons primarily control motor unit recruitment and de-recruitment. This presumption thus obviates any need to include consideration of any more central mechanisms that are related to motor control, such as the basal ganglia–thalamic-cortical system. It is highly likely, however, that the failure to consider the fundamental basis of motor physiology stems from the fact that nearly every theory of basal ganglia function is primarily an anatomical and neurochemical rather than a physiological theory (Montgomery 2012). Missing from a purely anatomical and neurochemical theory is any consideration of the dynamics at the time scale of motor unit recruitment and de-recruitment. It is an intriguing commentary on human nature that intuitively appealing theories are quite immune to contrary evidence (Johnson-Larid 2006), despite their failure to explain what ought to be considered relevant observations and considerations.

In many ways, consideration of movement disorders and the effects of DBS offer one advantage. The effects of central mechanisms are readily apparent in behavior of motor units. A relatively straightforward line of causal explanation extends from activities of the alpha motor units to muscles and observable behaviors manifested normally and pathologically, as well as in response to DBS.

Also, developing a causal explanation in the other direction—to the basal ganglia–thalamic-cortical system, for example—ought to be a relatively straightforward process. This is not to say that it is not difficult. Whether and when such an approach will be available for other neurological and psychiatric conditions is unknown. The difficulties in our current knowledge of motor physiology and pathophysiology, however, are in a sense self-inflicted as a consequence of a lack of realization that any theory must explain an entire chain of events. No theory of motor pathophysiology, such as applies to movement disorders, may be considered a success until it traces a complete causal chain from the pathoetiology, such as degeneration of the substantia nigra pars compacta neurons in Parkinson's disease, to the fundamental basis for clinical manifestations; that is, the physiological and dynamic orchestration of motor unit recruitment and de-recruitment.

What the fundamental basis will be for other neurological and psychiatric disorders is unknown. If one is to learn from the successes and failures of motor physiology, and pathophysiology particularly, however, one cannot not look to primarily anatomical and neurochemical theories, because they fail to address the relevant dynamics.

PATHOPHYSIOLOGICAL MECHANISMS

Pathophysiology is central to neuroscience and psychiatry for a number of reasons. Indeed, nearly every inference concerning normal functions of the nervous system is derived from notions of pathophysiology. For thousands of years, the only insight into the functioning of the nervous system was through observations of animals and humans that had suffered injury, accidental or otherwise (many insights were gained by observations of wounded Roman gladiators, for instance). Intact organisms are far too complex to permit an understanding of fundamental mechanisms at the neuronal level without exerting some control, which immediately renders the preparation pathological in a sense, if for no other reason than it becomes out of the ordinary. Understanding DBS's mechanisms of action—a therapeutic mechanism, particularly—greatly depends on the prior informing conception of pathophysiology. It is quite difficult to ascribe the many known brain responses to DBS (*see Chapter 6—Nervous System Responses to DBS*) to a therapeutic mechanism, if that which is supposed to be corrected is unknown.

DBS for patients with Parkinson's disease quite possibly exemplifies both the best and worst ways of developing theories of pathophysiological mechanisms from which may be drawn inferences about therapeutic mechanisms. Instances of errant efforts in treating Parkinson's disease should be taken as sobering precautions by those who are developing DBS for other neurological and psychiatric disorders—hence the value of including a discussion of pathophysiology of Parkinsonism in this book.

The therapeutic mechanism of action of DBS was initially attributed to a reduction of overactive neuronal activities in the GPi. This attribution rested on the *Fallacy of Pseudotransitivity* in that it posited an equivalence of the clinical similarity of pallidotomy to pallidal DBS to a similarity of underlying mechanisms (Montgomery 2012) and to animal studies that demonstrated increased neuronal activity in the GPi. The latter were primarily related to the method of producing the model rather than to actual pathophysiology (see discussion of pathophysiology as different from pathoetiology, below). In this author's opinion, this misconception hampered research into the mechanisms of action and continues to misinform research.

The notion of pathophysiology must be kept distinct from the notion of pathoetiology; that is, the sequence of events that leads to abnormal physiology. Parkinsonism is a case in point. There is the presumption that Parkinsonism is a dopamine deficiency because the correlation of symptoms and signs with dopamine levels in the brain suggests it. The symptom and signs constitute the syndrome, and in at least one form of Parkinsonism, there is degeneration of the substantia nigra pars compacta and consequent loss of dopamine neurotransmitters. Yet the same symptoms and signs are observed in patients who, though they clearly present with Parkinsonism, show no evidence of dopamine depletion. One such syndrome is known as *Symptoms Without Evidence of Dopamine Depletion* (SWEDD). Despite claims made by certain revisionists, patients with SWEDD were of sufficient clinical similarity to be thought of as having idiopathic Parkinson's disease by top movement-disorder neurologists. Other forms of Parkinsonism are associated with lesions of the globus pallidus, particularly the external segment, and others with lesions of the supplementary motor area. A multitude of insults may cascade, resulting in self-reorganization of neuronal dynamics that leads to common problems in driving motor units manifested in the motoric symptoms, signs, and disabilities of Parkinsonism.

THE GLOBUS PALLIDUS INTERNA RATE THEORY

This theory posits that excessive activity of the GPi is causal to akinesia and bradykinesia associated with Parkinsonism because it suppresses activity in the thalamic-cortical system (Figure 8.1). However, considerable evidence exists to challenge this theory. For example, delivery of relatively high doses of the Parkinsonism-producing neurotoxin n-methyl-4-phenyl-1, 2, 3, 6-tetrahydropyridine (MPTP) resulted in increased activity of GPi neurons, and delivery of low-to-moderate doses of MPTP produced Parkinsonism without increasing GPi neuronal activity (Wang et al. 2009). Similarly, Parkinsonism associated with electrolytic lesions of the medial forebrain bundle, which conveys dopaminergic axons from the substantia nigra pars compacta to the striatum and dopamine receptor–blocking neuroleptics, was not associated with increases in activity of the GPi (Percheron et al. 1993). Neuronal activity in the STN was posited as excessive activity and thus driving the GPi to excessive activity. The neuronal discharge frequencies and the variability of discharges, however, are no different in patients with Parkinson's disease than they are in patients with epilepsy (Montgomery 2008c).

The Globus Pallidus Interna Rate theory also extended to hyperkinetic disorders, such as dyskinesia owing to decreased neuronal activity in the GPi. However, it has long been known that pallidotomy improves dyskinesia, a result that runs contrary to the predictions of the Globus Pallidus Interna Rate theory.

EXCESSIVELY HIGH BETA OSCILLATIONS

The Excessively High Beta Oscillations theory posits that neuronal activities are periodic or oscillatory. The amount of oscillations at each frequency may be measured by a Fourier transform (*see Chapter 16—Oscillator Basics*). Applied to studies of local field potentials in various structures of the basal ganglia–thalamic-cortical system, increased amounts (power) in the high beta frequencies (15 HZ–30 Hz) were found. Though there are severe conceptual difficulties with inferring neuronal activities from local field potentials, studies have nonetheless shown that many patients with Parkinson's disease have increased beta power that is reduced with therapeutic interventions. Left unexplained—or explained in a vague way—is how an increase in high beta oscillatory activity interferes with the normal recruitment and de-recruitment of motor units, or how the high beta oscillations would interfere with movement in general. Even more fundamental, how does the theory explain increased high beta power based on any anatomical or physiological facts or principles?

Importantly, approximately 20% of patients with known Parkinson's disease do not have increased power in the high beta frequencies. The latter, then, cannot be a necessary condition for Parkinsonism. Also, stimulation in the high beta frequencies with DBS does not worsen Parkinsonism, if it is assumed that such stimulation drives neuronal activities at the high beta frequencies (Figure 8.2). High beta activity is thus probably not a sufficient condition. Neither a necessary nor sufficient condition, the high beta power observed in patients with Parkinson's disease must be epiphenomenal to Parkinsonism rather than causal. Though DBS may reduce high beta activity, it cannot be the mechanism of DBS's therapeutic action.

EXCESSIVE SYNCHRONIZATION OF NEURONAL ACTIVITIES

Both animal models and human cases of Parkinsonism show evidence of increased synchronization among neurons within a given structure of the basal ganglia–thalamic-cortical system. For example, under normal conditions, neurons within a specific structure have little interaction with each other, as measured by

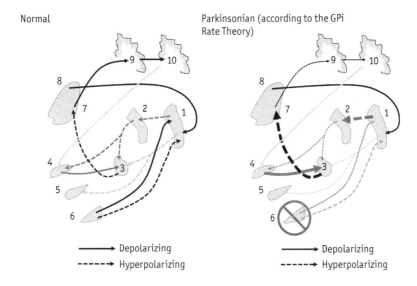

Normal

Parkinsonian (according to the GPi
Rate Theory)

Figure 8.1: Schematic representation of the basal ganglia–thalamic-cortical system in normal subjects and in Parkinsonism according to the Globus Pallidus Interna Rate (GPi) theory. Represented are the following various structures: 1—putamen (as representative of the striatum); 2—GPe; 3—GPi; 4—STN; 5—substantia nigra pars reticulata; 6—substantia nigra pars compacta (location of the cell bodies that utilize dopamine as their neurotransmitter); 7—Vop; 8—parafascicular and centromedian nuclei of the thalamus; 9—supplementary motor area; and 10—primary motor cortex. A primary assumption of the theory is that hyperpolarizing interactions, which are mediated by GABA, cause a net reduction in neuronal activities in the postsynaptic structures. Yet this is not entirely true; many neurons in the basal ganglia–thalamic-cortical system display post-hyperpolarization rebound excitation that may result in a net increase in neuronal activity in the postsynaptic structure. As it applies to Parkinson's disease, degeneration of dopamine neurons (structure 6) results in the loss of hyperpolarizing inputs to a group of neurons in the putamen (structure 1). These groups of putamen neurons are thought to increase their activities and thereby increase hyperpolarization of neurons in the GPe (structure 2), via what is known as the indirect pathway (red arrows), which is represented by the connecting arrow of greater thickness. The putative decrease of neuronal activity in the GPe is posited as reducing the hyperpolarization of the STN (structure 4) and the GPi (structure 3), represented by the thinner connecting arrows. The reduced hyperpolarization is thought to increase the activities in the STN, which then further increases the neuronal activities of the GPi, represented by the thicker connecting arrow. Similarly, loss of depolarizing inputs from the degenerated dopamine neurons of the substantia nigra pars compacta results in reduced activities in a portion of the putamen neurons that project to the GPi, via the direct pathway (green arrows). Thus, the reduction of activities in these putamen neurons decreased the hyperpolarization of the GPi neurons, leading to a posited increase in their activities. The net effect is an increase of GPi activities that results in the increased hyperpolarization of the Vop neurons (represented by the wide connecting arrow). Reduced activity in the thalamic relay neurons then reduces drive onto the neurons of the supplementary motor area (shown by the thin connecting arrow) and then onto the primary motor area, which presumably causes the bradykinesia and akinesia associated with Parkinsonism.

studies of cross-correlation. In Parkinsonism, cross-correlation between neurons is increased.

One potential explanation for abnormal motor function that follows increased synchronization between neurons is that the latter prevents neurons from processing information separately and thus differently. This reduces the complexities of neuronal activities by reducing degrees of freedom (Vyas et al. 2015). Consequently, information ultimately related to alpha lower motor neurons for execution does not have the complexity to properly orchestrate recruitments and de-recruitments of motor units (*see*

Chapter 7—DBS Effects on Motor Control). Though the above theory is quite plausible, de-synchronization is probably not a therapeutic mechanism of DBS. (This is reviewed in *Chapter 6—Nervous System Responses to DBS*.)

EXCESSIVE BURSTING

Some have posited that excessive bursting activities are causal to Parkinsonism. As information is entrained in a pattern of action potentials, excessive

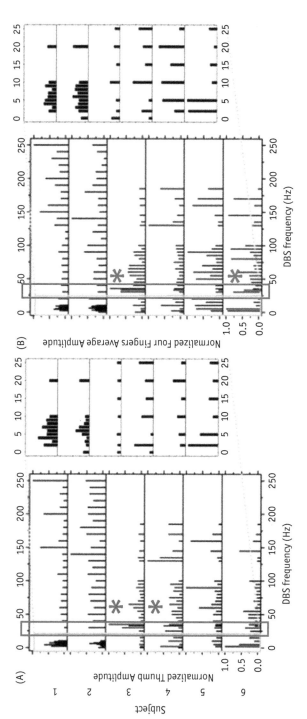

Figure 8.2: Mean-normalized movement amplitudes for (B) fingers (pooled) and (A) thumb for each of six subjects with Parkinson's disease who had DBS electrodes implanted in the vicinity of the STN. The subjects were asked to open and close their hands as wide and as rapidly as they could. Each subject was tested at each DBS frequency available. Absence of a column indicates that the associated stimulation frequency was unavailable with the subject's IPG (implanted pulse generator). There appear multiple peaks associated with large-amplitude movements across multiple frequencies, including low frequencies. The inserts show amplitudes for the lower range of stimulation frequencies. (Asterisks [*] indicate points at which DBS in the high beta frequencies significantly improved movement.)

Adapted from Huang et al. 2014, page 205.

bursting generates abnormal information and thus affects information processing elsewhere, ultimately to result in misinformation delivered to the motor units. Certainly, increasing bursting has been demonstrated in animal models of Parkinsonism, and bursting may be seen in neurons of the basal ganglia–thalamic-cortical system in humans. Of the animal studies it must be asked whether the animal model represents what occurs in humans relative to the phenomena studied. Of the human studies it must be asked, What is the comparison group? In one study, the incidence of bursting in the STN was no different in patients with Parkinson's disease than it was in patients with epilepsy (Vyas et al. 2015). At the very least, these issues require that one treat with skepticism the idea that excessive bursting is a causal mechanism of Parkinsonism, and indicate that any effect of DBS on bursting activity is not likely to be a therapeutic mechanism of action.

THE SYSTEMS OSCILLATORS THEORY

Proposed here is an alternative: the Systems Oscillators theory (Montgomery 2004a). It conceives of the basal ganglia–thalamic-cortical system as a network of coupled, polysynaptic, nonlinear oscillators

evidenced by the entrainment simultaneously of multiple frequencies in the spike train of neurons within the basal ganglia-thalamic-cortical system (Figure 8.3) and one such oscillator is depicted in Figure 8.4. The traditional anatomical structures form nodes of archetype oscillators. However, these archetype oscillators are replicated a very large number of times for specific ensembles of neurons within each node (Figure 8.5). The ensembles may be organized according to some common function, such as a specific component of the motor homunculus that is contained in each anatomical structure. The DBS system is also conceived of as another oscillator that becomes embedded in the network of neuronal oscillators within the basal ganglia–thalamic-cortical system and interacts with the neuronal oscillators. Evidence of the latter was presented in Chapter 6, Nervous System Responses to DBS, wherein it was demonstrated that the probability of a DBS pulse's producing an antidromic action potential in the STN varied as ~26 Hz and ~66 Hz oscillations in the neuron.

From the simplified general anatomy of the basal ganglia–thalamic-cortical system, a subset of the interconnections that form a closed or feedback loop is shown in Figures 8.3. Evidencing closed or feedback loops are resonance effects related to paired-pulse DBS in non-human primates. This evidence is reviewed in Chapter 6, Nervous System Responses to

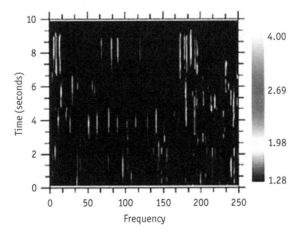

Figure 8.3: Spectrogram showing the appearance and disappearance of significant frequencies in the discharge of a neuron recorded in the GPe in a non-human primate. The circular statistical method is applied repeatedly over 10 s (vertical axis). The circular statistical method is applied to 2 s windows, which are then moved through time at 0.2 s increments. The circular statistics method is applied for periods (the inverse of the frequency) corresponding to frequencies from 1–250 Hz (horizontal axis). At every instant of time, multiple frequencies are observably represented in the neuronal spike train.
Verbatim from Montgomery and Gale 2008, page 403.

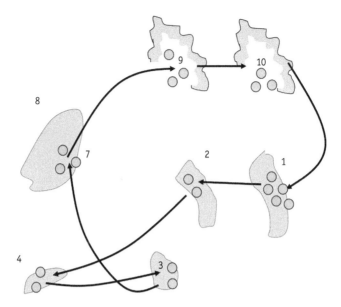

Figure 8.4: Schematic representation of one potential oscillator within the basal ganglia–thalamic-cortical system. Represented are the following various structures: 1—putamen (as representative of the striatum); 2—GPe; 3—GPi; 4—STN; 5—substantia nigra pars reticulata; 6—substantia nigra pars compacta (location of the cell bodies that utilize dopamine as their neurotransmitter); 7—Vop; 8—parafascicular and centromedian nuclei of the thalamus; 9—supplementary motor area; and 10—primary motor cortex. The lines do not indicate depolarization versus hyperpolarization, because these terms do not completely capture the nature of action potential generation. Specifically, hyperpolarization of some neurons results in post-hyperpolarization rebound excitation and the generation of action potentials. The oscillator shown above (just one of many possible oscillator configurations) contains seven nodes linked by seven connections. Each node is an ensemble of neurons in each traditional anatomical nucleus or cortex. Each node contains differing numbers of neurons.

DBS. . One possible oscillator has seven nodes linked by seven connections (Figure 8.4). If one assumes that the time delay for transferring a bit of information between two nodes is 3.5 ms, then it would take approximately 24.5 ms for the bit of information to traverse the oscillator corresponding to a frequency of 40.8 Hz. Other possible oscillator architectures derived from the basic anatomy appear in Figure 8.6.

Importantly, each node, which contains a number of neurons, does not generate action potentials with each cycle. Rather, whether an individual neuron in the ensemble discharges an action potential is probabilistic. The effect, then, is that neurons act as rate-dividers, the actual discharge frequency of an individual neuron being some fraction of the oscillators in which the neuron is embedded. There are observably the greatest number of neurons in each ensemble in the putamen, the fewest in the ensemble in the GPi and STN, and an intermediate number within the thalamus and motor cortex. The overall probability of a discharge with each cycle of

the oscillator will be less for putamen neurons, and their overall discharge frequency will be lower than the fundamental frequency of the oscillator, which in this hypothetical case is 40.8 Hz; and the average discharge frequency of a neuron in the GPi and STN will be much higher, as is the case in the biological condition. Though each neuron may not discharge with each cycle, the summed probability over the ensemble may be sufficient to sustain the oscillations, at least for some period of time. Should even a single oscillator cease because its nodes are likely to be shared among other oscillators, activations entering from other oscillators are able to restart the oscillator such as neurons in the motor cortex that participate in multiple oscillators (Figure 8.6).

Figure 8.7 depicts evidence of neurons acting as rate-dividers whose discharges are related to a behavioral event, but in a probabilistic manner. Neurons were recorded in the STN as a patient with Parkinson's disease voiced the phrase "*la, la, la, la, la*" in trials of the five syllables (Watson and Montgomery 2006).

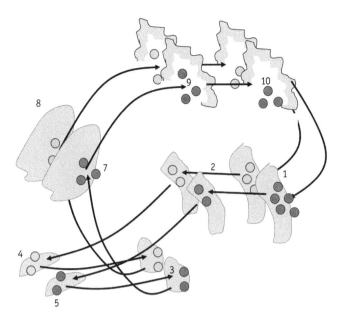

Figure 8.5: Schematic representation of two potential oscillators within the basal ganglia–thalamic-cortical system. Represented are the following various structures: 1—putamen (as representative of the striatum); 2—GPe; 3—GPi; 4—STN; 5—substantia nigra pars reticulata; 6—substantia nigra pars compacta (location of the cell bodies that utilize dopamine as their neurotransmitter); 7—Vop; 8—parafascicular and centromedian nuclei of the thalamus; 9—supplementary motor area; and 10—primary motor cortex. The two oscillators have the same general structure, but the nodes within each structure are different. The neurons that compose one oscillator are represented by solid blue circles, and the neurons of the other oscillator are represented by solid red circles. The blue set of neurons may ultimately be related to wrist-extensor motor neurons, and the red set of neurons to elbow-flexor motor units. The number of possible oscillators is thus quite large, particularly when it is multiplied by the number of oscillators with different architectures.

The neurons' discharge frequencies are modulated with the production of the syllables. Each neuron participates, however, neither in the voicing of each syllable nor in all trials.

Productive of a remarkable dynamic complexity is the network of interconnected oscillators whose different fundamental frequencies are based on the number of intervening nodes. Indeed, there is evidence that such networks demonstrate complexity. The remarkable number of oscillators that house neurons is suggested by the range of frequencies entrained in the neuronal spike train (Figure 8.3). These oscillators are discrete rather than continuous (*see Chapter 17—Discrete Neural Oscillators*) allowing different oscillators to simultaneously entrain multiple channels of information. Continuous oscillators resemble a single copper wire in a conductor from a television cable service provider, which is able to carry hundreds of different channels of video and audio simultaneously as long as the different frequencies have unrelated frequency

harmonics (non-commensurate frequencies). Discrete oscillators provide even more independent channels of information in shared medium, such as nodes of neurons shared among different oscillators. Shared nodes between different oscillators allow for the integration of different channels of information.

The Systems Oscillators theory suggests that the fundamental frequencies are relatively fixed and depend the number of nodes embedded within an oscillator. However, as discrete non-linear oscillators, there can be many action potentials during any single cycle and because each neuron acts as a rate-divider, the number and range of frequencies that can be entrained in the spike train of any neuron is very large (Figure 8.3). Moreover, each oscillator can change phase, depending on inputs into it from different sources (*see Chapter 16—Oscillator Basics*). Information is then encoded in the magnitude of the oscillations, which, according to the theory, is found in the probability that a neuron within the ensemble

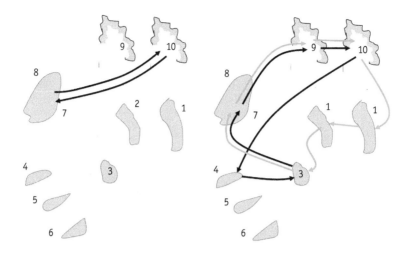

Figure 8.6: Schematic representation of the various components of the basal ganglia–thalamic-cortical system, demonstrating three other oscillator architectures. Represented are the following various structures: 1—putamen (as representative of the striatum); 2—GPe; 3—GPi; 4—STN; 5—substantia nigra pars reticulata; 6—substantia nigra pars compacta (location of the cell bodies that utilize dopamine as their neurotransmitter); 7—Vop; 8—parafascicular and centromedian nuclei of the thalamus; 9—supplementary motor area; and 10—primary motor cortex. The disynaptic oscillator shown in the figure to the left is consistent with the thalamic neuronal recordings during DBS of the GPi shown in Figure 8.5. Also, the figure to the right shows that the GPi participates in two different oscillators, each of which is associated with a different fundamental frequency, a 5-node loop, and a 6-node loop.

will discharge within a specific cycle of the oscillation. As shown in Figure 8.7, the probability of a neuron's discharge increases and decreases (modulates) over time as each "*la*" of the phrase is voiced.

Encoding information in the relative probability that a neuron across an ensemble will discharge with each cycle is analogous to encoding information in amplitude-modulated (AM) radio station. The radio

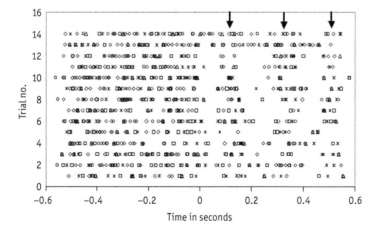

Figure 8.7: Raster of time of onset of action potentials for five neurons. Each neuron is represented by a different symbol. And each was simultaneously recording at a single site in the STN of a patient with Parkinson's disease during utterance of the phrase "*la la la la la*," the first three of which are associated with changes that are marked by the arrows. Each row represents a different trial. Each neuron's participation is inconsistent, but the aggregate activity is highly consistent with the behavior.

Adapted from Montgomery 2004, page 413.

station sends out a carrier signal at a specific frequency (Figure 8.8). The information is encoded in the amplitude of the carrier frequency. The Systems Oscillators theory posits that an increase in the amplitude of the information is directly related to the number of neurons in the ensemble that discharge with each cycle of the oscillator.

As information is encoded in oscillations of a wide range of frequencies, the information may span a range of time scales within the basal ganglia–thalamic-cortical system that are necessary for the orchestration of motor unit recruitment and de-recruitment of different orders, which are discussed in *Chapter 7—DBS Effects on Motor Control*. The range of oscillators available in the basal ganglia–thalamic-cortical system may also enable a type of holographic memory, as proposed by H. C. Longuet-Higgins, and may account for motor learning or skill acquisition (Longuet-Higgins 1968). Longuet-Higgins proposed that a bank of oscillators covering a range of frequencies may encode any periodic signal, such as the recruitment and de-recruitment of motor units.

Each oscillator could be coupled to all the other oscillators where the effect or connection strength could be changed. The system of oscillators is trained by varying the strength of the connection or coupling to reproduce any periodic signal. Subsequently, when presented with only an initial part of the original periodic signal, the system can reproduce the entire signal. Thus, the command for a specific movement may be just the initial piece of information that, when it enters the appropriate set of coupled oscillators, generates the entire information needed for the orchestration of motor unit recruitment and de-recruitment. This model in many ways is analogous to an inverse Fourier transform (*discussed in Chapter 16—Oscillator Basics*). The theory and mathematical derivations of it are analogous to actual physical phenomena (Korpel and Chatterjee 1981).

The Systems Oscillators theory provides an explanation of one possible mechanism of therapeutic action by DBS. DBS may be conceptualized as an additional "oscillator" that is embedded in a network of coupled neural oscillators and interacts

Signal from desired AM radio station

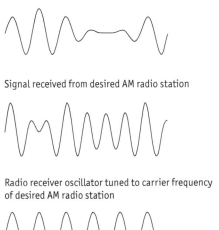

Signal received from desired AM radio station

Radio receiver oscillator tuned to carrier frequency of desired AM radio station

Signal heard when signal received from desired AM radio station and radio receiver's oscillators Are added

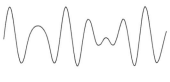

Figure 8.8: Schematic representation of independently encoded information among different oscillators that use the same medium. In this representation, the different oscillators are the electromagnetic waves generated in space at different fundamental frequencies unique to each radio station. The desired AM radio station transmits an electromagnetic wave of a specific frequency. The transmitted information is encoded in the various amplitudes of the same electromagnetic wave (signal from the desired AM radio station). The antenna of the AM radio receiver receives the signal from the desired AM station along with signals from all the other AM radio stations in the area. The AM receiver has an oscillator tuned to the carrier frequency of the desired AM radio station, which is added to the received signal. The result is then sent to the speaker, which renders the signal audible. The result is an acceptable replication of the original signal from the desired AM radio station.

with them. One mechanism of interaction is *positive resonance*, which is similar to a radio's reception of an AM radio signal (Figure 8.8). The broadcasting station's transmitter sends out electromagnetic waves of a single carrier frequency whose amplitude is modulated to encode information. The waves cause parallel motions of electrons in a radio receiver's antenna, as do the electromagnetic waves of every other radio station in the vicinity. A listener finds a specific radio station's broadcast by way of the radio receiver's own oscillator, which she can tune to a specific frequency so that it matches the carrier frequency of the desired radio transmission. The radio receives oscillator interacts and sums its oscillations with those of the desired radio transmission to increase the radio transmission's amplitude above all others.

As discussed in Chapter 6, Nervous System Responses to DBS, a DBS pulse interacts with oscillators by affecting changes in the membrane potential of neurons whose axons pass within the electrical field around the DBS electrode during the DBS pulse. The specificity of a DBS frequency for optimal benefit may relate to the fundamental frequency of a specific neural oscillator in the basal ganglia–thalamic-cortical system. One consequence is that the signal strength of information encoded in the neural oscillator increases in order to overcome noise resulting from disorder in basal ganglia–thalamic-cortical system. Another mechanism may be negative resonance in which the DBS oscillator reduces a signal—the signal that conveys misinformation, perhaps—in a specific oscillator.

The Systems Oscillators theory may also explain disorders associated with dyskinesia and other excessive or uncontrolled movement. The disorder of the basal ganglia–thalamic-cortical system could result in increased resonance interactions between some oscillators, such as production by stochastic resonance of an abnormal increased signal that inappropriately drives motor units. DBS may reduce abnormal resonance in the way discussed above.

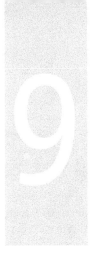

APPROACHES TO PROGRAMMING

Persistence and patience are the keys to successful DBS programming. Several studies show that one of the most common causes of unsuccessful DBS therapy is an inadequately programmed implanted pulse generator (IPG).

Note that, with the rapid increase in the types and manufacturers of DBS systems now and anticipated, precise statements about stimulation parameters are difficult to make. The responsibility for choice of stimulation parameters, electrode configurations, and pulse trains lies solely with the programmer. Specific examples of stimulation parameters, electrode configurations, and pulse trains provided in this text are for informational and educational purposes only.

Successful programming depends on several factors, including maximization of clinical benefit, minimization of adverse effects, extension of battery life (less of a concern with rechargeable IPGs), and efficient effort and use of time. Though published case series and clinical trials report average DBS frequencies, pulse widths, and the most common electrode configurations, the variability among patients limits the use of this information. These average or most common stimulation variables may be considered as starting points for programming rather than as endpoints. One must nevertheless be cognizant that reported electrode configurations—the arrangement of active negative and positive contacts (cathode and anodes, respectively)—may represent habit owing to

tradition or legacy. Basing the starting points on electroneurophysiological principles may be better. Such will be the basis to the approach taken in the present writing.

The thousands of possible stimulation parameters vary according to frequency, pulse width, current (voltage in constant-voltage IPGs), and electrode configurations. The recent capacity to interleave two or more different pulse trains (which differ in electrode configurations and some stimulation parameters) adds another variable to DBS programming that will be referred to as the *pulse train*. Development of a systematic approach to programming is therefore in both the programmer and the patient's best interests. Often, application of the principles of the above-mentioned electrophysiology and electronics and knowledge of regional anatomy around a DBS target (discussed below) will enable programmers to bypass many combinations and focus on those most likely to meet with success.

BATTERY LIFE

The advent of rechargeable IPGs has reduced consideration of battery life as the primary concern in approaches to DBS programming. The critical assumption is that a patient or a patient's family member or caregiver scrupulously adheres to a recharge schedule frequent enough to prevent loss of stimulation. Rechargeable IPGs also reduce the cost and risks associated with more frequent surgeries made necessary by non-rechargeable IPGs. For these reasons rechargeable IPGs are preferable. With each IPG replacement also comes increased risk of infection, owing perhaps to an increased amount of relatively avascular scar tissue at the surgical site.

IPGs eventually need to be replaced—rechargeable IPGs less frequently than non-rechargeable IPGs. Although IPG replacement is a fairly minor surgical procedure, it is not without risk and expense. Programmers must therefore attempt to select stimulation parameters and electrode configurations that will maximize battery life without compromising clinical effectiveness or increasing side effects. Yet optimization of battery charge is difficult, even when a rechargeable IPG is in use. Stimulation current not infrequently requires a voltage that exceeds the battery voltage of the IPG. Use of a constant voltage IPG makes this clear, but it is no less important with the use of constant current IPGs.

Though special electronics in most IPGs permit stimulation with voltages greater than the battery voltage, the capability may result in some loss of efficiency. For example, the current drained from the battery in increasing stimulation voltage in constant voltage IPGs or voltage necessary for stimulation current in constant-current IPGs from one volt below the battery voltage to the battery voltage is less than the amount of current drained in increasing the battery voltage to one volt above the battery voltage, for example. There is thus incurred a cost for stimulating that requires a voltage greater than the battery voltage. Compounding the problem is the fact that some IPGs have a battery voltage that is lower than stimulation voltages typically needed for clinical efficacy.

Largely unknown is degree of loss of efficiency when the voltage required for stimulation exceeds the battery voltage. Such information is apparently considered proprietary, notwithstanding its usefulness in helping physicians decide among competing DBS systems. An older IPG model, no longer commercially available, serves to illustrate the problem of battery efficiency at voltages required for stimulation. This model used a highly inefficient "voltage-doubling" circuit. That it did so was common knowledge, and it acknowledged various approaches to DBS programming.

DBS CONTACT NOMENCLATURE

Conventions for naming the DBS contacts are complicated and will grow increasingly more so. Even with currently available DBS leads that have similar general architectures, the naming of contacts varies widely and is a potential source of confusion. As there is no cross-manufacturer standardization of nomenclatures for DBS electrical contacts on DBS leads, the programmer needs to exercise care in documenting the various electrode configurations used. It is important to emphasize that documentation of DBS programming is not directed by the convenience of the programmer. Rather, the purpose is to convey to others the care that has been provided to the patient. Documentation that is ambiguous is of little use to others who at any point may assume responsibility for the patient's care.

It would be most helpful that any naming convention be intuitive. For example, one approach to a naming convention is based on the dimensions or axes that are particularly relevant, rather than on some arbitrarily applied label, such as a number. One important axis or dimension is along the long axis of the DBS lead (Figure 9.1). For systems that have four contacts (or set of contacts) at specific levels along the long axis of the DBS lead, one naming convention could be most ventral, ventral, dorsal, and most dorsal. The programmer should take the responsibility of exactly specifying the DBS lead manufacturer and model type of the DBS lead used in every piece of documentation related to the patient's care, particularly for DBS leads whose number of contacts or architectures prove cumbersome of intuitive naming.

In the case of leads whose contacts are segmented in the plane that is orthogonal to the long axis of a DBS lead, the naming becomes more difficult. It would be optimal to name each contact at a specific level by the angle in the plane orthogonal to the long axis of the lead. However, this presumes that the angle and reference point are known. The question is: What would an angle of 120 or 240 degrees mean relative to the orientation of the regional anatomy about the DBS lead or to the Cartesian reference frame relative to the anterior and posterior commissure? Were it even possible to precisely rotate the DBS lead so the spatial orientation of each segmented contact is known, the rotation about the long axis probably would be different for various DBS targets. For example, one may

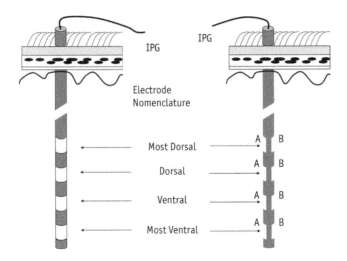

Figure 9.1: As there is no cross-manufacturer standardization of nomenclatures for DBS electrical contacts on DBS leads, the programmer needs to exercise care in documenting the various electrode configurations used. The convention suggested here presumes a DBS lead architecture in which the contacts are organized along the long axis of the DBS lead. This translates into a relative location within the brain as a function of the manner of DBS lead implantation. In the event segmented leads are utilized, the above suggestion can be generalized to identify each segment by some label but still organized by the relative anatomical position in the brain. The programmer should take the responsibility of exactly specifying the DBS lead manufacturer and the model type of the DBS lead used in every piece of documentation related to the patient's care, particularly for DBS leads whose number of contacts or architectures prove cumbersome for intuitive naming.

want to rotate the DBS lead to orient the segmented leads orthogonal (pointing away at 90 degrees) from the posterior limb of the internal capsule. However, depending on the specific architecture, this could place the minimal electrode surface area directed to the optimal target thereby limiting efficacy. The posterior limb of the internal capsule relative to the GPi runs from anterior and medial to posterior and lateral.

For the sake of discussion, it is assumed here that this line that forms the anterior border of the posterior limb of the internal capsule runs at 135 degrees in the axial plane relative to the line from the anterior commissure to the midpoint of the line connecting the anterior and posterior commissure. This means that an optimal orientation of the DBS lead is one that is 45 degrees, and thus pointing 90 degrees away from the posterior limb of the internal capsule, particularly in the case of DBS targeting the GPi (Figure 9.2). However, the remaining two segments would be directed towards the posterior limb of the internal capsule. Further, because of edge effects on the current densities, the edges of the two remaining contacts will be even closer to the posterior limb which then could prevent the use of these contacts because of the risk of adverse effects, such as tonic muscle

contraction. One could orient two contacts such that they are projecting away from the posterior limb of the internal capsule but note the posterior edges will be closer to the posterior limb of the internal capulse comparted to the orginal position described in Figure 9.2. In the case of DBS targeting the Vim, problems of speech, language, and swallowing are of concern. In this case, the optimal orientation in the plane orthogonal to the long axis of the DBS lead is a segment contact, which is oriented 180 degrees from the head-homuncular representation (Figure 9.3). In other words, it would be important to have a DBS lead segmented contact that points directly lateral.

It should not be assumed that the actual angle of the segmented contact can be known; consequently, some arbitrary label may be necessary. One kind of nomenclature would be to label the segmented contact first by its level in the long axis of the DBS lead and then use an arbitrary label to denote the segmented contact at the next level—most ventralt-A, for example.

Note that these suggestions are based on a DBS segmented lead in which the contacts are arranged as sectors around the circumference of the lead in the plane orthogonal to the long axis of the lead.

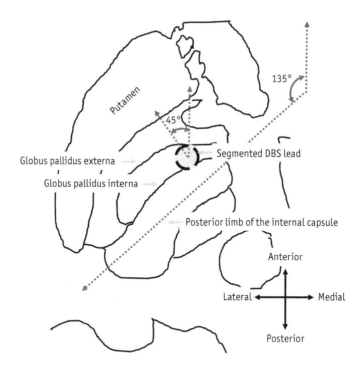

Figure 9.2: Hypothetical example of the importance of orientation of the contacts in a hypothetical segmented DBS lead, showing the structures in the vicinity of a DBS lead directed at the GPi (axial plane image). This orientation relates to the risk of producing tonic contractions when an electrical contact is too close to the posterior limb of the internal capsule. In such a case, the optimal orientation would be to have at least one contact oriented in such a way as to be maximally distant from the posterior limb of the internal capsule. One instantiation would be to have the contact oriented orthogonally (90°) relative to the plane of the posterior limb of the internal capsule. In this example, the posterior limb runs at an angle of 135° relative to the line connecting the anterior to posterior commissures. This means that at least one contact should be oriented to project (point) 45° relative to the anterior-posterior commissural line. (*Note:* images not to scale.)
Modified from Schaltenbrand and Wahren 1977.

These suggestions may not be appropriate for other segmented DBS lead architectures, but the general principle still may apply. It is important to note that changing from a continuous circumferential contact stimulation to a subset of contacts in a segmented lead can change the surface area of the electrical contacts over which the stimulation is applied. This could change the current densities and thus, affect safety (*see Chapter 5—DBS Safety*). These caveats apply to any and all discussions of segmented DBS leads in this book.

PRIOR TO DBS PROGRAMMING

At the beginning of any DBS programming session, is it important that electrode configurations, stimulation parameters, pulse train features, and measures of use such as percent time used and number of activations, are recorded first, because these may be changed during the course of programming. For example, in troubleshooting intermittent problems, it is often useful to know how many times the DBS system was deactivated or activated. However, these counters may be affected during the course of DBS programming, causing original information to be lost.

For most patients, several DBS programming sessions will be required before the most effective combination of parameters, electrode configurations, pulse trains, and medications can be determined. Because programmers will often need to refer to previous sessions in order to review patients' progress, they should assess symptoms and document clinical responses carefully (*see Chapter 15—Helpful*

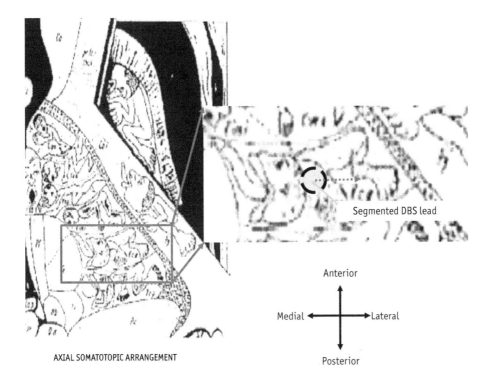

AXIAL SOMATOTOPIC ARRANGEMENT

Segmented DBS lead

Anterior

Medial ←——→ Lateral

Posterior

Figure 9.3: Hypothetical example of the importance of orientation of the contacts in a hypothetical segmented DBS lead, showing the structures in the vicinity of a DBS lead directed at the Vim (axial plane image). This orientation relates to the risk of producing speech, language, and swallowing complications when an electrical contact is too close to the head homuncular representation. In such a case, the optimal orientation would be to have at least one contact oriented in such a way as to be maximally distant from the head representation. One instantiation would be to have the contact oriented orthogonally (90°) relative to the anterior-posterior commissural line; in other words, directly lateral.

From Hassler R in Schaltenbrand and Wahren 1977.

Programming Hints). Templates of the forms used during programming sessions are available at *http://www.greenvilleneuromodulationcenter.com/DBS_Programming_forms/. /*. A hypothetical example of such use appears in Figure 9.4.

Prior to DBS programming, a survey of the patient's condition must be conducted, typically by a review of systems. An example of a review of systems that is relevant to patients undergoing DBS appears in the General Review of Systems for Patient's with Implanted DBS Systems, which are available at *http://www.greenvilleneuromodulationcenter.com/DBS_Programming_forms/.* It must be noted that, because every patient is different, a preformulated checklist alone must not be considered exhaustive or sufficient. It should serve, rather, as a starting point.

To consider DBS as a solo therapy that may be evaluated independently of all other therapeutic interventions is to cherish a mistaken conception. For some patients, such as those with Parkinson's disease, DBS works in synergy with other treatments, particularly medications. Optimal DBS programming therefore requires having a strong knowledge of other therapeutic modalities and paying conscientious attention to patients' responses to them. The ethical principle of justice dictates that patients' DBS must be managed by someone with expertise in all methods of management, rather than someone whose ability is limited to changing DBS electrode configurations, stimulation parameters, and pulse trains.

WHEN TO PROGRAM DBS

Because some patients may experience a synergistic effect between DBS and medications or other

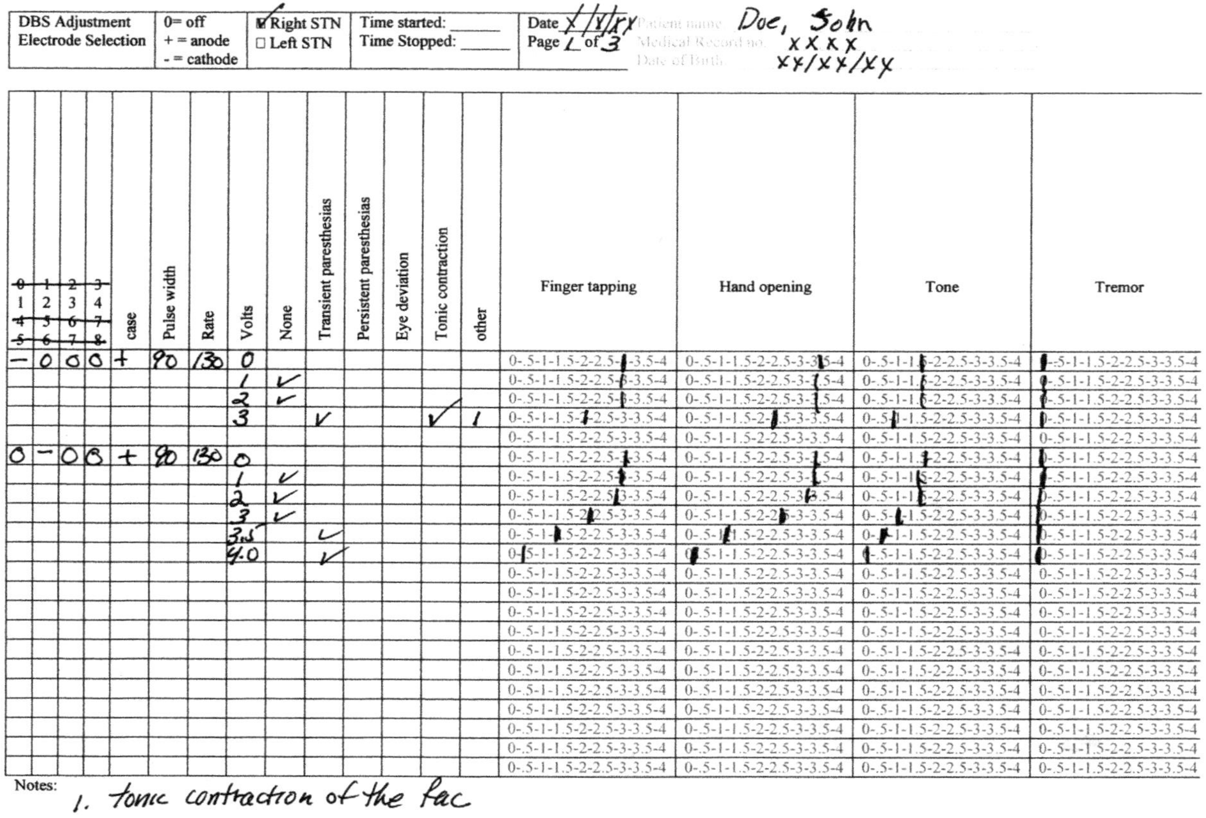

Figure 9.4: A hypothetical example of a programming session. As will be discussed subsequently in the text, the DBS lead used in this hypothetical example had a convention for naming contacts so that the first contact or most distal is contact 1, and the subsequent contacts (going proximally) are contacts 2, 3, and 4, respectively. These IPG naming conventions were entered into the form. DBS of the STN may be associated with potential side effects described as "transient paresthesias," "persistent paresthesias," "eye deviation," and "tonic contraction" of muscles. An additional category, "other," allows for identification of other different side effects or to specify one of the side effects checked. The patient in this hypothetical example has Parkinson's disease, so the following clinical signs were assessed using a grading scale described in Supplemental Tools - Aids to Programming: Paper Documentation, at http://www.greenvilleneuromodulationcenter.com/DBS_Programming_forms/. The scales are based on a 0–4 rating, with 0 being normal. As can be seen in this hypothetical example, the first electrode configuration, monopolar with contact 1 negative, produced tonic muscle contraction. Consequently, a new electrode configuration was determined. In this second configuration, the subject was able to have good control of the symptoms. However, the most-optimal control required 4 volts, which was above the IPG battery voltage. Therefore, trial of another set of stimulation parameters would be indicated. These templates have the advantage of a visual analogue scale that is easy to interpret. In addition, the data for multiple settings can be seen at once.

treatments, the synergistic effects of the other treatments must be controlled for. Doing so requires that the endpoint or targets for the DBS programming first be defined. For example, DBS may be used to treat adverse effects of other treatments. In such cases, DBS programmers must titrate electrode configurations, stimulation parameters, and pulse trains to the adverse effects produced by the medications. This means that the medications' effects ought to be at their maximum, which is usually reached at the peak nervous system concentrations of the medications. For example, DBS in the vicinity of the GPi is quite effective at reducing dyskinesias secondary to levodopa therapy in patients with Parkinson's disease, often enabling them to tolerate levels of medications necessary for sufficient control of symptoms and disabilities directly due to the underlying disease being treated. If reduction of levodopa-induced dyskinesia is the primary goal, then a patient needs to be dyskinetic, because this allows programmers to evaluate the effectiveness of the DBS electrode configurations, stimulation parameters, and pulse trains. Depending on the formulation of the medications that contain the levodopa, peak levels in the brain may not be reached until 30–60 minutes following administration of immediate-release levodopa compounds. In the case of slow or extended release, the latency may be 60–120 minutes. Similarly, dopamine agonists may have latencies of 60–120 minutes. DBS programming should commence at the moment at which it is expected that peak nervous system levels will be reached.

If the primary goal of the DBS programming session is that of treating underlying symptoms and disabilities proper to the disorder in question, then those symptoms and disabilities must be manifest. It does little good to attempt DBS programming when, for example, symptoms and disabilities are minimal or absent secondary to prior administration of medications. Symptoms and disabilities are most observable when medications are at their minimum in the nervous system. From this perspective, the symptoms and disabilities are likeliest to be at their maximum following a prolonged fast from medications—overnight as a patient sleeps, for example. Therefore, the optimal time for DBS programming is in the morning prior to a patient's first daily dose of medications. However, caution is necessary, because a patient's disabilities may be such as to create significant risk. The time that

a patient postpones taking her first dose of medications must therefore be kept to a minimum. Other drug-minimal states may be a patient's state immediate prior to her taking a subsequent dose of medications, particularly the medications whose short durations of action lead to fluctuations of symptoms and disabilities throughout the day.

This author's experience has shown him that the practice—past, if not present—of arbitrarily reducing medications following implantation of a DBS system places the patient at risk. Sometimes done in anticipation of eventual reductions that typically follow DBS therapies for some patients under some conditions places patients at considerable risk for worsened symptoms and disabilities of the disorder being treated. Most frequently, the extent and time course of subsequent medication adjustments cannot be predicted.

CONCEPTUAL APPROACHES

Simply advocating reasoning from concepts risks a serious backlash from Evidence-Based Medicine (EBM) proponents, particularly those who, in violation of the original conception, regard randomized controlled trials as the only true form of EBM (Montgomery and Turkstra 2003). The very basis of randomized controlled trials renders use of their results in the management of individual patients highly problematic and therefore requires reasoning from concepts (Montgomery and Turkstra 2003). In reasoning, for example, one does not need to repeat experiments that prove Newton's laws of motion (analogous to randomized controlled trials) each time he wishes to throw a ball, or Maxwell's equations for electromagnetism each time he wishes to use a computer. In any event, to this author's knowledge, there has not been nor is there likely to be any randomized controlled trial of DBS programming techniques; preventing them are practical issues, cost, and the absence of any organization that stands to realize a return on the investment. Therapeutic nihilism, therapeutic adventurism, a coin toss, and reason are thus the only options remaining. This author employs reason, which he tempers with experience.

The conceptual approach distinguishes maximization of clinical benefit from minimization of adverse effects directly attributable to stimulation. The distinction is drawn because, not infrequently, clinical benefit may be difficult to achieve without producing adverse effects. In such cases, attempts at increasing clinical benefit, experience has shown, often worsen adverse effects. Similarly, attempts at relieving adverse effects can reduce clinical benefit.

Clinical benefit usually requires generation of action potentials in a sufficient number of axons in the vicinity of a negative contact (cathode). One possible reason is that activations of large networks of neurons required by DBS make it necessary to drive activations across multiple synapses among a network's neurons (*see Chapter 6—Nervous System Responses to DBS*). The act of driving responses across synapses may involve the use of temporal and spatial summation (*see Chapter 3—Principles of Electrophysiology*). Temporal summation depends on the DBS stimulation frequency. In order for temporal summation to be effective, each successive DBS pulse must activate a neuron that is postsynaptic to the axon directly stimulated and thus add to the previous pulse's effect. Though temporal summation depends on a number of factors, increasing frequency also usually increases it. Yet the major driver of clinical benefit is likely to be related in a more complex way to DBS frequency, and the resonance effects associated with DBS frequency are likely to be the most important (*see Chapter 6—Nervous System Responses to DBS*). Were frequency-dependent temporal summation the controlling variable, the experiments conducted by Huang and colleagues (Huang et al. 2014), which are described in Chapter 7, DBS Effects on Motor Control, would have been different in that the response in the hand-opening and hand-closing task's amplitude would have increased monotonically with increasing DBS frequencies.

DBS's effectiveness may be increased by spatial summation in situations in which different axons whose action potentials are generated directly by a DBS pulse converge on the same postsynaptic neuron. Increasing the number of axons in which action potentials are generated increases spatial summation on a postsynaptic neuron and thus propagates further activations of neural systems necessary for producing a clinical benefit.

As outlined in *Chapter 4, Controlling the Flow of Electrical Charges*, with use of a single negative contact (cathode) there are three ways of increasing the number of axons in which a DBS pulse generates an action

potential. The first way is by increasing the volume of an electrical field created by a DBS pulse. The volume of the electrical field must be distinguished from the volume of tissue activation. The volume of the electrical field represents the field's spread consistent with the principles of physics. The primary factors are the impedance of the surrounding tissues and the voltage applied. The volume of tissue activation relates to the biophysics of neuronal responses to the electrical fields—particularly to the biophysical mechanisms of action potential generation. Illustrative of this are two volumes—a volume of large myelinated axons and a volume of electrical field containing only small unmyelinated axons—that are otherwise identical. For the same volume of electrical field, more axons will have action potentials in the volume containing large, myelinated axons than will neurons in the volume containing small, unmyelinated axons. The volume of tissue activation—that is, the volume containing axons generating action potentials—is thus greater in the volume containing large myelinated axons than it is in the volume containing small unmyelinated axons for the same volume of electrical field.

Within the volume of the electrical field, one may increase the current density at a particular point in the volume by using bipolar stimulation with increasing distance between the negative contact (cathode) and positive contact (anode) (*see Chapter 4—Controlling the Flow of Electrical Charges*). Though the volume of the electrical field may not change significantly, the intensities within the electrical field may vary with different efficacy in generating action potentials. The volume of tissue activation for the same relative volume of the electrical field may thus be greater in wide bipolar configurations than it is in other configurations. Finally, one may increase the pulse width. Though changing the pulse width will not change the volume of the electrical field generated by each DBS pulse, increasing pulse width can increase the number of axons in which an action potential can be generated. For the same volume of the electrical field, then, the volume of tissue activation can increase with increasing pulse width. Again, the distinction between volume of the electrical field and volume of tissue activation must be maintained.

Another means of increasing the volume of an electrical field and, secondarily, tissue activation is by using multiple negative contacts (cathodes). The approaches for increasing the number of axons in which an action potential is generated for each of the multiple negative contacts (cathodes) are the same as they are for the above-mentioned individual contact.

The axons that are critical to DBS's clinical benefit must be within reach of the volume of tissue activation. For example, the optimal axon location may be closer to one negative contact (cathode) than to another. Moving the volume of tissue activation toward the contact that lies closer to the optimal axon location may increase the clinical benefit.

Adverse effects most often result from stimulation of unintended axons. In the case of DBS in the vicinity of the STN, for example, inadvertent expansion of the volume of tissue activation to include the medial lemniscus will result in paresthesias that may limit tolerable DBS intensities and result in insufficient clinical benefit. Methods of countering adverse effects are the converse of those that increase clinical benefit. These counters include reduction of the volume of tissue activation via reduction of the volume of the electrical field and reduction of stimulation intensity, which in turn reduces the intensity within the volume of the electrical field by changing to bipolar configurations with shorter distances between the negative and positive contacts (cathodes and anodes, respectively) or changing from bipolar electrode configurations to monopolar. The volume of tissue activation, relative to the volume of the electrical field, may be reduced by decreasing the efficiency of generating action potentials in axons by decreasing the pulse width. Decreasing the DBS frequency can reduce temporal summation and thus decrease the propagation of action potentials through the neural network though this likely is not a significant factor.

In addition to changing the volume of the electrical field and the volume of tissue activation, one may move the volume of tissue activation further from axons whose activation results in adverse effects. This method depends on the regional anatomy around the DBS lead and is described in the chapters that cover DBS in the vicinity of the STN, GPi, and Vim.

Many DBS systems have additional features that enable one to shape with greater precision the volume of tissue activation in order to make it better conform to the regional anatomy (Figure 9.5). Though such shaping usually involves multiple negative contacts (cathodes), different stimulation currents may be applied to each contact. Thus, there are multiple volumes of tissue activation but of different sizes. The contact nearest the axons whose stimulation causes adverse effects may be assigned a stimulation current that creates a small volume of tissue activation in order to avoid eliciting an adverse effect, while also stimulating as many axons associated with clinical benefit as possible, even if that number is insufficient. Another contact further from the axons associated with adverse effects may be assigned a larger stimulation current for generating a large volume of tissue activation in order to activate a greater number of axons associated with clinical benefit. Though axons activated in the larger volume of tissue activation may be insufficient on their own, they may be combined with the axons from the smaller volume of tissue activation to deliver sufficient clinical benefit. A hypothetical example in the case of DBS in the vicinity of the Vim appears in Figure 9.5.

A number of methods may achieve multiple volumes of tissue activation, allowing shaping of the electrical fields in greater conformity to the regional anatomy about a DBS lead. Some are able to partition different currents on different contacts simultaneously. Others interleave multiple DBS pulse trains, each having a different electrical current and perhaps different active contacts. For those that implement multiple and different volumes of tissue activation by means of interleaving, the question becomes: What is the timing relationship between pulses in the interleaved trains? In some implementations, the DBS pulse of one train is delivered midway between a pair of pulses delivered in the other train (Figure 9.5). Yet the efficacy of such interleaving versus simultaneous delivery of different pulses comes into question. Simultaneously delivered pulses of different currents would optimize spatial summation. Whether interleaving is able take advantage of spatial summation is as yet unknown. The potential for spatial summation depends on the duration of postsynaptic potentials induced by the prior pulse and on the length of delay to the next pulse.

THE GROWING IMPORTANCE OF MONOPOLAR SURVEYS

DBS systems' marked improvement in functionality since the publication of this text's first edition, and the pace of development of further functionalities, have greatly increased the complexity of

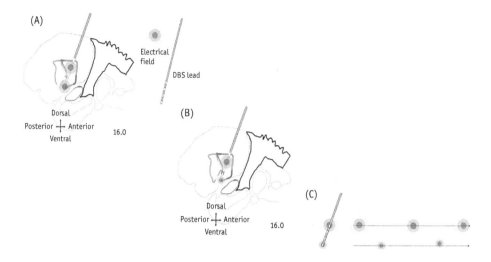

Figure 9.5: Schematic representation of DBS lead that is too posterior in the Vim. In this case, stimulation through the most-ventral contact produced intolerable paresthesias because of the proximity to the medial lemniscus posteriorly. Stimulation through the most dorsal contact did not produce paresthesias; however, alone it did not provide sufficient relief of tremor (A). One option is to apply a smaller stimulation current through the most ventral contact so as to reduce the volume of tissue activation that would not affect axons in the medial lemniscus, in addition to a higher stimulation current through the most dorsal contact (B). Thus, while each active negative contact (cathode) alone fails to provide sufficient clinical benefit, the combination has a synergistic effect that is sufficient. In one commercially available system, the two different negative contacts (cathodes) operate as two independent pulse trains with the same frequency but different stimulation currents. The two pulse trains are combined into an interleaved single pulse train where each set of pulses alternate. Note that the pulse in one contact is delivered halfway between a pair of pulses in the other contact. Thus, the phase delay is 50% of the interval between pulses on one contact. The delay will vary, based on the overall frequency of DBS. Note that, in some commercially available systems, the maximum DBS frequency is less than when no interleaved stimulation is used and therefore may not be optimal.

DBS programming. Even with older, more limited systems, the number of combinations of electrode configurations and stimulation parameters (the parameter space) is overwhelmingly large. For this reason, an approach in which every combination is tried becomes virtually impossible. Some means of economically navigating the parameter space—by use of algorithms, for example—is critical. However, current and predicted advances make construction of a single specific algorithmic approach difficult.

One approach to reducing the parameter space for testing potential candidates post-operatively is that of conducting a monopolar survey. A successful survey may identify specific negative contacts (cathodes) that suggest possible clinical benefit or risk of adverse effects. For example, production of adverse effects with what have been low-stimulation currents (or voltage), historically speaking, suggests that use of this contact may not be feasible. Similarly, the negative contact (cathode) with the best clinical

improvement at the lowest stimulation current (or voltage) is a place to begin, once it is identified.

Warranted here is some comment that anticipates segmented DBS leads. In currently commercially available DBS leads (at least in the United States), each contact is continuous around the circumference of the long axis of the DBS lead. In the future, contacts may be divided into segments that extend radially in the plane that is orthogonal to the long axis of the DBS lead (Figure 9.6).

Much subsequent discussion of the monopolar stimulation presumes that a stimulation current has been applied to the entire circumference of the contact that lies in the single plane orthogonal to the DBS lead's long axis. Discussed below is stimulation restricted to a subset of contacts to direct radially a volume of tissue activation. In cases in which segmented DBS leads are used, "continuous circumferential stimulation" (Figure 9.6) denotes stimulation through a set of all of those contacts that constitute

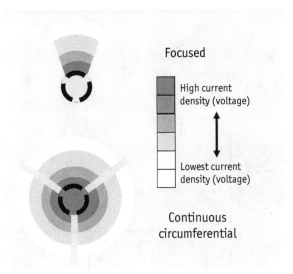

Figure 9.6: In the future, the contacts may be broken into segments that extend radially in the plane that is orthogonal to the long axis of the DBS lead. When stimulation current is applied to one segment, the volume of the electrical field is said to be *focused*. When all segments at a specific level along the long axis of the DBS lead are active, the stimulation is said to be *continuously circumferential*.

the DBS lead's circumference. In cases in which a non-segmented lead is used, "continuous circumferential stimulation" denotes stimulation in all directions in the plane that are orthogonal to the DBS lead (Figure 9.7).

The critical task becomes that of stimulating each contact in the monopolar survey in a way that sufficiently inspires confidence. For example, a monopolar survey at ineffective DBS frequencies might falsely suggest that stimulation through a contact will be ineffective in the future. Yet, as discussed in *Chapter 6—Nervous System Responses to DBS*, stimulation at a slightly higher frequency at the same contact may be quite effective. One of the first and most important steps in the monopolar survey is therefore that of testing a range of DBS frequencies at small, incremental changes. Though the incremental steps between sequential DBS frequencies tested are largely determined by the DBS system in use, this author's experience has shown that increments of no fewer than 5 pulses per second (pps), if possible, are recommended.

Though a range of closely spaced DBS frequencies is critical, the points at which the range begins and ends must be determined. Testing every DBS frequency available on most DBS systems during the initial monopolar survey is infeasible. Clinical practice thus faces a conundrum. The study by Huang and colleagues (Huang et al. 2014) (Figure 9.8) suggests that frequencies on the order of less than 30 pps may be effective. Low-frequency DBS reduces battery current drainage, thus also reducing the frequency of non-rechargeable IPG replacement and the risk of a failed recharging of rechargeable IPGs. Yet Huang and colleagues (Huang et al. 2014) evaluated only a hand-opening and hand-closing task. Despite the fact, then, that low-frequency DBS was effective in reducing bradykinesia, as measured in that task, it is unclear whether this measure predicts clinically optimal benefit generally.

Clinical studies of lower-frequency DBS are limited and have been applied to special cases to overcome adverse effects, such as speech and gait problems. These reports are thus not directly comparable to optimal clinical benefit, which is assumed to be the case with higher-frequency DBS in all but a few cases. One such case involves patients with dystonia for whom the typical high-frequency DBS was ineffective. Experience has shown that DBS's efficacy lies at high frequencies. This is not to say that lower DBS frequencies will prove ineffective. It is to say that their efficacy is unknown.

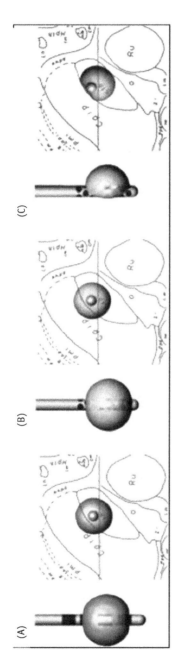

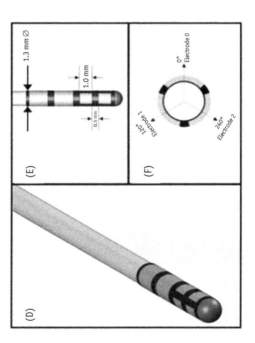

Figure 9.7: Schematic representations of two types of segmented DBS leads whose use in human studies have been reported, A–C (Contarino et al. 2014) and D–F (Pollo et al. 2014). Figure A shows a typical, currently available unsegmented DBS lead. D, E, and F show a DBS lead whose two upper circumferential contacts are unsegmented and whose bottom two circumferential contacts are segmented. B and C show another lead that consists solely of segments that lack any continuous circumferential contact. As shown in B, however, the active negative contacts (cathodes) may be configured to approximate a continuous circumferential contact.

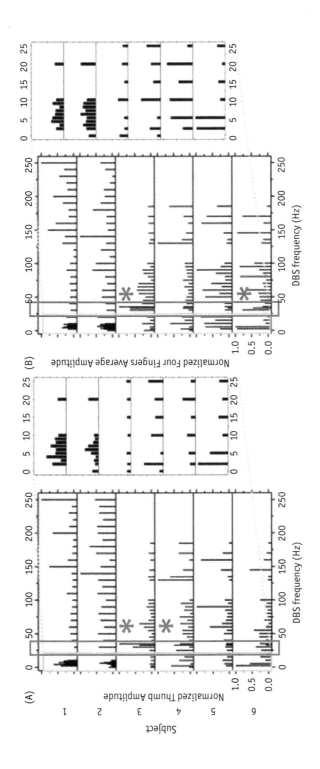

Figure 9.8: Mean-normalized movement amplitudes for (B) fingers (pooled) and (A) thumb for each of six subjects with Parkinson's disease who have had DBS electrodes implanted in the vicinity of the STN. The subjects were asked to open and close their hand as widely and as rapidly as they could. Each subject was tested at each DBS frequency available. (Absence of a column indicates that the associated stimulation frequency was unavailable with the subject's IPG.) There appear multiple peaks associated with large-amplitude movements across multiple frequencies, including low frequencies. The inserts show amplitudes for the lower range of stimulation frequencies. (Asterisks indicate points at which DBS in the high beta frequencies significantly improved movement.)

Adapted from Huang et al. 2014, page 204.

This author believes that the actions and recommendations in clinical practice require reasoned justification. Until such time as definitive studies are published in greater numbers, this author recommends that the range of DBS frequencies begin at approximately 120 pps before increasing by 5 pps up to approximately 200 pps, if doing so is feasible with the particular DBS system in use.

The same concerns for DBS frequency also attend pulse width. Unmyelinated axons of smaller diameters respond by generating an action potential if the duration of the negative (cathodal) phase of the DBS pulse is sufficiently long. Larger-diameter myelinated axons have a threshold to generation of action potentials at shorter pulse widths, compared to small-diameter unmyelinated axons. This phenomenon is related to the concept of *chronaxie*, which involves the threshold to some response as a function of pulse width. Maximization of the probability of generating action potentials requires a pulse width of sufficient length for activating as many axons as possible. The axons in which generation of an action potential produces clinical benefit and axons that are associated with adverse effects may be different (Groppa et al. 2014).

The optimal pulse width is unknown. Determination of the initial pulse width and the range over which to sample a pulse width during DBS programming is difficult and may depend on the DBS target. Chronaxie in patients with Essential tremor whose tremor was abolish by the voltage (by means of a constant voltage IPG) was studied allowing estimation of the chronaxie to tremor suppression (Groppa et al. 2014). The study's results were of limited help in determining the appropriate pulse width to assure a maximal response. In a re-analysis of the study's data, there came to light a logarithmically decaying function whose minimum threshold determined the point at which the plot of threshold voltage to pulse width became asymptotic, which occurred at 150 microseconds. This subsequent finding suggests that the point of becoming asymptotic is the minimum pulse width that assures the minimum voltage threshold necessary for producing an effect (Figure 9.9). Whether these findings may be generalized to other DBS targets and disorders is unclear. Holsheimer and colleagues presented similar results for DBS in the vicinity of the Vim for patients with tremor secondary to Essential tremor and Parkinson's disease (Holsheimer et al. 2000).

Moro and colleagues (2002) examined the results of varying the pulse width, while leaving DBS frequency and stimulation voltage (used constant voltage IPGs) unvaried, on hand-tapping and on rigidity in 11 patients with Parkinson's disease undergoing DBS in the vicinity of the STN. The results are shown in Figure 9.10. In the case of rigidity, the greatest improvement reached its maximum between 120 and 190 microseconds. This is consistent with the suggestion that 150 microsecond pulse widths are those with which it is best to begin. Unfortunately, the study was probably underpowered relative to the assessment of the hand-tapping task, owing to the very large variance evidenced by the standard deviation bars. Therefore, no claim may be made about the effect of pulse width in this study.

The concern has been raised that a pulse width of 150 microseconds would more quickly exhaust an IPG battery than would a pulse width of 60 microseconds. Yet, were the required stimulation current higher as a consequence of the use of a 60 microsecond pulse width, little would be gained. Reduction from 150 microseconds to 60 microseconds, for example, would preserve approximately as much battery charge as would be lost with increasing the stimulation intensity from 2 mA to 3.2 mA. If beginning at 60 microseconds required a stimulus intensity of 3.2 mA, and beginning at 150 microseconds only 2 mA, no conservation of battery charge is realized.

A monopolar survey also affords an opportunity for assessing risk of adverse effects. Most adverse effects depend on the regional anatomy around a DBS target. Consequently, the likeliest specific adverse effects are covered in the chapters devoted to specific DBS targets. Discussed here is the general approach to assessing the risk for adverse effects.

Critical during a monopolar survey is demonstration of a therapeutic window. In pharmacology, a "therapeutic window" is defined as the difference between a dose of medication that produces benefit and a dose that causes adverse effects. For DBS programming, the term is defined as the difference in a stimulation intensity that produces clinical benefit and a stimulation intensity that produces adverse effects. The therapeutic window may be assessed during a monopolar survey. The DBS negative contact (cathode) that is associated with the greatest therapeutic window often serves as a starting point for subsequent DBS programming. It must be noted

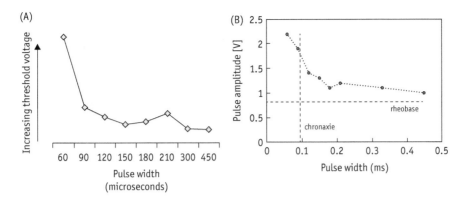

Figure 9.9: In (A) appears a graph that relates the voltage threshold to abolish tremor in patients with essential tremor and DBS in the vicinity of the STN created by reanalysis of data presented by Groppa et al. (2014). These results are similar to those of Holsheimer et al. (2000), which appear in (B). The voltage thresholds first become minimal at 150 microsecond pulse widths, which suggests that longer pulse widths are unlikely to reduce the voltage necessary for tremor suppression.

that, in situations in which stimulation produces no adverse effects, the contact with the lowest threshold stimulation intensity to producing clinical benefit is selected as the contact whose therapeutic window is the widest.

In cases in which above-mentioned a segmented DBS lead is used, an initial monopolar survey is conducted with all contiguous contacts at or near the same level (plane) along the long axis of a DBS lead being stimulated simultaneously, depending on the lead's construction (Figures 9.6 and 9.7). In this manner, continuous circumferential stimulation will be applied. In cases in which adverse effects occur within a relatively narrow therapeutic window on the order of 2 mA (2 volts with constant voltage IPGs), the therapeutic window ought to be assessed for each segmented contact individually, because subsequent use of an individual segment may become necessary

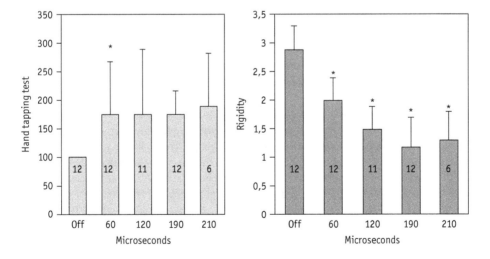

Figure 9.10: Changes in rating scores on the hand-tapping task (where increase is improvement) and rigidity (decrease is improvement), respectively, in patients undergoing DBS in the vicinity of the STN. The numbers in the bars are the numbers of patients studied at that condition. The pulse width was varied while the patient's DBS frequency and stimulation voltage were held constant modified.

From Moro et al. 2002, pages 708–709.

for projecting an electrical field generated by a DBS pulse away from the structures that are responsible for the adverse effect when stimulated.

DETECTION OF A RESPONSE IS CRITICAL

Determining what constitutes a response thus becomes the issue. The initial intent of a monopolar survey is not that of achieving optimal clinical benefit. It is that of comparing responses at different negative contacts (cathodes).

Evaluations must be sensitive to changes and of sufficiently high resolution. Causal observation may be insufficient. Clinical rating scales, such as the Unified Parkinson Disease Rating Scales (UPDRS), are ordinal: The evaluation is in rank order; the intervals between ranks convey little information. For example, changes in finger-tapping task scores on the UPDRS are rated on a scale of 0–4, and half units between. Yet a change in the UPDRS score from 3–4 is not comparable to a change from 1–2. Nonetheless, rating scales, such as the UPDRS, are based on performance. Therefore, they are perhaps less subjective.

There are systems available that use objective measures, such as accelerometers to measure movement speed. These may be useful during a monopolar survey. However, these quantitative measures are often insufficient for determining the clinical significance of the responses produced. Consequently, these objective measures may be less valuable than the judgement of experienced clinicians when DBS undergoes programming for clinical benefit, particularly judgements that predict quality of life.

Responses to DBS may be subtle and confusing (*see Chapter 10—Clinical Assessments*). For example, patients may describe an unusual feeling localized to a part of the body. In the case of DBS targeting the Vim or the STN, such a symptom could be interpreted as the volume of tissue activation encompassing the posterior ventral caudal nucleus of the thalamus or the ascending fibers of the medial lemniscus. However, these symptoms also may stem from unobservable slight muscle contractions. Similarly, abnormalities of speech induced by stimulation may be related to the volume of tissue activation that encompasses the homuncular head representation in the targeted nuclei, or to spread of stimulation to the corticobulbar fibers in the posterior limb of the internal capsule.

It is important that sufficient stimulation current be applied in order to determine the precise nature of the symptom or sign associated with the adverse effect. For example, failing to produce frank muscle contraction at higher stimulation intensities in a patient who initially complained of unusual feelings in a limb suggests that the complaint was unrelated to muscle contraction. Similarly, if higher stimulation intensities produce contraction of muscles about the face in an individual who initially noted speech difficulties at lower stimulation intensities, then the likely cause of the adverse effect was unintended spread of stimulation current to the corticobulbar fibers in the posterior limb of the internal capsule. Stimulation intensities usually increase until an adverse effect is encountered and clearly characterized, or until stimulation intensities reach approximately 4 mA (5 volts with constant voltage IPGs). However, a programmer must ensure that stimulation intensities do not exceed the accepted safety limit of 30 microcoulombs/cm^2/phase.

PROGRAMMING FOR OPTIMAL BENEFIT IN THE ABSENCE OF ADVERSE EFFECTS

As discussed above, this author approaches DBS programming by distinguishing programming for optimal clinical benefit from programming to avoid adverse effects. In each case, the DBS frequency that is found during a monopolar survey to deliver greatest clinical benefit at the lowest stimulation intensity is chosen for use for in all subsequent programming (certain exceptions will be noted when relevant).

Step 1. Programming for adverse effect—free optimal clinical benefit begins with the contact found to have the lowest threshold to any improvement during a monopolar survey. The initial electrode configuration is monopolar. It consists of a single active negative contact (cathode), with the IPG serving as the positive contact (anode). In the case of segmented DBS leads, the system would be used in continuous circumferential mode. (Note that these suggestions are based on a DBS segmented lead in which the contacts are arranged as sectors around the circumference of the lead in the plane orthogonal to the long axis of the lead. These suggestions may not be appropriate for other segmented DBS lead architectures, but the general principle still may apply. It is important to note that changing from a continuous circumferential contact stimulation to a subset of contacts in a segmented lead can change the surface area of the electrical contacts over which the stimulation is applied. This could change the current densities and thus, affect safety [*see Chapter 5—DBS Safety*]. These caveats apply to any and all discussions of segmented DBS leads in this textbook.) Choice of the initial pulse width is problematic, for reasons discussed above. Early studies usually involve use of pulse widths on the order of 60 microseconds. Yet, as presented in the studies cited above, use of a pulse width 60 microseconds in duration demands stimulation intensities that are considerably higher than those associated with pulse widths of 150 microseconds.

DBS with pulse widths of 60 microseconds may well deliver clinical benefit. Yet if observations in the studies cited above are accurate and generalizable to the patient's circumstance, the stimulus intensity required is likely to be much higher. Extension of battery life involves a tradeoff between the use of narrower pulse widths and higher stimulation intensities and the use of wider pulse widths and lower stimulus intensities. The combination that drains an IPG battery less rapidly is unknown. DBS at twice the stimulation intensity and half the pulse width, for example, may draw just as much current from an IPG battery as does half the stimulation current at twice the pulse width. However, stimulation intensities that require voltages that are greater than an IPG battery's voltage may actually deplete the battery's charge more rapidly.

Though use of an initial 60-microsecond DBS pulse width followed by progressive increases as necessary is certainly consistent with many current standards of practice, simplification in service of programming efficiency has its merits. Initiating DBS programming at 150 microseconds may reduce the need for subsequent increases in pulse width. A possible exception is in the case of DBS in the vicinity of the GPi for dystonia, for which has been reported use of DBS pulse widths that are considerably greater than 150 microseconds.

Step 2. From initial electrode configurations and stimulation parameters, the volume of tissue activation is increased until the patient gains sufficient, adverse effect–free clinical benefit. This is usually accomplished via an increase in stimulation intensity until a clinically sufficient benefit is obtained, or

the stimulation intensity reaches, for example, 4 mA (5 volts with constant voltage IPGs) or the maximal safe stimulation intensity, whichever is lower. A patient who realizes sufficient clinical benefit and experiences no adverse effects is prepared for exiting the programming session, which is discussed below.

Step 3. A stimulation intensity that has been increased to 4 mA without delivery of sufficient clinical benefit (5 volts for constant-voltage IPGs) or arrival at the safety limit prompts many programmers to begin increasing DBS frequency. This is the conventional response, and it is predicated on the idea that in the range of high frequencies beneficial clinical response increases with increasing DBS frequencies in a monotonic fashion. A number of observations have suggested that an increase in DBS frequency may not improve clinical benefit. The study by Huang and colleagues (Huang et al. 2014) has shown that the relationship of benefit to DBS frequency is not a monotonically increasing function (Figure 9.8). Other studies, whose authors had examined correlations in the total electrical energy delivered (TEED), failed to find any correlation between TEED and benefit, which would be inconsistent with a monotonically increasing relationship between DBS frequency and clinical benefit. However, the issue has not been rigorously studied. Current convention thus remains that of progressively increasing DBS frequency.

Step 3A. An alternative to increasing DBS frequency is increasing the intensity within the volume of the electrical field in response to the DBS pulse. Doing so also increases the volume of tissue activation by changing the electrode configuration from monopolar to wide bipolar (discussed below are certain caveats about changing the stimulation intensity prior to changing electrode configurations and pulse widths). The deepest, or most ventral, contact is thus negative (cathode); and the shallowest, or most dorsal, contact is positive (anode). As discussed in *Chapter 4, Controlling the Flow of Electrical Charges,* the electrical field's intensity decreases by the square of the distance of the axons from the negative contact (cathode), and it increases by the square of the length between the negative and positive contacts (cathode and anode, respectively). Once a bipolar electrode's configuration has been established, the stimulation intensity may be increased until a clinically sufficient benefit is achieved, or until the intensity reaches, for example, 4 mA (5 volts using a constant voltage IPG) or approaches the safety limit. Each outcome assumes an absence of adverse effects.

Step 4. Should clinical benefit prove inadequate and limiting adverse effects remain absent, a programmer may increase the pulse width. Though increasing the pulse width does not change the volume and spatial distribution of the electrical field generated by a DBS pulse, it does increase the number of axons within the electrical field in which action potentials are generated. Increasing the pulse width effectively increases the volume of tissue activation. Longer pulse widths may progressively recruit unmyelinated axons, smaller diameter axons, and neuronal cell bodies. Determination of an initial pulse width and the range over which a pulse width ought to be sampled during DBS programming are problematic (see discussion above).

At least in the case of DBS in the vicinity of the STN and Vim, the above-mentioned chronaxie experiments suggest that pulse widths greater than 150 microseconds probably do not reduce the threshold intensity for tremor control. It must be recognized that the data presented are group data. As such, they do not account for individual variability. Unfortunately, studies to date have not reported sample variance. It cannot be known, therefore, whether some individuals would have an even lower threshold to tremor suppression at pulse widths greater than 150 microseconds. Testing higher pulse widths is altogether reasonable, then, and beginning at 150 microseconds reduces the number of pulse widths in need of testing.

Step 5. Should increased pulse widths or wide bipolar DBS stimulation fail to deliver optimal, adverse effect–free clinical benefit, a programmer may repeat the steps described above at higher stimulation currents than the examples given above (or voltages, if a constant voltage IPG is in use). Such high currents, if they are associated with voltages that are higher than an IPG's battery voltage, raise the concern that they would more quickly exhaust it. Alternatively, a programmer may resort to multiple negative contacts (cathodes) in a typical monopolar electrode configuration. Yet multiple negative contacts (cathodes) accelerate battery exhaustion as well. Unfortunately, there is insufficient information on comparisons between the exact consequences of high stimulation intensities (in light of the issue of IPG efficiency) and multiple negative contacts (cathodes). Should it be

decided to increase the stimulation intensities beyond 4 mA (5 volts in constant voltage IPGs), for example, a programmer may return to *Step 1*. In conducting a new monopolar survey, a programmer may select the contact with the next-lowest threshold to clinical benefit as the second negative contact (cathode).

A caveat: The preceding discussions presume that the DBS system is intact and functioning properly. Certainly, the absence of any clinical response or adverse effects with more aggressive increases in stimulation should alert a programmer to the possibility of an IPG failure or poor DBS lead location. Methods of determining IPG failure are somewhat peculiar to a particular IPG's manufacturer. Programmers are advised to review user manuals or contact manufacturers directly. The electrical integrity of a DBS system may usually be evaluated by testing the electrical impedances and the current passing through it. Very high impedances suggest a break in electrical continuity—a conclusion that is supported by electrical currents that are less than nominal. Very low impedances, particularly those that are associated with electrical currents that are higher than nominal, suggest the possibility of a short circuit, which shunts electrical current away from the DBS contacts. Sometimes there may be an intermittent electrical discontinuity or short circuit, owing perhaps to positional factors. Pressing on the IPG or its connectors during testing may produce results that suggest electrical discontinuity or a short circuit.

Should clinical response fail despite an appearance of electrical integrity of the DBS system, a programmer ought to consider the possibility of lead migration, in which DBS contacts move to a location where stimulation produces no observable effects. In DBS targeted at the GPi, for example, lead migration may pull the contacts toward non-motor regions and further from the posterior limb of the internal capsule and the optic tract. Consequently, few observable effects are produced.

Currently, brain shift occurring during DBS lead implantation surgery is perhaps the most common cause of lead migration, particularly if the migration is due to tension pneumocephaly. Even if the DBS lead is placed in the proper location during the surgery, the brain will move as intracranial air is reabsorbed, pulling and displacing the DBS lead as it does so. For guarding against possible lead migration over subsequent post-operative days and weeks as intracranial air is reabsorbed, this author recommends that a series of skull X-rays be obtained immediately following implantation. Thus, if at any time in the post-operative period no adequate clinical benefit is realized, another skull X-ray series may serve as a simple and relatively inexpensive means of confirming DBS lead migration.

PROGRAMMING TO PREVENT ADVERSE EFFECTS

A programmer must consider several issues should his patient experience adverse effects during DBS. First, he must consider whether the specific adverse effects have localizing value that he may leverage by selecting *electrode configurations*, defined here as the set of active negative (cathodal) and positive (anodal) contacts. For example, DBS in the vicinity of the Vim may affect speech. The effect on speech may be mediated by unintended propagation of electrical charge to the corticobulbar fibers in the posterior limb of the internal capsule, or it may be due to mechanisms that are intrinsic to the thalamic nucleus. If the effect on speech is attributable to stimulation in the thalamus, it may stem from the spread of electrical stimulation current to the head region in the homunculus within the thalamus. Yet it is also possible that the effect on speech is not attributable to any exact location. Clearly, an adverse effect that is possibly localized in anatomy surrounding the DBS lead presents an opportunity for redirecting the volume and location of tissue activation by changing electrode configuration.

Latency to the onset of the adverse effects represents a second dimension by which to consider adverse effects. Because many adverse effects become apparent within seconds—paresthesias and tonic muscle contractions, for example—they permit continuous real-time adjustments. Other adverse effects, such as gait and balance adverse effects, take several minutes to develop. Though these adverse effects are difficult to use for titration of DBS electrode configurations and stimulation parameters, they nonetheless ought to be assessed before a patient exits the clinic.

Other adverse effects such as depression, euphoria, and impulse-control problems may not become apparent for many days or weeks. These symptoms become much more difficult to titrate accurately. In other words, even if a programmer makes the appropriate changes in electrode configurations and stimulation parameters, the impact of these changes may not become detectable until well after a patient has left the clinic. Specific maneuvers exist for dealing with these symptoms. For example, in treating mood disturbances or impulse control problems in patients undergoing DBS in the vicinity of the STN, a programmer may move the volume of tissue activation dorsally.

Electrode configuration and stimulation parameters that present the widest therapeutic window are selected, no matter whether the mode is segmented or continuously circumferential. It must be noted that, in the absence of any adverse effects on the monopolar survey, the electrode configuration with the lowest stimulation-intensity threshold to producing clinical benefit is chosen and in the continuous circumferential mode is typically used in situations where a segmented DBS lead is employed. DBS programming proceeds as described above (see Programming for Optimal Benefit in the Absence of Adverse Effects, this chapter). Otherwise, the electrode configuration with the widest therapeutic window is chosen. DBS programming proceeds as described above (see Programming for Optimal Benefit in the Absence of Adverse Effects, this chapter) in the hope that a sufficient clinical benefit is achieved without creation any limiting side effect. If this fails, a programmer must change the shape, size, efficiency for action potential generation, and location of the volume of the electrical field generated by the DBS pulse so as to maximize clinical benefit and minimize the risk of adverse effects.

Step 1. If persistent adverse effects make it necessary to change the shape, size, or location of the volume of an electrical field, a programmer may maintain the initial use of monopolar stimulation while moving to different negative (cathodal) contacts in order to avoid adverse effects. It so happens that adverse effects are usually more associated with stimulation of the deepest, most ventral negative (cathodal) contacts in the STN, GPi, and ventral intermediate thalamus (see chapters specific to those DBS targets: *Chapter 11—Approach to Subthalamic Nucleus*, *Chapter 12—Approach to Globus Pallidus Interna*, and *Chapter 13—Approach to Thalamic DBS*). Unfortunately, the same is true of clinical benefit. However, by moving the volume of the electrical field dorsally, a programmer may obviate many adverse effects. If a programmer moves a volume of the electrical field by selecting a different negative contact or sets of negative contacts in the case of multiple negative contacts (cathodes), and if this move effectively avoids adverse effects, she may pursue the procedure for programming for optimal benefit in the absence of adverse effects until a sufficient clinical response is achieved without producing adverse effects.

Step 2. In monopolar electrode configuration with continuous circumferential stimulation, if the volume of an electrical field is moved and fails to obviate adverse effects, a possible next step is that of reducing the volume of tissue activation relative to the volume of the electrical field. This can be accomplished in non-segmented DBS systems by changing the electrode configurations to bipolar (*see Chapter 4—Controlling the Flow of Electrical Charges*). Current DBS leads typically feature four continuous circumferential electrical contacts that are organized in a linear array along the long axis of the DBS lead. This design accommodates varying degrees of bipolar stimulation—active most ventral and most dorsal contacts, for example, in which there are two contacts and three inter-contact spaces between the negative (cathodal) and positive (anodal) contacts. Such a configuration is *wide bipolar*. Other configurations may have one inactive contact and two inter-contact spaces between the active contacts. These configurations are known as *close bipolar*. Finally, *narrow bipolar* denotes a single space between active contacts.

As in the case of monopolar DBS, the location of the active negative contact (cathode) may be moved along the long axis of the DBS lead to find the position that delivers sufficient clinical benefit without creating adverse effects. These maneuvers, which depend on the regional anatomy around a DBS lead, are specific to the DBS target and are covered in detail in the chapters devoted to each DBS target (*Chapter 11—Approach to Subthalamic Nucleus, Chapter 12—Approach to Globus Pallidus Interna,* and *Chapter 13—Approach to Thalamic DBS*).

Step 2A. In cases in which a segmented DBS lead is in use, a programmer may take a monopolar or bipolar approach. In case in which a segmented contact in a monopolar configuration is in use, the approach outlined in *Step 1* may be taken. The approach in *Step 2* may be taken when using a segmented lead in a bipolar configuration.

Step 3. Should there arise the need to relocate and reduce the volume of an electrical field that is generated by each DBS pulse by a lead that is in a bipolar configuration, a programmer may use a *tripolar configuration*. A typical configuration is one in which the middle of three contiguous contacts is negative (cathodal) and the outer contacts of the trio are positive (anodal). Yet the negative (cathodal) contact may only be moved along the long axis of the DBS lead for a limited distance. A tripolar configuration moreover generates a considerably smaller volume of the electrical field. It therefore activates a smaller volume of tissue.

Step 4. It may be that no combination of negative (cathodal) contacts in a single pulse train produces sufficient clinical benefit at adverse effect–free stimulation parameters. Yet some combinations of negative contacts (cathodes) produce benefit at tolerable stimulation parameters. These negative contacts may be combined in an interleaved pulse train (Figure 9.5). For example, the most ventral contact produces significant benefit, but its stimulation parameters also produce adverse effects. The ventral contact produces clinical benefit that is nonetheless insufficient. However, the threshold to adverse effects is higher with the ventral contact than it is with the most ventral contact. It is possible to construct two pulse trains. In pulse train A, the most ventral contact stimulation parameters are just below those that produce adverse effects. Pulse train B, which involves the ventral contact, is set at higher stimulation intensities, because its threshold to adverse effects is higher. Pulse trains A and B may then be combined in an interleaved pulse train that produces adequate clinical benefit with no attendant adverse effects. It must be noted, however, that some IPGs have limited frequencies in an interleaved mode, and that other limitations attend the use of a single pulse train.

Step 5. Should relocation and reduction of the volume of the electrical field generated by the DBS pulse fail to obviate adverse effects, a programmer may reduce the number of axons that are activated by the electrical field. This serves to reduce the volume of tissue activation, which a programmer may do by reducing the pulse width in such a way as to avoid increasing stimulation intensity.

Step 6. If a reduction of pulse width fails to obviate the onset of adverse effects at stimulation intensities that are necessary for achieving adequate clinical benefit, a programmer may reduce the DBS frequency. There is evidence, however, that suggests that the range of effective DBS frequencies is quite narrow. For example, the study by Huang and colleagues (Huang et al. 2014), which appears in Figure 9.8, suggests that simply a reduction in stimulation frequency from 150–145 pps results in marked reduction in the amplitude of a hand-opening and hand-closing task. A programmer may alleviate adverse effects somewhat by reducing DBS frequency, which in turn reduces temporal summation of the postsynaptic electrical potentials that are necessary for propagating activations through the polysynaptic pathways that mediate adverse effects. Unfortunately, reduced efficiency of trans-synaptic activations may also diminish clinical benefit.

Programmers are advised to set stimulation intensities at zero before they change any electrical configurations, because doing so may significantly lower the threshold to adverse effects. Though stimulation intensity with one configuration may produce no adverse effects, an equal intensity with another configuration may do so. Also, programmers must return stimulation parameters to initial conditions, such as those set in the last instance of monopolar survey, before they implement any new electrode configuration.

Should no combinations of electrode configurations and stimulation parameters prove able to deliver adequate adverse effect–free clinical benefit, a programmer must evaluate the location of the DBS lead. If a skull X-ray series was obtained from the patient immediately following lead implantation, a second series may be obtained to discover possible lead migration.

Though a lead may not have migrated, it may nonetheless be misplaced. Additional imaging may be necessary to establish its true position. A computed tomography (CT) scan alone is usually unhelpful, because metal in the DBS lead scatters X-rays, producing artifact. If it is merged with a preoperative MRI scan, however, it may be of use. Alternatively, a second MRI scan may be obtained. It must be obtained according to DBS manufacturer's recommendations for safety.

EXITING THE DBS PROGRAMMING SESSION

Once a programmer has completed DBS programming, he must concern himself with what to do with other treatments, particularly medications. If a DBS system was programmed while the patient was in a medication-minimal state, the patient may experience a negative synergistic interaction that produces adverse effects once the patient takes her medication. A newly programmed patient, once she has gone off her medications, must therefore be observed for a period that is sufficient for her medication's effects to have reached maximal effect.

Any observed synergistic adverse effect must be managed. A programmer must resist the temptation of returning to previous and perhaps relatively ineffective DBS electrode configurations, stimulation parameters, and pulse trains because these were the last variables changed. He must also resist the temptation of attributing an adverse effect solely to the DBS rather than to the medications (this affects particularly DBS programmers who lack a strong understanding of medication management of the treated disorder). In most cases, the appropriate response is that of adjusting medications rather than backtracking on the DBS. After all, the medications are known to have failed, because it is unlikely the patient would otherwise be undergoing DBS.

If DBS programming is performed while a patient is in a medication-maximum state, as it would be when the primary focus is that of reducing medication-induced side effects, he must later be observed while he is in a medication-minimal state in order to ensure that his symptoms and disabilities that stem directly from the underlying disease are effectively controlled. The time to a medication-minimal state from peak nervous system medication levels varies greatly with the particular medication and formulation. Nonetheless, patients and their family members and caregivers may often offer some insight into the time course of the medication's effects.

The concern has been raised that some programmers may too aggressively reduce medication, often in an *a priori* routine manner. In light of the iterative process between adjustments to DBS and medication (as well as other forms of therapy), the concern becomes that of knowing when to stop. There are two general issues. One argument is that the programmer stops when the patient has reached satisfactory control. The question becomes: What constitutes "satisfactory control?" Any notion of satisfactory control must be patient-centered. That is, it must be what a patient or her family member or caregiver considers satisfactory.

Ideally, it is not what the programmer would consider satisfactory control that should drive the DBS programming. Doing so verges on violation of the ethical principle of autonomy and may constitute a form of paternalism. In the real world, there is a cost to pursuing satisfactory control—expense, effort, allocation of resources, and so on. These issues affect everyone involved with a patient, including clinicians. Thus, as is common in medical decision making, a cost–benefit analysis is made, either explicitly or implicitly. The question is: Who determines the cost–benefit ratio? There is a natural inclination for the treating clinician to do so, either out of a sense of protecting the patient (which can dangerously approach paternalism) or per consequences to reimbursement issues, putting the treating clinician in a significant conflict of interest.

These questions are vexing and their answers elusive. However, no answers will be forthcoming if the questions are not asked. In such situations, what may be considered effective resolution is usually best achieved by consensus rather than conflict. The interactions between programmers and a patient or family member or caregiver are in partnership with shared goals and shared appreciation of the practical implications. In the situations in which there may be some conflict, it is far better to seek resolution short of litigation, either legal or extralegal.

There is another issue in how aggressively medication reduction is pursued. In many ways, DBS avoids many of the problems medications entail by virtue of pharmacokinetic and pharmacodynamics principles. Unlike medications, problems caused by the nature of absorption, distribution, and metabolism of medications are not problems to the same degree for DBS. For many patients, DBS provides constant and consistent effects as long as the DBS system is on. Just that inherent advantage would be justification to maximize DBS allowing minimization of medications. Thus, in this author's practice in the case of Parkinson's disease, following successful DBS programming, medications are reduced, expecting there to be some worsening of symptoms and disabilities. These are attended to in the subsequent DBS programming session. Thus, there is a continual iterative process of DBS optimization and medication reduction.

Once the optimal electrode configurations and stimulation parameters have been determined and the DBS IPG is appropriately programmed, there are other issues that need to be reviewed prior to the patient's exit from the clinic.

1. A decision needs to be made regarding what control is given to a patient or their family member or caregiver over DBS pulse trains, electrode configurations, and stimulation parameters. The DBS IPG is then configured appropriately. It is important to assure that, whatever the changes that can be implemented by the patient or their family member or caregiver, they will not produce adverse effects or unsafe operation.

2. Potential late-occurring adverse effects, such as mood changes, impulse control problems, gait, postural stability, and speech, language, or swallowing difficulties, should be reviewed and patients or their family members or caregivers given information regarding what to do and how to contact appropriate medical personnel should the patients experience an adverse effect.

3. Precautions regarding the electrical environment the patients may reasonably be exposed to should be reviewed with the patients, family members, and caregivers.

4. The patients should keep on their persons some notification that the they have an implanted electrical medical device.

5. The patients should be encouraged to keep their controller in their immediate possession at all times. For example, emergency medical personnel may not have access to a knowledgeable clinician or to the clinician programming systems used to interrogate and control the DBS system. In those situations, the emergency medical personnel may have to resort to using the patient's controller.

6. Skin over an implanted system should be inspected for evidence of infection, inflammation, and erosion.

7. Battery status should be checked. A clinician should assure herself that a patient or his family member or caregiver understands and can demonstrate the proper use of the patient controller and any recharging system.

8. Indicators in use that are affected by the DBS programming session, such as the number of activations, should be reset so that any changes during the subsequent time prior to the next DBS programming session can be reviewed.

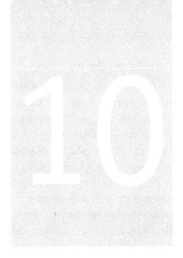

CLINICAL ASSESSMENTS

Titration of DBS is outcomes-based as there is no surrogate marker as yet to predict benefit and the absence of adverse effects (*see Supplemental essay—Automated Assisted DBS Programming, at http://www.greenvilleneuromodulationcenter.com/DBS_Programming_essays//*). Thus, the DBS electrode configurations, stimulation parameters, and pulse trains are evaluated based on the efficacy of the symptoms and disabilities being treated and the range of possible adverse effects, particularly those related to the regional anatomy around the DBS lead.

In assessing symptom and disability relief as well as adverse effects, it is important to recognize the time course of these effects. Any particularly DBS programming session has to be executed in a reasonable time frame. It may not be possible to directly observe for benefit or adverse effects within the time constraints of a DBS programming session. Indeed, for disorders such as dystonia or Obsessive Compulsive Disorder (OCD), the latency to clinical benefit may be months. Similarly, latencies to adverse effects, particularly non-motor such as mood and impulsivity, may take weeks. While always assessing for long-term effects, it is necessary to be judicious in selecting items to assess within the time frame of a DBS programming session.

The quality of clinical examination determines the quality of the information gained from DBS programming sessions. Some symptoms of the disorders treated may respond to stimulation, albeit in a manner that fails to predict subsequent beneficial or adverse effects. Propagation of the stimulation current to the corticospinal tract, for example, may reduce tremor and thus create the impression of symptomatic benefit. The involvement of the corticospinal tract, however, limits benefit, because it is likely to interfere with normal use of the limb. One must establish that tremor reduction stems from the therapeutic mechanisms, known or unknown, rather than involvement of the corticospinal tract. In order to do so, one must distinguish the first sort of reduction from the second.

CLINICAL ASSESSMENTS BY DISEASE

The following sections review the clinical assessments of the symptoms of diseases targeted for DBS, before proceeding to a discussion of the clinical assessments specific to the DBS anatomical or physiological target that is particularly relevant to assessing adverse effects. DBS of more than one target improves symptoms of various disorders. For example, stimulating both the GPi and the STN relieves a wide range of symptoms related to Parkinson's disease. Conventional wisdom holds that DBS of the thalamus is effective solely for tremor. However, in the past, patients were selected primarily based on tremor, and less attention was paid to motor symptoms such as bradykinesia. Consequently, it is unknown what effect Vim DBS would have on symptoms other than tremor.

CLINICAL EVALUATION
OF PARKINSON'S DISEASE

DBS fulfills its primary purpose when it relieves the symptoms and disabilities characteristic of Parkinson's disease without adverse effects. Numerous and varied, symptoms and signs of Parkinson's disease include slow movement and other motor symptoms, as well as depression, cognitive decline, and other non-motor symptoms. Though the current use of DBS is directed primarily towards alleviating motor symptoms, the programmer may detect depression and impulse control problems, two potential complications.

The primary motor symptoms of Parkinson's disease include bradykinesia (slowness of movement), akinesia (absence of movement), tremor, rigidity (resistance to passive joint rotations), and postural and gait abnormalities. These last two do not lend themselves to testing in the time allotted for programming. It is recommended to quantify these symptoms by use of the Movement Disorders Society–Unified Parkinson's Disease Rating Scales Part III (Goetz et al. 2008). Doing so allows comparisons over subsequent DBS programming sessions and conveys useful information to others involved in the care of the patient.

While bradykinesia may affect speech, respiration, and nearly every movement, convenient movements tested to assess bradykinesia in the clinic include rapid repetitive finger tapping—the index finger to the the the thumb, for example. The DBS programmer notes this activity's frequency (speed), amplitude, and whether there is a reduction in amplitude or halting of the movement as the effort continues. Unique to Parkinson's disease is the finger-tapping amplitude, which tends to decrease as it continues yet preserved ability to individuate the tapping fingers. This decrease in amplitude helps distinguish bradykinesia owing to Parkinson's disease from similar symptoms owing to inadvertent stimulation of the corticospinal tract.

Two phenomena—the relative lack of finger-tapping amplitude reduction with corticospinal tract stimulation, and frank muscle contractions with progressive increase in the stimulation current (voltage)—may allow distinguishing slowness of movement owing to Parkinson's disease from the spread of the stimulation current to the corticospinal tract in the posterior limb of the internal capsule. Patients with Parkinson's disease also make normal individuated finger movements. A clinician can test for this by having the patient tap each finger to the thumb in succession. Patients with Parkinson's disease move all fingers independently except the ulnarmost two. Corticospinal tract involvement diminishes the independence of the finger movements; all fingers tend to move together (Figure 10.1). However, this observation needs further testing. Bradykinetic finger-tapping quantities correspond to the following scale: a grade of 0 = normal; a grade of 1 = slight slowing with disintegration of the normal rhythm (one or two possible interruptions, or diminishing amplitude after approximately 10 taps); a grade of 2 = three to five interruptions or prolonged arrest, mild slowing, or

Bradykinesia
individuated movements
retained

Corticospinal tract stimulation
individuated movements lost

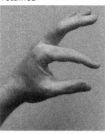 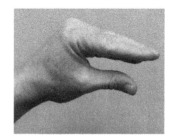

Figure 10.1: Demonstration of the effects of Parkinson's versus stimulation of the corticospinal tract on finger tapping. Patients with Parkinson's disease may be slow in their finger-tapping frequency and diminished in amplitude, as will be patients with spreading of stimulation to the corticospinal tract in the posterior limb of the internal capsule. However, patients with Parkinson's disease can make individuated movements, whereas spreading of stimulation to the corticospinal tract tends to make the fingers move together.

amplitude reduction midway in a ten-tap sequence; a grade of 3 = more than five interruptions or at least one prolonged arrest, moderate slowing, or decreased amplitude following the commencement of tapping; a grade of 4 = finger tapping that proves extremely difficult or impossible to perform.

One may assess bradykinesia in a hand-opening and -closing task according to a similar rating scale, which consists of the following values: a grade of 0 = normal; a grade of 1 = slight slowing with disintegration of a normal rhythm (one or two interruptions, or diminishing amplitude as the task approaches completion); a grade of 2 = three to five interruptions during tapping, prolonged arrest, mild slowing, or amplitude reduction mid-task; a grade of 3 = more than five interruptions, at least one prolonged arrest, moderate slowing, or decreased amplitude immediately following the task's commencement; a grade of 4 = finger tapping that proves extremely difficult or impossible for the patient to perform. The importance of testing both finger tapping and hand-opening and -closing owes to different degrees of patient sensitivity to DBS. Experience has shown this author that, although hand-opening and -closing is more responsive to DBS, finger-tapping response more effectively

predicts subsequent therapeutic effect. (This observation requires additional study.)

Typical of Parkinson's disease, tremor during rest is assessed as the patient lies still and has her upper extremities supported against gravity. Tremor amplitude determines ratings that correspond to the following scale: a grade of 0 = an absence of tremor; a grade of 1 = an amplitude less than 1 cm; a grade of 2 = an amplitude greater than 1 cm but less than 3 cm; a grade of 3 = an amplitude greater than 3 cm but less than or equal to 10 cm; a grade of 4 = an amplitude greater than 10 cm. Patients displaying little tremor while at rest may display pronounced tremor when holding their upper extremity in a particular position—just ask the patient. Intraoperative assessment in such instances involves testing DBS effects on the postural tremor resulting from the patient's assuming that position. Rating proceeds according to the same grading scale as that listed for resting tremor.

The examiner assesses rigidity by noting the amount of resistance he encounters when rotating various joints on the patient's body. He typically holds the patient's hand as he rotates the patient's wrist to observe the manner in which the patient's elbow pronates and supinates (Figure 10.2). The examiner must

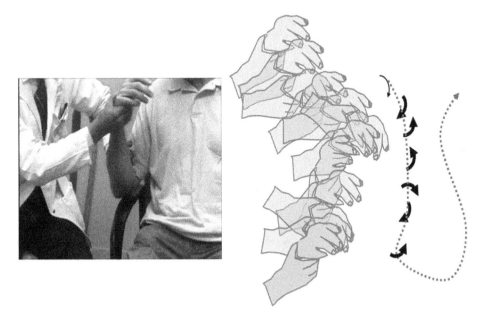

Figure 10.2: Representation of the assessment of rigidity. The key issue is to prevent the patient's unconscious assistance with the joint rotation, which would result in an underestimation of the degree of rigidity. The patient's upper extremity is moved by rotations about several joints simultaneously and asynchronously. For example, the elbow can be flexed and extended at the same time that the forearm is pronated and supinated.

take care that the rotations do not follow the same pattern. Rather, he must make these rotations as varied and random as possible. Should the patient anticipate the rotations, he may unknowingly begin to assist the examiner's manipulations, resulting a misleading reduction in resistance. The reader may discover this for herself by rotating the limb of a person with normal tone in the manner described above. The degree of resistance encountered in this instance rates a 0 according to the Movement Disorders Society–Unified Parkinson's Disease Rating Scales Part III. The reader may then rotate her own arm, using her other arm to do so. She will notice that her own arm resists far less than another person's, because, unbeknownst to her, the rotated arm yields to the arm rotating it. The examiner might thus be tempted to rate her own resistance –1. To avoid this, normal rigidity scores a 1 in order to reserve 0 for lower tone. This is important because intraoperative DBS may reduce resistance to a level less than what is normally encountered even in normal subjects.

A 0 rating goes to any patient mustering resistance similar to what the examiner felt when rotating her own limb. A score of 1 indicates that the patient offers normal resistance. A score of 2 indicates that the patient offers increased resistance but remains capable of a full range of motion. A score of 3 indicates that the patient offers greater resistance and remains capable of a full range of motion, albeit at considerably greater effort. A score of 4 = the patient is incapable of a full range of motion.

Clinical Evaluation of Essential Tremor and Cerebellar Outflow Tremor

The examiner assesses tremor under specific conditions. These conditions include the patient's remaining at rest, maintaining a particular posture, touching a finger to his chin, and lifting a cup to his lips (Figure 10.3). This last action is known as the "cup task." Magnitudes of tremor under each condition correspond to the following rating scale: a grade of 0 = absence of tremor; a grade of 1 = tremor amplitude of 1 cm or less; a grade of 2 = tremor amplitude of more than 1 cm but less than 4 cm; a grade of 3 = tremor amplitude of more than 4 cm that does not prevent the patient from completing the task; a grade of 4 = tremor of such pronounced amplitude that it prevents the patient from performing the task. The examiner may hold a measuring device or her index finger 4 cm apart from her thumb as a way of measuring tremor amplitude (Figure 10.4).

The examiner assesses resting tremor by having the patient rest quietly and supporting his extremities against gravity. The examiner assesses postural tremor by having the patient hold his upper

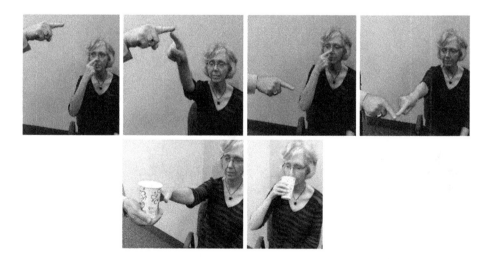

Figure 10.3: Examples of examining tremor on the finger-to-nose test in the upper row of images. It is important that the examiner vary the position of the target, in this case the examiner's fingertip. In addition it is important to position the target so that the patient's upper extremity is fully extended. The lower row of images demonstrates the cup task. Again, the cup is positioned so that the subject must fully extend with upper extremity in order to reach the cup.

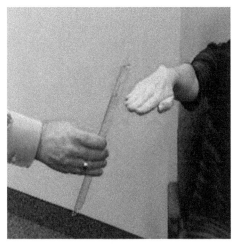 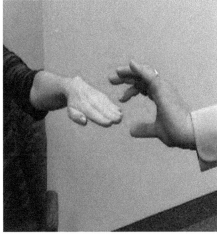

Figure 10.4: The examiner can quantify the patient's tremor, in this case postural tremor, by holding a measuring ruler next to the extended limb. Alternatively, the examiner can position his fingers to estimate a 4 cm gap between the forefinger and the thumb to estimate the amplitude of the tremor.

extremity outstretched. The examiner assesses action tremor by having the patient hold outstretched his upper extremity and touching the index finger on the hand of that outstretched extremity to his nose. The patient performs this task several times. In the cup task, the patient reaches for a cup held out to him by the examiner. The patient takes the cup from the examiner and brings it to his lips as if to drink from it.

The measures of tremor appear to vary in terms of their degree of sensitivity to DBS. Rest tremor appears the most responsive, and cup task–associated tremor the least. Though it is important to test rest tremor in order to discern some effect of DBS, the examiner must bear in mind that reduction of cup task–associated tremor indicates probably the most significant functional improvement. Cerebellar outflow tremors, such as those owing to multiple sclerosis, present a challenge. DBS in this situation would be considered a standard and accepted "off-label" use of an FDA-approved device. It appears that tremor in distal-most musculature responds better to DBS than does tremor in proximal musculature.

As it is for Parkinson's disease–associated tremor, it is necessary to distinguish between tremor suppression attributable to the therapeutic mechanisms of action of DBS and suppression attributable to stimulation current's having spread to the corticospinal tract. The key is to increase the stimulation intensity

to determine whether tonic contraction is produced, thus indicating suppression of tremor secondary to spread of stimulation current into the posterior limb of the internal capsule.

Clinical Evaluation of Dystonia

A host of challenges greets the examiner when he attempts to evaluate clinical response to intraoperative DBS. Many dystonic symptoms may fail to respond within the time frame of a DBS programming session, because their improvement often requires months of stimulation. Tremor and some other phasic symptoms of dystonia, however, may demonstrate an acute response to intraoperative DBS. In such cases, an examiner may evaluate the tremor according to the ratings described for Essential tremor and cerebellar outflow tremor. In other instances, a phasic dystonic symptom may appear as hyperkinesia, as it does in chorea. An examiner may evaluate these symptoms according to the ratings for hyperkinetic syndromes listed below.

An examiner may assess persistent posturing, a static feature of dystonia, by estimating—as a percentage of the normal range of motion in the direction of the departure from a neutral position at rest due to dystonia (Figure 10.5). As the normal upper extremity remains at rest, the wrist is extended to

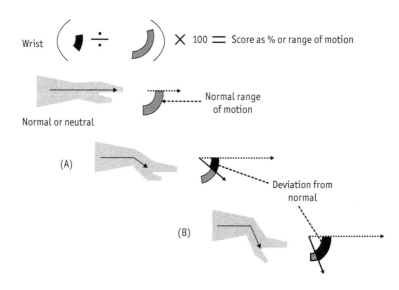

Figure 10.5: Schematic representation of estimating the degree of departure from neutral position of the wrist in dystonia. First, the neutral position must be determined, which in this case is when the wrist is at approximately 10% of extension. The patient's position at rest (i.e., when the patient is not attempting to straighten the wrist) is determined. The angle of departure is divided by the normal range of motion in the direction the wrist is turned. In example (A), the deviation is slightly less than 50%, resulting in a grade of 2. In example (B), the deviation is more than 75%, resulting in a grade of 4.

approximately 10 degrees and has a normal range of motion of 70 degrees in extension and 75 degrees in flexion. The metacarpal-phalangeal joints are flexed to an angle of approximately 30% and have a normal range of motion of 45 and 90 degrees, in extension and flexion, respectively. The proximal interphalangeal joints are flexed to an angle of approximately 30% and have a normal range of motion of 70 and 175 degrees, in extension and flexion, respectively. The wrist is pronated to an angle between 30% and 60% and has a normal range of motion of 70 degrees. The elbow is flexed approximately 30% from full extension and has a normal range of motion of 70 and 80 degrees in pronation and supination, respectively.

Neutral position (while supine) in the lower extremity is typically at 180% at the hip and has a normal range of motion of 100 degrees (Figure 10.6). The neutral position (while supine) of the knee is 180 degrees, and it has a normal range of motion of 150 degrees. The ankle is laterally rotated to approximately 30 degrees from the vertical and has a normal range of motion of 30 and 45 degrees in extension and flexion, respectively.

According to this author's definition, the neutral position of the head is directed and extended such that the eyes are centered in the orbit in order to direct

the gaze straight ahead. The normal range of motion for lateral rotation is 80 degrees in each direction. For neck flexion and extension, the range of motion is 50 and 60 degrees, respectively. For the neck, lateral flexion is 50 degrees in each direction. Schematic examples are shown in Figure 10.7.

Translating the degrees of departure from neutral position is as follows: 0 = no departure; 1 = < 25%; 2 = between 25% and 50%; 3 = > 50% but ≤ 75%; and 4 = >75%. The examiner can observe her own neutral position and range of motion with which to compare to the patient by imitating the patient's position, and subsequently, can estimate the grade of departure from normal (assuming that the examiner is normal).

Stimulation of the corticospinal tract may affect the assessment of dystonia. The examiner must distinguish the former from the latter if the latter appears to have worsened. Stimulation of the corticospinal tract is evident when frank tonic contraction of muscles originally unaffected by the dystonia results from increasing the stimulation voltage or current. In the event that the tonic posturing is caused by stimulation of the posterior limb of the internal capsule, reexamination with stimulation switched off ought to improve it.

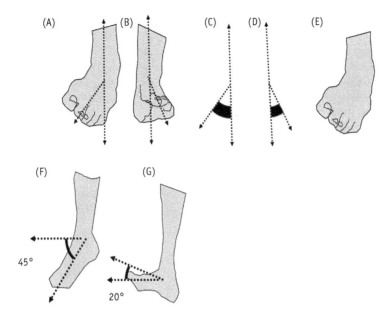

Figure 10.6: Schematic representation of range of motion of the ankle. With respect to eversion and inversion of the ankle, the patient's relaxed position was as illustrated in (A) whereas the normal relaxed position is shown in (B). The range of motions are shown in (C). E, The deviation of the patient's ankle is estimated as a percentage of the noromal range (E); the deviation from neutral clearly is greater than 75%, resulting in a grade of 4. The normal ranges for dorsiflexion and plantar flexion are shown in (F) and (G).

Clinical Evaluation of Hyperkinetic Disorders

Characteristics of hyperkinetic disorders are the following four features: (1) the portion of the body affected; (2) the speed of the involuntary movement; (3) the coarseness of the movement; and (4) the degree of stereotypy. For example, athethosis, which tends to affect more distal musculature, is more

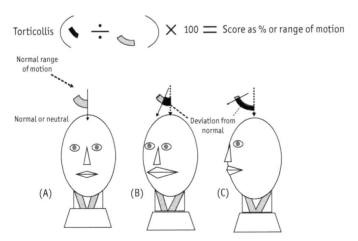

Figure 10.7: Schematic representation of estimating the degree of departure from the neutral position in torticollis in cervical dystonia. First, the neutral position must be determined, which in this case is when the head is straight ahead (A). The patient's position at rest (the patient is not attempting to straighten the head) is determined. The angle of departure is divided by the normal range of motion in the direction the head is turned. In example (B), the deviation is slightly more than 50%, resulting in a grade of 3. In example (C), the deviation is more than 75%, resulting in a grade of 4.

graceful; whereas chorea, which tends to affect proximal musculature, is jerkier.

This author considers changes in the amplitude and frequency of involuntary movements to be most important. Again, the range of motion through joints allows one to estimate the degree of movements. Most examiners, however, rely on a qualitative scale ranging from 0 (no involuntary movements) to 4 (the worse possible or maximal involuntary movements). Though this qualitative assessment is reasonable, its scale lacks anchoring as well as fixed intervals, the critical issue being the degree of change under two conditions: stimulation and no stimulation. Examiners using the qualitative scale must take care that they maintain their subjective reference points (anchors) and intervals. As discussed above, the effects of inadvertent stimulation of the corticospinal tract need to be assessed.

This author uses the following scale: 0 = no dyskinesia; 1 = slight dyskinesia that does not interfere with the patient's attempting a volitional task that utilizes the joint rotations involved by the dyskinesia; 2 = the dyskinesia does interfere but can be overcome without great difficulty; 3 = the dyskinesia does interfere but can be overcome with great difficulty; 4 = the dyskinesia does interfere and cannot be overcome.

Clinical Evaluation of Tic Disorders

DBS for tic disorders, such as Tourette's syndrome, is considered a standard and accepted "off-label" use of an FDA-approved device. These disorders are assessed according to the tics' frequency and location. A patient may have multiple tics. There are multiple rating scales for tic disorders, Tourette's syndrome, for example. Most are retrospective and developed primarily to access the degree to which the symptoms interfere with the quality of life. Generally, they are not suited to the clinic. This author suggests rating based on the frequency of the tics such that 0 = no tics; 1 = < 3 tics per minute; 2 = 3–6 tics per minute; 3 = 7–10 tics per minute; and 4 = > 10 tics per minute.

CLINICAL ASSESSMENT OF CORTICOSPINAL AND CORTICOBULBAR STIMULATION

The corticospinal and corticobulbar tracts, within the posterior limb of the internal capsule, may be stimulated as a consequence of DBS of the GPi, the thalamus, and the subthalamic nucleus. The effects of stimulation of the corticospinal and corticobulbar tracts will therefore be discussed independently.

The corticobulbar fibers innervate the lower motor neurons in the brainstem that subsequently innervate muscles of the face, the tongue and pharynx, and the extraocular muscles of the eyes. Typically, stimulation of the corticobulbar fibers effects a conjugate, rather than a disconjugate, gaze owing to involvement of the fronto-pontine fibers that originate in the frontal eye fields and descend to the centers in the pons for conjugate horizontal eye movements (Figure 10.8).

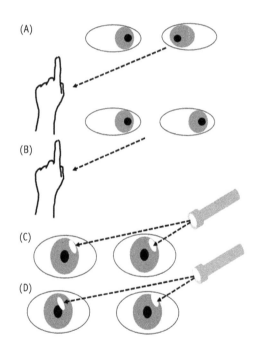

Figure 10.8: Schematic representation of possible effects of stimulation on eye movements. Figure (A) demonstrates disconjugate gaze. The patient is instructed to look at the examiner's finger. As can be seen, one eye is able to do so, but the other eye is being pulled by the medial rectus muscle due to spread of stimulation to the fascicles of the oculomotor nerve. In 9B), again the patient is instructed to look to the examiner's finger, but now both eyes are deviated away, owing to stimulation of the fronto-pontine fibers that descend in the corticobulbar tract. Figures (C) and (D) demonstrate testing for disconjugate gaze by examining the reflection of a focused beam of light, such as from a flashlight. In figure (C), the reflection falls on the same point (homologous) on the iris, consistent with normal gaze. In figure (D), the reflection falls on non-homologous points, suggesting disconjugate gaze.

Though the nature and severity of the symptoms produced is related to the intensity of stimulation, the mechanisms' nonlinearity complicates the relationship. One of the earliest symptoms described by patients is a "funny feeling," which is localized somewhere on the body. Though many patients report the sensation as one of being "pulled," others are unable to describe it in such terms. Care must therefore be taken to assure that the "funny feelings" are not caused by the medial lemniscus's involvement in the stimulation as in the case of the STN DBS, or the posterior or tactile ventral caudal thalamus in the case of DBS in the vicinity of the ventral intermediate nucleus.

Increasing stimulus intensity allows one to distinguish a "funny feeling" owing to corticobulbar or corticospinal tract involvement from a funny feeling owing to involvement of the medial lemniscus or posterior tactile ventral caudal thalamus. At some point, contraction of the muscle may become evident; thus, it is important to increase the intensity within reasonable limits to assure that the "funny feeling" has neither a corticobulbar nor corticospinal origin.

An early sign of underlying muscle contraction, "dimpling" of the skin surface, aids in distinguishing muscle-pulling from corticobulbar or corticospinal tract activation from dystonia, because, at relatively lower intensities, not all the muscles contract in response to stimulation of the internal capsule's posterior limb. By shining a beam of light across the patient's skin surface and looking for shadows, one may observe such dimpling (Figure 10.9).

Reduced tremor and worsening dexterity also indicate corticobulbar or corticospinal tract involvement prior to demonstrating frank tonic contractions. The latter is most apparent in finger movements and speech. As discussed above, the loss of manual dexterity manifests as a reduction in the individuated finger movements (Figure 10.1). Speech may be slurred. Patients are often best able to judge the quality of their speech, and thus they ought to be asked whether it sounds normal to them (speech and language are discussed in greater detail below).

Assessing patients with facial dystonia for facial contractions owing to stimulation of the corticobulbar tract within the posterior limb of the internal capsule may prove difficult. (Patients with Meige's syndrome are notable examples.) Stimulation of the corticobulbar fibers sufficient ffect muscle contraction typically do so on one side of the patient's face. Facial dystonias, on the other hand, often affect muscles bilaterally.

CLINICAL ASSESSMENT OF SPEECH, LANGUAGE, AND SWALLOWING

There are numerous ways speech may be affected by DBS; consequently, each must be assessed through careful examination. Affects include: aphonia, inability to produce any sound; word-finding difficulty; changes in prosody, the melodic changes in intonation; and dysarthria, slurring of words. It is important to have the patient speak phrases that are not routinely

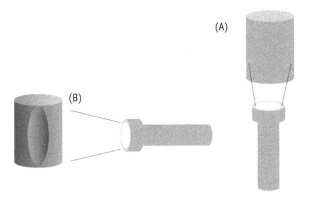

Figure 10.9: A subtle sign of may be contraction of small groups of muscle fibers, causing a dimpling of the skin that may be difficult to see, particularly if a diffuse light is shown on the muscle (A). The dimpling may be seen if a focused beam of light is shown tangentially on the surface of the muscle (B).

used (such as the patient's name) and to use phrases that stress a range of speech articulators. This author has patients say "Today is a lovely day," "British constitution," and "Methodist episcopal." Patients often are better judges of effects on speech, so asking the patient's impressions of his speech is helpful.

Stimulation of the posterior limb of the internal capsule may affect speech and language. Speech abnormalities may be due to the stimulation current's propagation to the corticobulbar fibers within the posterior limb of the internal capsule, or they may be caused by other mechanisms intrinsic to the targeted structure. Continuing to increase the stimulus intensities to a reasonable extent may demonstrate observable muscle contractions of the face and head and thus suggest that the speech involvement is due to electrical current spread to the corticobulbar fibers in the posterior limb of the internal capsule.

In the case where speech and language involvement is not associated with frank facial muscle contractions at reasonable stimulation intensities, speech and language involvement may relate to stimulation of the head homuncular representation within the Vim or GPi (although speech and language functions typically are less affected by DBS in the vicinity of the GPi). It may be possible to move the volume of tissue activation by DBS away from the head homuncular regions. The subthalamic nucleus's relatively small size renders it difficult to reposition the volume of tissue activation to alleviate effects on speech and language. There are cases in which it is difficult to attribute speech and language involvement to a specific volume of tissue activation position. In such cases, volume of tissue activation repositioning fails to avoid effects on speech and language. Bilateral DBS occurrence may significantly increase the risk of speech and language impairment; therefore, effects on speech and language need to be assessed with stimulation through each DBS lead, and then both in situations where the patient has bilateral DBS.

DBS that affects speech and language has a high probability of affecting swallowing. However, patients may have difficulty swallowing even in the absence of speech or language problems. Impaired swallowing not associated with speech or language impairment may be difficult to assess during the DBS

programming session, but it should be reviewed during the review of systems. When there is sufficient concern, a modified barium swallow with the DBS on and off may be indicated. Unfortunately, a fiberoptic endoscopic evaluation of swallowing (FEES) lacks sufficient sensitivity.

HINTS FOR CLINICAL EVALUATIONS

The purpose of DBS is to improve the disability of neurological and psychiatric disorders—in this case, particularly movement disorders—through postoperative programming of the implanted pulse generator (IPG). Postoperative programming can be complex; consequently, the physicians and healthcare professionals need to be confident that the DBS lead was placed in an optimal location. Lack of confidence can lead to premature abandonment of the therapy or to drawing a premature conclusion that DBS lead revision surgery is needed. Providing that confidence is the responsibility of the surgeon and the intraoperative neurophysiologist.

One must increase stimulation until effects clear. As discussed above, multiple mechanisms can produce a specific adverse effect detectable by clinical assessment during postoperative programming. Effective DBS of the target may relieve tremor but may also cause inadvertent propagation to the corticospinal tract. All cases require that one confidently understand the mechanisms. The examiner must consequently increase, within safe limits, stimulation current (voltage) until he clearly determines the nature of the adverse effect. He must also repeat the test stimulation until he becomes confident of the results.

ACKNOWLEDGMENT

This chapter was modified from Chapter 12, Clinical Assessments During Intraoperative Neurophysiological Monitoring, in E. B. Montgomery, Jr., *Intraoperative Neurophysiological Monitoring for Deep Brain Stimulation: Principles, Practice and Cases*, Oxford University Press, 2015.

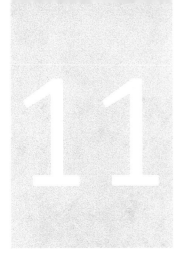

APPROACH TO DBS IN THE VICINITY OF
THE SUBTHALAMIC NUCLEUS

DBS REGIONAL ANATOMY OF
THE SUBTHALAMIC NUCLEUS (STN)

The subthalamic nucleus (STN) lies near the junction of the diencephalon and mesencephalon. It is just ventral to the thalamus, just lateral to the brachium conjunctivum and red nucleus, and posterior, medial and dorsal to the internal capsule. These structures are important because inappropriate stimulation of them causes adverse effects. For example, just dorsal and posterior to the STN lie the Vim and ventrocaudal (Vc) nuclei of the thalamus. The thalamic nuclei relay somatosensory information from the periphery through the medial lemniscus and spinothalamic tracts, which ascend just posterior to the STN, and thence to the cerebral cortex. Electrical fields spreading to ascending sensory medial lemniscus and spinothalamic pathways behind the STN produce paresthesias. The brachium conjunctivum contains fibers running from the deep cerebellar nuclei to the Vim of the thalamus. Inadvertent stimulation of the brachium conjunctivum can cause ataxia and loss of balance. The red nucleus lies in the brachium conjunctivum, and the exiting axons from the oculomotor nucleus run within the red nucleus. Electrical fields spreading to these structures can result in disconjugate gaze and diplopia. Stimulating the internal capsule laterally, anteriorly or ventrally can cause tonic muscle contractions.

It is unclear where stimulation in the vicinity of the STN is optimal for clinical benefit. The presumption

has been that the beneficial effects are related to stimulation of structures intrinsic to the STN. However, this probably is not the case. An excellent study by Eisenstein and colleagues plotted the spatial distribution of sites that produced clinical benefit, and is shown in Figure 11.1 (Eisenstein et al. 2014). The region is very large and extends beyond the anatomical boundaries of the STN. This has several important implications. For DBS leads that are too ventral, stimulation through the dorsal contacts still may provide clinical benefit, provided the contacts are spaced sufficiently appart or example, 1.5 mm. Use of DBS leads with widely spaced contacts is more likely to cover the regions associated with clinical benefit than are leads with more closely spaced contacts. The ability to cover a wider anatomical region as well as the ability to generate more intense volumes of electrical fields are strong arguments against using DBS leads with more closely spaced contacts.

ADVERSE EFFECTS CREATED BY THE
POSITION OF THE DBS LEAD RELATIVE
TO THE STN

DBS Lead Too Medial

The adverse effects of DBS are related directly to stimulation of structures near the STN. If the DBS lead is too medial, the electrical current will spread to the

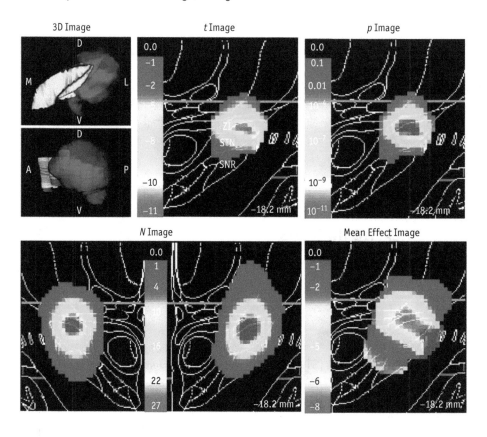

Figure 11.1: Results of a study of the effects sites of stimulation in the vicinity of the subthalamic nucleus (STN). The analyses are complex and the reader is referred to the original article (Eisenstein et al. 2014). For the purposes here, attention is drawn to the images labled "*t* Images" and "*p* Images". The *t* Image indicate the contribution of location corresponding to each voxel to the improvement in the Unified Parkinson Disease Rating Scale III (UPDRS III) motor scores while the *p* Image indicates the p value of each voxel with respect to the voxel in the *t* Image. Note, the results to do not indicate the degree that the patients improved with DBS in the vicinity of the STN as all improved to a similar degree. What the *t* Image suggests, is that DBS in a great many locations including those outside the anatomical confines of the STN contribute to the improvement following DBS. *Abbreviations*: A = anterior; D = dorsal; L = lateral; M = medial; P = posterior; SNR = substantia nigra; V = ventral; ZI = zona incerta.

From Eisenstein et al. 2014, page 286.

brachium conjunctivum, which is the cerebellar outflow to the Vim and motor cortex. The symptoms will include ataxia. Also, the nerve roots of the oculomotor nucleus run from the midline laterally past the red nucleus before turning medially to exit in the interpeduncular fossa. Stimulation of the oculomotor nerve roots can result in diplopia.

The effects of the DBS lead's being too medial can often be corrected by using the more dorsal contacts in either a monopolar or a bipolar configuration, because the DBS lead is often runs lateral and dorsally to medial and ventral in the coronal plane (Figure 11.2). Using more dorsal contacts pulls the current laterally as it moves dorsally. Alternatively, initially wide

bipolar, or if necessary, narrower bipolar, configurations can be used to shrink the electrical field to pull it away from the brachium conjunctivum, the oculomotor nerve roots, or both. However, the value of such approaches may be limited, as the most effective stimulation site may be more ventral.

If these measures fail and the efficacy is insufficient, another approach would be to use multiple cathodes in an interleaved fashion such that a lower stimulation current/voltage is applied to the more ventral contact (Figure 11.3) (note this does not necessarily mean the "most ventral" contact—see figure 6.8) and a greater stimulation current/voltage is applied to more dorsal contacts (note this does

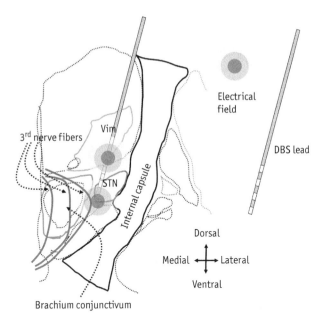

Figure 11.2: DBS lead too medial. Coronal view of the STN 4 mm anterior to the midpoint of the line connecting the anterior and posterior commissure (AC–PC line). The STN is outlined in red, Vim is outlined in blue, the brachium conjunctivum (also containing the red nucleus) in orange, and the internal capsule is outlined in solid black. The Vc (not shown) thalamic nuclei are dorsal and posterior to the STN. The brachium conjunctivum is just medial and slightly posterior to the STN, and the internal capsule is lateral and ventral. Also shown are the nerve fibers exiting the oculomotor nucleus to form the third cranial nerve. The DBS lead in this case is too medial, causing activation of the third nerve and producing diplopia when the most ventral contact is used as the negative contact. In addition, spread of electrical activation could affect the cerebellar outflow fibers, causing ataxia. One response would be to move the electrical field more dorsal away from the third nerve fibers and the brachium conjunctivum. However, cathodal stimulation of the most dorsal contact could activate the thalamus, leading to paresthesias.

Modified from Schaltenbrand and Wahren 1977.

---

not necessarily mean the "most dorsal" contact—see Figure 9.1 in *Chapter 9—Approaches to Programming*).

For patients implanted with DBS leads with segmented contacts, current can be applied to the contact that is directed laterally (Figure 11.4). Note that these suggestions are based on a DBS segmented lead in which the contacts are arranged as sectors around the circumference of the lead in the plane orthogonal to the long axis of the lead. These suggestions may not be appropriate for other segmented DBS lead architectures, but the general principle still may apply. It is important to note that changing from a continuous circumferential contact stimulation to a subset of contacts in a segmented lead can change the surface area of the electrical contacts over which the stimulation is applied. This could change the current densities and thus, affect safety (*see Chapter 5—DBS Safety*). These caveats apply to any and all discussions of segmented DBS leads in this textbook.

DBS Lead Too Anterior

The internal capsule borders the STN on the lateral, ventral, and anterior sides. Stimulation spreading to the internal side can produce contralateral tonic muscle contractions. The results of the monopolar survey can help determine whether the DBS lead is too deep, too lateral, or too anterior. For a DBS lead that is too anterior, the threshold of tonic contraction through the most-dorsal cathode is similar to the threshold through the most-ventral cathode because the DBS lead often is parallel to the internal capsule anteriorly (Figure 11.5). The most effective way to prevent muscle contractions when the DBS lead is too anterior is to use bipolar configurations, beginning with wide bipolar and progressing to narrow bipolar as necessary. For patients implanted with DBS leads with segmented contacts, current can be applied to the contact that is directed posteriorly (Figure 11.6).

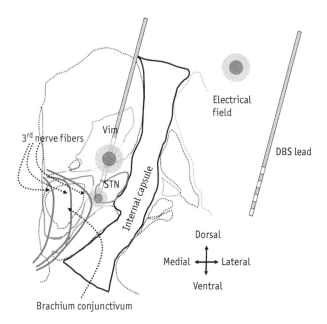

Figure 11.3: DBS lead too medial. Coronal view of the STN 4 mm anterior to the midpoint of the AC–PC line. The STN is outlined in red, Vim is outlined in blue, the brachium conjunctivum (also containing the red nucleus) in orange, and the internal capsule is outlined in solid black. The Vc (not shown) thalamic nuclei are dorsal and posterior to the STN. The brachium conjunctivum is just medial and slightly posterior to the STN, and the internal capsule is lateral and ventral. Also shown are the nerve fibers exiting the oculomotor nucleus to form the third cranial nerve. The DBS lead in this case is too medial causing activation of the third nerve, producing diplopia when the most ventral contact is used as the negative contact. In addition, spread of electrical activation could affect the cerebellar outflow fibers, causing ataxia. In situations where stimulation through the most ventral contact is important for clinical benefit but has a low threshold to adverse effects, interleaved stimulation can be applied. A stimulation intensity just below the threshold for adverse effects can be applied to the most ventral contact, note that the size of the electrical field is smaller, and a higher intensity applied to the ventral contact. Modified from Schaltenbrand and Wahren 1977.

DBS Lead Too Ventral

To prevent muscle contractions when the DBS lead is too ventral, stimulation should be delivered through the more dorsally located contacts (Figure 11.7). Most often, you would start with monopolar stimulation and progress to wide bipolar and then to narrow bipolar stimulation, as necessary. This circumstance may be appropriate for partitioning the stimulation current/voltage among the electrode contacts. For example, stimulation through the most ventral contact may be most the effective in producing a clinical response but produce adverse effects. Stimulation through the more-dorsally placed contacts may not produce sufficient benefit but also not produce as many adverse effects. One could stimulate both through the most-ventral contact at a reduced stimulation current/voltage and then through a most dorsal contact at a higher

stimulation current/voltage. Sometimes, if the DBS lead is too ventral and every electrode configuration continues to result in tonic muscle contraction, the entire DBS lead can be moved dorsally with surgery performed under local anesthetic and fluoroscopic control. Surgery should be done with the stimulator on to monitor adverse effects and efficacy. If these measures fail and the efficacy is insufficient, another approach would be to use multiple cathodes in an interleaved fashion such that a lower stimulation current/voltage is applied to the more-ventrally located contacts (Figure 11.8).

DBS Lead Too Lateral

Tonic contraction also can occur if the DBS lead is too *lateral* (Figure 11.9). To prevent these muscle contractions, stimulation should be administered through the

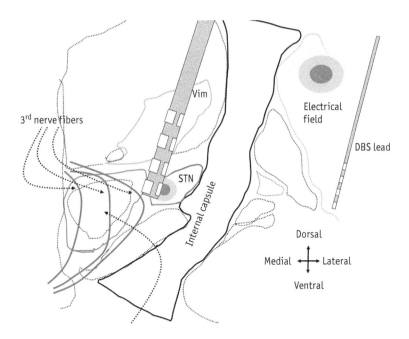

Figure 11.4: DBS lead too medial. Coronal view of the STN 4 mm anterior to the midpoint of the AC–PC line. The STN is outlined in red, the Vim is outlined in blue, the brachium conjunctivum (also containing the red nucleus) in orange, and the internal capsule is outlined in solid black. The Vc (not shown) thalamic nuclei are dorsal and posterior to the STN. The brachium conjunctivum is just medial and slightly posterior to the STN, and the internal capsule is lateral and ventral. Also shown are the nerve fibers exiting the oculomotor nucleus to form the third cranial nerve. The DBS lead in this case is too medial causing activation of the third nerve, producing diplopia when the most ventral contact is used as the negative contact. In addition, spread of electrical activation could affect the cerebellar outflow fibers causing ataxia. For patients implanted with DBS leads with segmented contacts, current can be applied to the single contact that is directed laterally relative to the DBS lead.

Modified from Schaltenbrand and Wahren 1977.

more-dorsally located contacts. You would typically start with monopolar stimulation and then progress to wide bipolar and to narrow bipolar stimulation, as necessary. However, such approaches may be of limited benefit, as the most effective stimulation site may be more ventral. If these measures fail and the efficacy is insufficient, another approach would be to use multiple cathodes in an interleaved fashion such that a lower stimulation current/voltage is applied to the more-ventrally located contacts. For patients implanted with DBS leads with segmented contacts, current can be applied to the contact that is directed medially.

DBS Lead Too Posterior

The ascending fibers of the medial lemniscus and spinothalamic pathways run posterior to the STN. If the DBS lead is too posterior, stimulating the medial lemniscus and spinothalamic pathways, it can produce paresthesias (Figure 11.10). *Transient* paresthesias are not a problem; however, *persistent* paresthesias are. The most effective way to prevent paresthesias when the DBS lead is too posterior is to use bipolar configurations, beginning with wide bipolar stimulation and progressing to narrow bipolar stimulation as necessary. Alternatively, you can stimulate through the more dorsally placed contacts because the lead is typically anterior dorsally to posterior ventrally in the sagittal plane. Moving the electrical field dorsally also moves the field anteriorly. However, the value of such approaches may be limited, as the most effective stimulation site may be more ventral. If these measures fail and the efficacy is insufficient, another approach would be to use multiple cathodes in an interleaved fashion such that a lower stimulation current/voltage

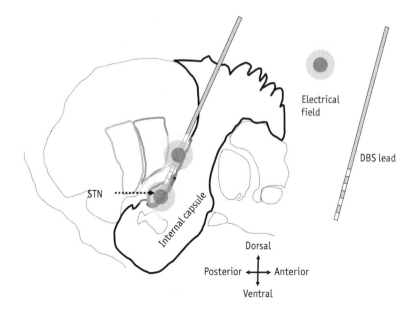

Figure 11.5: DBS lead too anterior. A sagittal section 17 mm lateral to the AC–PC line of the subthalamic nucleus (STN, outlined in red) with a DBS lead that is too anterior. Electrical stimulation spreads to the internal capsule (outlined in black), causing muscle contractions. Note that the distance between the most ventral contact and the internal capsule and the distance between the most dorsal contact and the internal capsule are nearly the same. This similarity means that the threshold for muscle contraction will be approximately the same for monopolar stimulation through the dorsal and ventral contacts, and suggests that a DBS lead is too anterior. The most effective way to prevent muscle contractions when the DBS lead is too anterior is to use bipolar configurations, beginning with wide bipolar and progressing to narrow bipolar stimulation, as necessary.

Modified from Schaltenbrand and Wahren 1977.

is applied to the more ventrally placed contact and a greater stimulation current/voltage is applied to more dorsally placed contacts. For patients implanted with DBS leads with segmented contacts, current can be applied to the contact that is directed anteriorly (Figure 11.11).

Patients can experience psychological adverse effects from DBS in the vicinity of the STN, including depression, mania, and impulse-control problems. Although the exact mechanisms for these adverse effects are unclear, they most often occur with stimulation through the more ventrally placed contacts. Moving the electrical field dorsally often resolves these problems.

APPROACH TO DBS IN THE VICINITY OF THE STN FOR PARKINSON'S DISEASE

DBS programming has to be understood in the larger context of the entire treatment program, particularly in Parkinson's disease. Programmers have to be expert, not only in DBS, but also in managing medications and other treatments. Consequently, postoperative DBS management should not be undertaken by those without expertise in the total management of Parkinson's disease.

The primary purpose of STN DBS is to improve symptomatic control. One measure of success is the degree to which medications can be reduced. Continued dependence on medications may indicate that DBS is not optimal. The goal of treatment is not necessarily to reduce or eliminate the concurrent use of medications (except when medications are causing significant adverse effects), but some programmers tend to abandon further DBS programming too quickly and resort to using medications more aggressively. However, this strategy is a poor choice because, by definition, patients would not have had DBS surgery had medications been effective.

DBS programming is complex for multiple reasons, not least of which are the synergistic effects

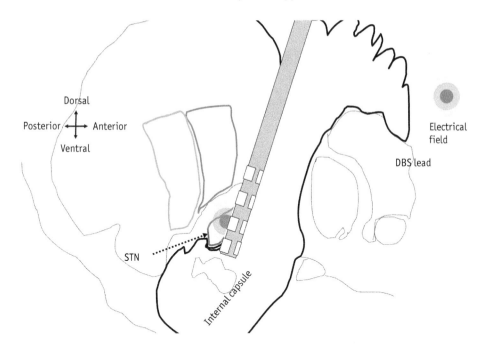

Figure 11.6: DBS lead too anterior. A sagittal section 17 mm lateral to the AC–PC line of the STN (outlined in red) with a DBS lead that is too anterior. Electrical stimulation spreads to the internal capsule (outlined in black), causing muscle contractions. Note that the distance between the most ventral contact and the internal capsule and the distance between the most dorsal contact and the internal capsule are nearly the same. This similarity means that the threshold for muscle contraction will be approximately the same for monopolar stimulation through the dorsal and ventral contacts and suggests that a DBS lead is too anterior. For patients implanted with DBS leads with segmented contacts, current can be applied to the contact that is directed posteriorly, note the segmented contacts with the electrical field posterior to the lead.
Modified from Schaltenbrand nd Wahren 1977.

between DBS and anti-Parkinson medications. Some programmers arbitrarily reduce the medications when DBS is started, which may result in precipitous worsening of the patient's symptoms and putting the patient at risk for complications. Instead, consider an iterative approach of first improving the patient's symptoms with DBS programming, followed by reducing the medications, followed by further DBS programming, and so on, until optimal symptom control is achieved. This approach takes time, patience, and commitment on the part of patients, caregivers, and programmers alike. Particularly important is the commitment to see the patient frequently enough to provide a thorough exploration of the programming options within a reasonable time frame. One of the most common mistakes is to quit too early.

The choice of which of the often-numerous anti-Parkinson medications to reduce first depends on which medication-related adverse effect is worse. For example, if dyskinesias are the most troublesome, then the medications most likely to cause dyskinesias are reduced first. In order of greatest to least risk of dyskinesia, these medications are (1) catecholamine-o-methyl transferase (COMT) inhibitors, such as entacapone or tolcapone; (2) immediate-release carbidopa-levodopa; (3) controlled-release carbidopa-levodopa; (4) duodenal L-dopa/carbidopa infusion; (5) the dopamine agonists, such as pramipexole, transdermal rotigotine, and ropinirole; and (6) anticholinergics, such as benztropine and trihexyphenidyl. If cognitive or psychiatric problems are the most troublesome, then medications with the greatest risk of these complications should be reduced first. They are, in decreasing order: (1) anticholinergics; (2) pramipexole; (3) ropinirole; (4) controlled-release carbidopa-levodopa; (5) duodenal L-dopa/carbidopa infusion; (6) COMT inhibitors; and (7) immediate-release carbidopa-levodopa.

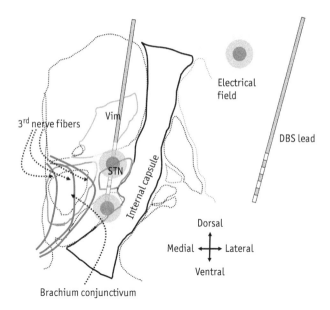

Figure 11.7: DBS lead too ventral. Coronal view of the STN 4 mm anterior to the midpoint of the AC–PC line. The STN is outlined in red, Vim is outlined in blue, the brachium conjunctivum (also containing the red nucleus) in orange, and the internal capsule in solid black. The Vc (not shown) thalamic nucleus is dorsal and posterior to the STN. The brachium conjunctivum is just medial and slightly posterior to the STN, and the internal capsule is lateral and ventral. Also shown are the nerve fibers exiting the oculomotor nucleus to form the third cranial nerve. The DBS lead in this case is too ventral, causing activation of the internal capsule and tonic muscle contraction when the most ventral contact is used as the negative contact. One response would be to move the electrical field dorsally, away from the internal capsule.

Modified from Schaltenbrand and Wahren 1977.

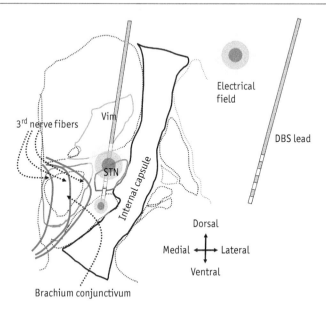

Figure 11.8: DBS lead too ventral. Coronal view of the STN 4 mm anterior to the midpoint of the AC–PC line. The STN is outlined in red, Vim is outlined in blue, the brachium conjunctivum (also containing the red nucleus) in orange, and the internal capsule in solid black. The Vc (not shown) thalamic nucleus is dorsal and posterior to the STN. The brachium conjunctivum is just medial and slightly posterior to the STN, and the internal capsule is lateral and ventral. Also shown are the nerve fibers exiting the oculomotor nucleus to form the third cranial nerve. The DBS lead in this case is too ventral, causing activation of the internal capsule and tonic muscle contraction when the most-ventral contact is used as the negative contact. Multiple cathodes in an interleaved fashion can be used such that a lower stimulation current/voltage is applied to the more-ventral contact. Note the smaller electrical field around the most ventral contact.

Modified from Schaltenbrand and Wahren 1977.

Because the primary purpose of DBS in the vicinity of the STN is to improve symptoms, the symptoms should be readily apparent during the programming session. Thus, patients should be asked to forego their anti-Parkinson medications overnight, to allow their symptoms to surface during the programming session. However, medications need to be withheld cautiously. Patients may be highly symptomatic and at risk for complications, such as falls and a rare neuroleptic-malignant-like syndrome. Ask patients how they function first thing in the morning. If their functioning is poor enough that they would be at risk, have them continue to take their medications. An alternative is to advise patients to take their first morning dose and schedule the programming session just prior to their next dose of anti-Parkinson medications. Presumably, the effects of the medications would thus be minimal, and any symptoms not controlled by DBS would be apparent at this time.

Synergistic effects between the anti-Parkinson medications and DBS require you to assess the patient for interactions after the DBS programming session. Typically, patients take their medications after the programming session and, an hour later, when the medications have reached their maximal effects, they are assessed for any medication-related adverse effects. If adverse effects worsen, avoid the temptation to reduce electrical stimulation; rather, reduce the medications.

Different symptoms respond to changes in stimulation at different times. Tremor and muscle tone are affected within seconds and bradykinesia within seconds to minutes. However, postural stability and gait may take tens of minutes to change. Consequently, the initial DBS parameters are based primarily on tremor, muscle tone, bradykinesia, and adverse effects, but you should also observe the patient after about 20 minutes, to assess postural stability and gait.

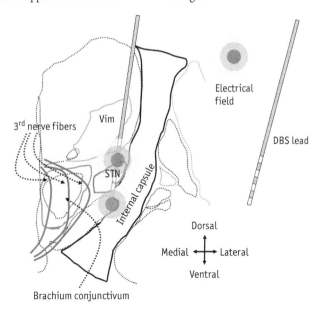

Figure 11.9: DBS lead too lateral. Coronal view of the STN 4 mm anterior to the midpoint of the AC–PC line. The STN is outlined in red, Vim is outlined in blue, the brachium conjunctivum (also containing the red nucleus) in orange, and the internal capsule is outlined in solid black. The Vc (not shown) thalamic nucleus is dorsal and posterior to the STN. The brachium conjunctivum is just medial and slightly posterior to the STN, and the internal capsule is lateral and ventral. Also shown are the nerve fibers exiting the oculomotor nucleus to form the third cranial nerve. The DBS lead in this case is too lateral, causing activation of the internal capsule and tonic muscle contraction when the most-ventral contact is used as the negative contact. Evidence that the DBS lead is too lateral is that the threshold to tonic muscle contraction might be higher with the most-dorsal contact as the negative contact compared to the threshold when the most ventral contact is used as the negative contact. One response would be to move the electrical field more dorsally, away from internal capsule. For patients implanted with DBS leads with segmented contacts, current can be applied to the contact that is directed medially (not shown).

Modified from Schaltenbrand and Wahren 1977.

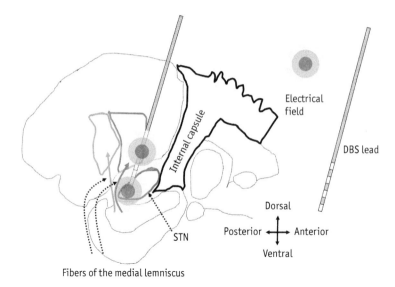

Too posterior

Figure 11.10: DBS lead too posterior. A sagittal section 16 mm lateral to the AC–PC line of the STN (outlined in red) with a DBS lead that is too posterior. Electrical stimulation spreads to the fibers of the medial lemniscus, causing paresthesias. Ways to prevent paresthesias include moving the electrical field upwards by using more-dorsal contacts as the negative contacts, because the typical trajectory slopes from anterior to posterior as it descends. Other approaches include the use of bipolar configurations, beginning with wide bipolar and progressing to narrow bipolar stimulation, as necessary.

Modified from Schaltenbrand and Wahren 1977.

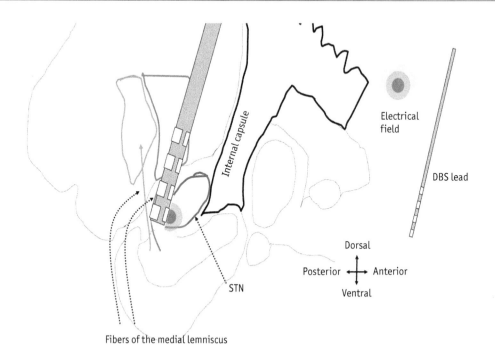

Figure 11.11: DBS lead too posterior. A sagittal section 16 mm lateral to the AC–PC line of the STN (outlined in red) with a DBS lead that is too posterior. Electrical stimulation spreads to the fibers of the medial lemniscus, causing paresthesias. For patients implanted with DBS leads with segmented contacts, current can be applied to the contact that is directed anteriorly. Note the smaller electrical field anterior to the DBS lead.

Modified from Schaltenbrand and Wahren 1977.

Some commercially available and anticipated IPGs are rechargeable. While a significant advantage in reducing surgeries for IPG replacement, there are the concerns regarding the consequence of IPG failure due to lack of recharge. This is particularly an issue for patients with Parkinson's disease. Many patients are able to substantially reduce their medications and consequently, depend greatly on DBS for symptomatic control. This means that in the event of an IPG failure, the patient's parkinsonism could worsen dramatically and expose the patient to serious consequences.

APPROACH TO DBS IN THE VICINITY OF THE STN FOR OTHER DISORDERS

DBS in the vicinity of the STN is being used for an increasing array of neurological disorders and clinical trials are underway for psychiatric disorders. These additional indications include dystonia and Essential tremor. Adverse effects directly related to stimulation are very much the same as described here for Parkinson's disease and the approaches to countering the adverse effects also apply.

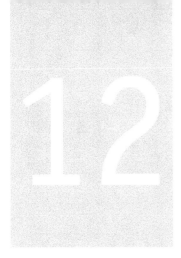

APPROACH TO DBS IN THE VICINITY OF THE GLOBUS PALLIDUS INTERNA

REGIONAL ANATOMY OF THE GLOBUS PALLIDUS INTERNAL (GPi)

Just ventral to the sensorimotor region of the GPi is the optic tract. Spread of stimulation to the optic tract can produce *phosphenes* (the experience of seeing light without light actually entering the eye). The internal capsule lies just posterior to the globus pallidus, and stimulation there can cause tonic muscle contractions. Anteriorly lies the non-motor region, and stimulation of this region could cause changes in cognition and personality, although the incidence of these problems is much less than with DBS in the vicinity of the STN.

ADVERSE EFFECTS RESULTING FROM THE POSITION OF THE DBS LEAD RELATIVE TO THE GPi

DBS Lead Too Ventral

If the DBS lead is too *ventral*, electrical current will spread to the internal capsule, causing tonic muscular contraction; and to the optic tract, causing phosphenes (bright, flashing lights in the visual fields; Figure 12.1). The usual response is to move the electrical field dorsally, first in a monopolar configuration and subsequently in a bipolar configuration.

This circumstance may be appropriate for partitioning the stimulation current/voltage among the electrode contacts. For example, stimulation through the most-ventral contact is most effective in producing a clinical response but produces adverse effects. Stimulation through the more-dorsally placed contacts dos not produce sufficient benefit but does not produce as many adverse effects. One could stimulate through the most-ventral contact at a reduced stimulation current/voltage and then through a more-dorsally placed contact at a higher stimulation current/voltage (Figure 12.2).

Another option for patients with segmented DBS leads and only experience phosphenes as an adverse effect, the segment that is directed posteriorly. Note that these suggestions are based on a DBS segmented lead in which the contacts are arranged as sectors around the circumference of the lead in the plane orthogonal to the long axis of the lead. These suggestions may not be appropriate for other segmented DBS lead architectures, but the general principles still may apply. It is important to note that changing from a continuous circumferential contact stimulation to a subset of contacts in a segmented lead can change the surface area of the electrical contacts over which the stimulation is applied. This

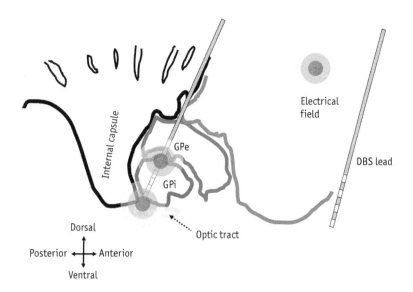

Figure 12.1: A sagittal section 22 mm lateral to the AC–PC line of the GPi (GPi, outlined in red) with a DBS lead that is too ventral. Also shown is the GPe in blue, the optic tract in green, and the internal capsule in black. In this case, electrical stimulation spreads to the fibers of the optic tract, causing such visual disturbances as phosphenes. Ways to prevent phosphenes include moving the electrical field upwards by using more dorsal contacts as the negative contacts. Other approaches include the use of bipolar configurations, beginning with wide bipolar and progressing to narrow bipolar stimulation, as necessary.
Schaltenbrand and Wahren 1977.

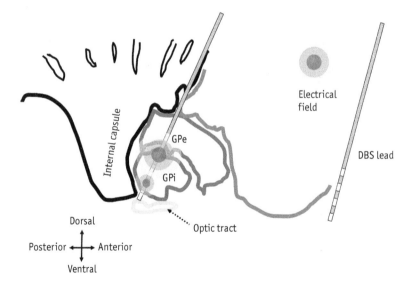

Figure 12.2: A sagittal section 22 mm lateral to the AC–PC line of the GPi (GPi, outlined in red) with a DBS lead that is too ventral. Also shown is the GPe in blue, the optic tract in green and the internal capsule in black. In this case, electrical stimulation spreads to the fibers of the optic tract, causing visual disturbances such as phosphenes; and to the posterior limb of the internal capsule, to produce tonic contraction. Ways to prevent phosphenes and tonic contractions while maintaining optimal clinical benefit would be to partition the stimulation current between multiple, continuous, circumferential contacts. In this case, a higher stimulation intensity on the more-dorsal contacts did not produce adverse effects; however, there was insufficient clinical benefit. Adding a lower-intensity electrical field in the more-ventral contacts added to the clinical benefit without causing adverse effects. Note the smaller electrical field about the most ventral contact.
Schaltenbrand and Wahren 1977.

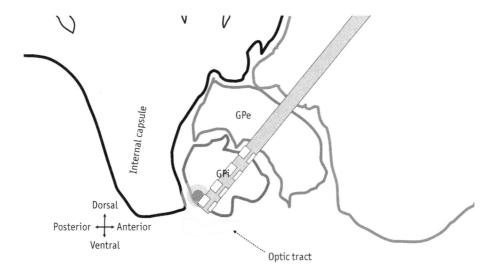

Figure 12.3: A sagittal section 22 mm lateral to the AC–PC line of the GPi (GPi, outlined in red) with a DBS lead that is too ventral. Also shown is the GPe in blue, the optic tract in green, and the internal capsule in black. In his case, electrical stimulation spreads to the fibers of the optic tract, causing visual disturbances such as phosphenes. In this case, a segmented DBS lead was used. Because of the orientation of the DBS lead, the posterior segment of the most ventral set of contacts is also more dorsal, and thus, farther from the optic tract. This would increase the threshold for the production of phosphenes. Note the smaller electrical field above the DBS segment projecting posteriorly and dorsally.
Modified from Schaltenbrand and Wahren 1977.

could change the current densities and thus, affect safety (*see Chapter 5—DBS Safety*). These caveats apply to any and all discussions of segmented DBS leads in this textbook.

Given that the typical trajectory in the sagittal plane is from dorsal and anterior to ventral and posterior, the posteriorly directed contact also would be directed dorsally as well (Figure 12.3). If this change fails, patients can be taken to the operating room and, under local anesthesia with continual DBS testing, the DBS lead can be pulled back under fluoroscopic control.

DBS Lead Too Posterior

If the DBS lead is too posterior, electrical current will spread to the internal capsule, causing tonic muscle contraction, as described above (Figure 12.4). Leads that are too medial often are close to the posterior limb of the internal capsule, as the posterior limb of the internal capsule moves forward as it moves medially. Often the DBS lead moves from anterior, dorsally, to posterior, ventrally, in the sagittal plane. For DBS leads that are

too medial or too posterior, moving the electrical field more dorsally also may move the electrical field more anteriorly. However, the benefit of such approaches may be limited, as the most effective stimulation site may be more ventral and posterior. If these measures fail and the efficacy is insufficient, another approach would be to use multiple cathodes in an interleaved fashion such that a lower stimulation current/voltage is applied to the more-ventrally placed contacts and a greater stimulation current/voltage is applied to more- dorsally placed contacts.

Another option for patients with segmented DBS leads is to use the segment that is directed anteriorly (Figure 12.5). If this change fails, patients can be taken to the operating room and, under local anesthesia with continual DBS testing, the DBS lead can be pulled back under fluoroscopic control.

DBS Leads Too Anterior or Too Lateral

When DBS leads are too anterior or too lateral, most often symptomatic benefits are lost. In these cases, large volumes of stimulation may be required to

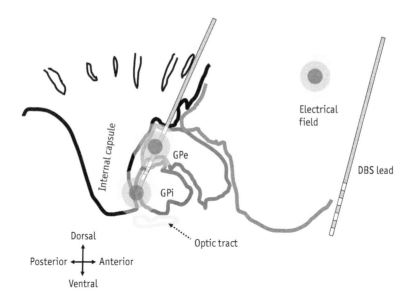

Figure 12.4: A sagittal section 22 mm lateral to the AC–PC line of the GPi, outlined in red, with a DBS lead that is too posterior. Also shown is the GPe in blue, the optic tract in green, and the internal capsule in black. In his case, electrical stimulation spreads to the fibers of the internal capsule, causing tonic muscle contractions. Ways to prevent tonic muscle contractions include moving the electrical field upwards by using more-dorsal contacts as the negative contacts, as the trajectory typically moves anterior with more-dorsal contacts. Other approaches include the use of bipolar configurations, beginning with wide bipolar and progressing to narrow bipolar stimulation, as necessary.

Modified from Schaltenbrand and Wahren 1977.

extend the field posteriorly and medially to reach the appropriate targets. Monopolar, wide bipolar, and multiple cathodes may be necessary.

APPROACHES TO DBS IN THE VICINITY OF THE GPI FOR PARKINSON'S DISEASE

Two strategies are often applied when administering DBS to the vicinity of the GPi. The point of differentiation is the remarkable efficacy of DBS in the vicinity of the GPi in suppressing dyskinesia. One approach is to use DBS to suppress dyskinesia, allowing a more aggressive use of medications. Alternatively, one can use DBS in the vicinity of the GPi to improve the Parkinsonian symptoms and hopefully reduce medications that could help reduce dyskinesia. Thus, these strategies are based on the intentions of the medications' use. The principle consideration is to determine how to direct the DBS programming relative to the patient's medications.

In some patients, the primary intention of DBS is to allow more aggressive treatment with medications. For example, patients with otherwise good symptom control may still have disabling dyskinesias and no other adverse effects. For these patients, the primary goal of DBS could be to reduce the dyskinesia, allowing the patient to benefit from the medications. That is, medication reduction is not a goal for these patients, and DBS is primarily directed at suppressing the dyskinesia directly. For other, symptomatic, patients, DBS reduces dyskinesia, allowing increases in medications to treat the other symptoms.

An alternative approach is directed at decreasing the need for medications; consequently, the DBS is directed at reducing symptoms, either because of a lack of symptomatic efficacy or because of medication-related adverse effects. In these patients, symptomatic improvement is the main goal, and medication reduction would be a secondary goal.

For patients in whom controlling dyskinesia is a primary goal, the initial DBS programming sessions should occur when the patient is experiencing

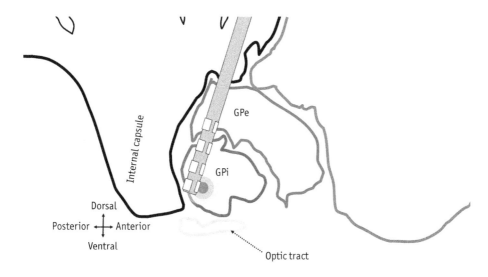

Figure 12.5: A sagittal section 22 mm lateral to the AC–PC line of the GPi, outlined in red, with a DBS lead that is too posterior. Also shown is the GPe in blue, the optic tract in green, and the internal capsule in black. In this case, electrical stimulation spreads to the fibers of the internal capsule, causing tonic muscle contractions. In this case a segmented DBS lead was used. Because of the orientation of the DBS lead, the anterior segment of the most-ventral set of contacts would place the electrical field farther from the posterior limb of the internal capsule. This would increase the threshold for production of tonic contraction. Note the smaller electrical field anterior to the DBS lead.

Modified from Schaltenbrand and Wahren 1977.

the full effect of the medications, particularly the medication-induced dyskinesias. Typically, this time is about an hour after the usual medications are taken. Observations at this time allow you to assess medication effects that may be synergistic with DBS. For example, if the patient is in the medication maximum state and is having dyskinesia, you may want to adjust the DBS to the point that the dyskinesias are suppressed.

Also, you should also observe the patient when the effects of medication are minimal, typically just before the next dose of anti-Parkinson medications is to be taken. The patient's condition at this time should help you decide how to adjust the medications because, in the medication-minimum state the primary effect may be from the DBS. This will allow you to see what the DBS is doing and then judge how to change the medications in order to obtain additional benefit.

For patients in whom symptomatic control is the primary goal, you should program the DBS parameters when the effects of medication are minimal. The approach is analogous to that described for the STN in chapter 11.

As before, different symptoms respond to changes in stimulation at different times. Initial DBS parameters should be based primarily on tremor, muscle tone, bradykinesia, and adverse effects, but postural stability and gait should be assessed after about 20 minutes.

Some commercially available and anticipated IPGs are rechargeable. While these have a significant advantage in reducing surgeries for IPG replacement, there are the concerns regarding the consequence of IPG failure due to lack of recharging. This is particularly an issue for patients with Parkinson's disease. Many patients are able to substantially reduce their medications; consequently, they depend greatly on DBS for symptomatic control. This means that, in the event of an IPG failure, the patient's Parkinsonism could worsen dramatically and expose the patient to serious consequences. For patients in whom the DBS in the vicinity of the GPi is used to suppress dyskinesia, a sudden failure of the IPG could result in markedly worse dyskinesia that could pose a serious threat to their health and safety (*see Chapter 5—DBS Safety*).

TREATING DYSTONIA WITH DBS IN THE VICINITY OF THE GPI

DBS for dystonia is complicated by the fact that, although dystonic symptoms may be affected immediately after stimulation, the maximal response may not be seen for weeks or months. For Parkinson's disease, begin DBS with the parameters that create the least current drain on the IPG, then increase the electrical current/voltage, because the response to the DBS is relatively fast and can be assessed during the DBS programming session. However, taking this approach to dystonia is problematic. Alternatively, increasing the current/voltage at intervals of several weeks takes too long to control symptoms of dystonia.

One approach is to begin with the maximum tolerated parameters that can be expected to provide reasonable symptom control. For example, you might begin with a wide pulse width, typically about 150-180 μs and a DBS rate of about 150 pps; a voltage near that of the IPG battery in the case of constant voltage DBS, or a current whose associated voltage is near the battery voltage for the constant current IPGs; and monopolar stimulation through the more-ventrally placed leads, which are more likely to be in the sensorimotor region of the GPi. These initial parameters should be modified as indicated by the patient's adverse effects. Observe the patient for at least three weeks, or until the symptomatic response appears to plateau. At that point, the parameters can be changed, often by increasing the voltage or current or going to multiple cathodes.

Some dystonia patients require high stimulation current/voltage, pulse widths, and/or frequencies (rates), which may dramatically shorten battery life. In these circumstances, a rechargeable system may be an advantage. However, the potential consequences of an IPG failure because of lack of recharge must be considered.

Medication adjustments or intramuscular botulinum toxin injections generally are not a major concern in dystonia. Most medications are relatively ineffective, and lack of response to drug therapy is a prerequisite for DBS surgery. Generally, medications are not changed until the patient has experienced maximal therapeutic benefit from DBS.

TREATING HYPERKINETIC DISORDERS

Although DBS treatments for hyperkinetic disorders, such as Tourette's syndrome, Huntington's disease, and tardive dyskinesia, have not been FDA-approved, substantial evidence supports the efficacy of DBS in the vicinity of the GPi for these conditions (Montgomery 2015). The multitude of hyperkinetic disorders responding to DBS is itself a strong argument to consider DBS a symptom-specific therapy, rather than a disease-specific one. The implications are substantial. Typically, clinical trials are not conducted for each and every conceivable cause of pain, with the presumption that pain-relief medications are relevant to the symptoms, regardless of cause. Extending that logic to hyperkinetic disorders would mean that clinical trials of every conceivable cause of hyperkinesia should not be a prerequisite to using DBS therapy. However, some caution is necessary. DBS for Parkinsonism cannot be considered, at the time of publication, a symptomatic therapy, because the same symptoms that improve in idiopathic Parkinson's disease are not improved in atypical Parkinsonism. The DBS programming approach in hyperkinetic disorders is similar to the approach with GPi DBS in the vicinity of the GPi to suppress dyskinesia in patients with levodopa-induced dyskinesia, which often complicates idiopathic Parkinson's disease, as described above.

APPROACH TO DBS IN THE VICINITY OF THE VENTRAL INTERMEDIATE NUCLEUS OF THE THALAMUS DBS

REGIONAL ANATOMY OF THE VENTRAL INTERMEDIATE THALAMUS (VIM)

Key structures in the regional anatomy of thalamus Vim include the Vim, which is the target of therapeutic DBS. The ventrocaudal nucleus of the thalamus (Vc) lies posterior to the Vim. Electrical stimulation of the Vc can cause treatment-limiting paresthesias. The corticospinal and cortical bulbar tracts in the internal capsule lie lateral and ventral to the Vim. Electrical stimulation of the internal capsule can cause tonic muscle contractions. There are multiple nomenclatures of the subnuclei of the thalamus. Previously, I have referred to the ventrolateral thalamus (VL). Although this term is commonly used in the physiology literature, the alternative, ventral intermediate thalamus (Vim), is used in the DBS literature. Technically, "VL" refers to both regions of the thalamus that receive inputs from the GPi and cerebellum, whereas "Vim" refers to the cerebellar-receiving area of the thalamus and is thus a subdivision of what is otherwise referred to as "the VL" and is the target of DBS for tremor-related disorders (note other thalamic subnuclei have been targeted for DBS in other conditions such as Tourette's syndrome, epilepsy, and minimally conscious state patients).

ADVERSE EFFECTS RESULTING FROM THE POSITION OF THE DBS LEAD RELATIVE TO THE VIM

DBS Lead Too Posterior

If the thalamic lead is placed too *posterior*, electrical current can affect the Vc and produce intolerable paresthesias (Figure 13.1). Although transient paresthesias are not a problem, persistent paresthesias are. Moving the electrical field dorsally by using more-dorsally placed electrical contacts as cathodes may reduce these paresthesias. This maneuver is frequently effective because the lead often has an anterior, dorsally, to posterior, ventrally, orientation in the sagittal plane (Figure 13.1). Thus, moving the electrical field dorsally has the effect of moving the DBS lead anteriorly. However, this maneuver depends on the orientation of the lead in the sagittal plane. For example, if the angle of the lead in the sagittal plane is too shallow, moving the electrical field more dorsally along the long axis of the DBS lead may move the electrical field too anteriorly (see discussion below). However, the value of such approaches may be limited, as the most effective stimulation site may be more ventral, particularly if the angle of the DBS lead relative to the regional anatomy is too shallow. If these measures fail and the efficacy is insufficient, another approach

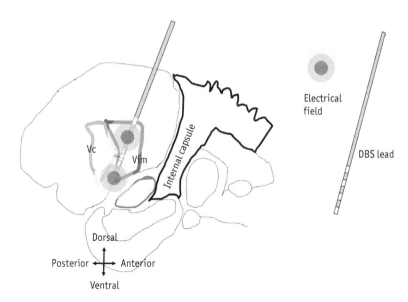

Figure 13.1: A sagittal section 16 mm lateral to the AC–PC line of the Vim (outlined in red) with a DBS lead that is too posterior. Electrical stimulation spreads to the ventrocaudal nucleus of the thalamus (VC), causing paresthesias. Ways to prevent paresthesias include moving the electrical field upwards by using more-dorsal contacts as the negative contacts because the typical trajectory slopes from anterior to posterior as it descends. Other approaches include the use of bipolar configurations, beginning with wide bipolar and progressing to narrow bipolar stimulation, as necessary.
Modified from Schaltenbrand and Wahren 1977.

would be to use multiple cathodes in an interleaved fashion such that a lower stimulation current/voltage is applied to the more-ventral contact and a greater stimulation current/voltage is applied to more-dorsal contacts. Another approach is to go to progressively narrower bipolar active contact configurations.

In cases where a segmented DBS lead is in place, the anterior contact on the most-ventral set of contacts will move the electrical field anteriorly and away from the posterior ventral caudal thalamus, thereby reducing the risk of treatment-limiting paresthesia. Using the anterior contact of the most-ventral set of contacts also has the advantage of not moving the electrical field too anteriorly, particularly in cases where the angle in the sagittal plane is shallow. Note that these suggestions are based on a DBS segmented lead in which the contacts are arranged as sectors around the circumference of the lead in the plane orthogonal to the long axis of the lead. These suggestions may not be appropriate for other segmented DBS lead architectures, but the general principles still may apply. It is important to note that changing from a continuous circumferential contact stimulation to a

subset of contacts in a segmented lead can change the surface area of the electrical contacts over which the stimulation is applied. This could change the current densities and thus affect safety (*see Chapter 5—DBS Safety*). These caveats apply to any and all discussions of segmented DBS leads in this textbook (Figure 13.2).

Poor Orientation of the DBS Lead

If its angle is too great (shallow) with respect to the vertical in the saggital plane, the position of the lead may be such that one or none of the cathodes are actually in Vim while the rest of the contacts may be too deep in the Vc or too shallow in the basal ganglia receiving area of the thalamus (Vop). (Figure 13.3). Contacts more ventrally placed to Vim may be in Vc, where stimulation may cause paresthesias, and the more dorsally placed contacts may be in Vop, which is the pallidal receiving area where DBS may be less effective. Consequently, the surgeon should attempt to place the DBS lead as vertically as possible in the saggital plane. DBS leads in too shallowly often have to be re-placed.

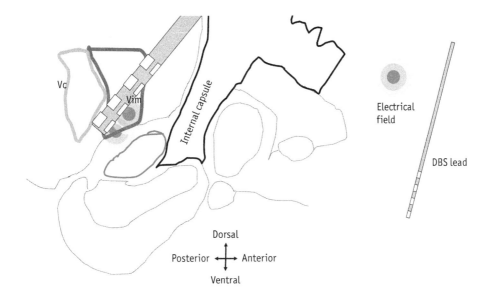

Figure 13.2: A sagittal section 16 mm lateral to the AC–PC line of the Vim (outlined in red) with a DBS lead that is too posterior. Electrical stimulation spreads to the Vc, causing paresthesias. In this case where a segmented DBS lead is in place, the anterior contact on the most ventral set of contacts will move the electrical field anteriorly and away from the posterior ventral caudal thalamus, thereby reducing the risk of treatment-limiting paresthesia. Note the smaller electrical field anterior to the DBS lead. Using the anterior contact of the most-ventral set of contacts also has the advantage of not moving the electrical field too anterior, particularly in cases where the angle in the sagittal plane is shallow.

Modified from Schaltenbrand and Wahren 1977.

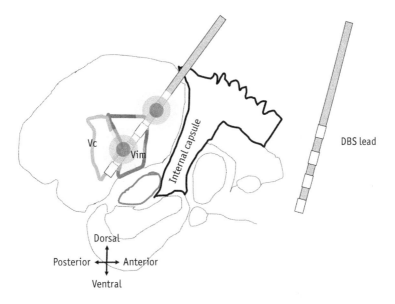

Figure 13.3: A sagittal section 16 mm lateral to the AC–PC line of the Vim (outlined in red) with a DBS lead that is angled too swallow. This results in the most ventral and ventral contact in or near Vc where electrical stimulation causes paresthesias. The dorsal and most dorsal contacts are not optimally positioned in Vim, resulting in poor clinical efficacy. Often DBS leads in this position have to be re-placed.

Modified from Schaltenbrand and Wahren 1977.

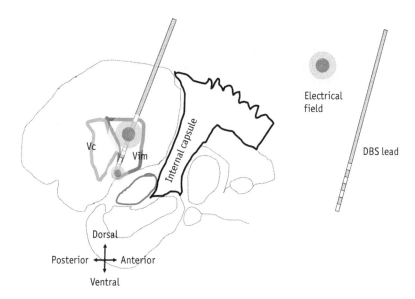

Figure 13.4: A sagittal section 16 mm lateral to the AC–PC line of the Vim (outlined in red) with a DBS lead that is angled too swallow. This results in the most ventral and ventral contact in or near Vc where electrical stimulation causes paresthesias. The dorsal and most dorsal contacts are not optimally positioned in Vim, resulting in poor clinical efficacy. Often DBS leads in this position have to be replaced. However, interleaved stimulation can be attempted with the smaller stimulation current applied to the most ventral contact. Note the smaller electrical field aroung the most ventral contact.
Modified from Schaltenbrand and Wahren 1977.

The circumstance where the DBS lead is placed too shallowly in the saggital plane may be appropriate for partitioning the stimulation current/voltage among the electrode contacts. For example, stimulation through more ventrally placed contacts are most effective in producing a clinical response but produces adverse effects. Stimulation through the more-dorsal contact does not produce sufficient benefit but does not produce as much adverse effects. One could stimulate both through the ventrally placed contacts at a reduced stimulation current/voltage and then through a more dorsally placed contacts at a higher stimulation current/voltage (Figure 13.4).

In cases where a segmented lead is used, applying the electrical field to the anterior contact of the more ventrally placed contacts would move the electrical field anteriorly, while making the posterior contacts of more dorsally placed levels would project the current posteriorly so to maximize the volume of tissue activation within Vim (Figure 13.5). This is particularly an advantage when the DBS lead angle is very shallow in the sagittal plane. In circumferentially continuous contacts, the more ventrally placed contacts may be too posterior to avoid treatment-limiting paresthesias,

yet more dorsally placed contacts are anterior to Vim and less effective. Using the anterior contacts in the most-ventral or the ventral set of segmented contacts still can retain the electrical field in Vim.

DBS Lead Too Lateral

The internal capsule borders Vim on the lateral and ventral sides. Stimulating the internal capsule can produce contralateral tonic muscle contractions. The monopolar survey can help determine whether the DBS lead is too deep or too lateral (Figure 13.6). For a lead that is too lateral, the threshold to tonic contraction through the most-dorsal cathode is similar to the threshold through the most-ventral cathode, because the lead often is more parallel to the internal capsule anteriorly. The most effective way to prevent muscle contractions when the DBS lead is too lateral is to use bipolar configurations, beginning with wide bipolar and progressing to narrow bipolar stimulation as necessary. In cases where a segmented DBS lead is used, another approach for a lead that is too lateral and causing tonic muscle contractions is to use contacts that are directed medially (Figure 13.7).

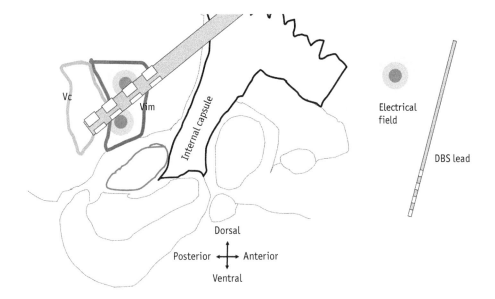

Figure 13.5: A sagittal section 16 mm lateral to the AC–PC line of the Vim (outlined in red) with a DBS lead that is angled too swallow. This results in the most ventral and ventral contact in or near Vc where electrical causes paresthesias. The dorsal and most dorsal contacts are not optimally positioned in Vim, resulting in poor clinical efficacy. In this hypothetical case using a segmented DBS lead, the anteriorly directed contact of the ventral set of contacts and the posteriorly directed contact in the dorsal set of contacts can be used to avoid stimulation of the posterior Vc and maintain stimulation in Vim.

Modified from Schaltenbrand and Wahren 1977.

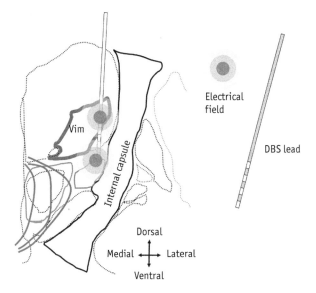

Figure 13.6: DBS lead too lateral. A coronal section 4 mm anterior to the midpoint of the AC–PC line of Vim (outlined in red) with a DBS lead that is too lateral. Electrical stimulation spreads to the internal capsule (outlined in black), causing muscle contractions. The internal capsule is closer to the most ventral contact, and is less than the distance between the most dorsal contact and the internal capsule. This difference means that the threshold for muscle contraction will be less for monopolar stimulation through the dorsal contacts compared to stimulation through the ventral contacts. The most effective way to prevent muscle contractions when the DBS lead is too lateral is to move the electrical field higher or to use bipolar configurations, beginning with wide bipolar and progressing to narrow bipolar stimulation as necessary.

Modified from Schaltenbrand and Wahren 1977.

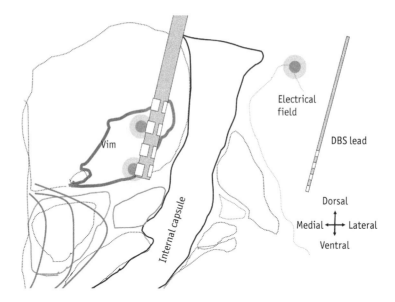

Figure 13.7: A coronal section 4 mm anterior to the midpoint of the AC–PC line of Vim (outlined in red) with a DBS lead that is too lateral. Electrical stimulation spreads to the internal capsule (outlined in black), causing muscle contractions. In this case, where a segmented DBS lead is used, another approach for a lead that is too lateral and causing tonic muscle contractions is to use contacts that are directed medially. Note the smaller electrical field medial to the DBS lead.
Modified from Schaltenbrand and Wahren 1977.

DBS Lead Too Ventral

If the DBS lead is placed too deep or *ventral,* the threshold for tonic muscle contraction will be less with the ventrally placed active contacts than with the more dorsally placed contacts (Figure 13.8). To prevent muscle contractions when the DBS lead is too ventral, stimulation should be done through the more dorsally placed contacts. You can start with monopolar stimulation and then progress to wide bipolar and to narrow bipolar stimulation as necessary. This circumstance may be appropriate for partitioning the stimulation current/voltage among the electrode contacts. For example, stimulation through the more ventrally placed contacts are most effective in producing a clinical response, but it produces adverse effects. Stimulation through the more dorsally placed contacts does not produce sufficient benefit but does not produce as many adverse effects. One could stimulate both through the more ventrally placed contacts at a reduced stimulation current/voltage and then through a more dorsally placed contacts at a higher stimulation current/voltage (for an example of the concept, see Figure 13.4). If the DBS lead is too ventral

and every electrode configuration continues to result in tonic muscle contraction, the DBS lead can be moved more dorsally with surgery performed under local anesthetic and fluoroscopic control. The patient should be stimulated during surgery to monitor adverse effects and the efficacy of the new placement.

EFFECTS OF DBS ON SPEECH, LANGUAGE, AND SWALLOWING

Speech, language, and swallowing problems sometimes occur in patients receiving thalamic DBS. Consequently, a relative exclusion criterion for thalamic DBS is a marked preexisting speech or swallowing problem. The mechanisms by which thalamic DBS affects speech and swallowing are unknown. Problems can occur in patients without other DBS adverse effects, suggesting that DBS can affect speech and swallowing without directly affecting Vc or the internal capsule. Sometimes increasing the stimulation intensity will initiate tonic muscle contractions, in which case the lead may be too lateral, with stimulation spreading to the corticobulbar fibers in the

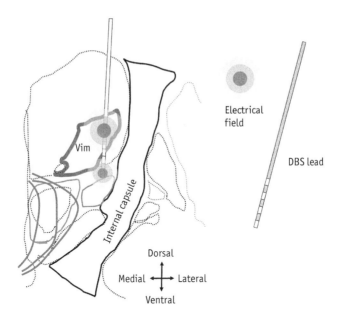

Figure 13.8: A sagittal section 16 mm lateral to the AC–PC line of the (outlined in red) with a DBS lead that is too ventral. This circumstance may be appropriate for partitioning the stimulation current/voltage among the electrode contacts. For example, stimulation through the most ventral contact is most effective in producing a clinical response but produces side effects. Stimulation through the more dorsal contact does not produce sufficient benefit, but it does not produce as many side effects. One could stimulate both through the most ventral contact at a reduced stimulation current/voltage and then through a more dorsal contact at a higher stimulation current/voltage.

Modified from Schaltenbrand and Wahren 1977.

posterior limb of the internal capsule. The general presumption is that placing the thalamic DBS in the head homuncular representation in Vim (more medial) is more likely to cause these problems.

For patients in whom a segmented DBS lead is used, it may be possible to use the medially directed contact (for an example of the concept, see Figure 13.4). Using the medial contact could direct the electrical field laterally and, presumably, away from the head homuncular representation, thereby reducing speech, language, and swallowing problems.

Often there is no programming method to reduce speech and swallowing complications without simultaneously reducing therapeutic benefit. Consequently, some centers routinely use IPGs that allow the patient or caregiver to adjust the stimulation voltage or current. Thus, when speech or swallowing control are relatively more important than suppressing tremor, the patient or caregiver can set the IPG to a lower voltage or current. Conversely, when tremor control is relatively more important, the IPG can be set to a higher voltage or current. Most IPGs allow patients

and/or caregivers to switch among predefined electrode configurations and stimulation parameters, thereby reducing ambiguity. *Caution:* in some commercial stimulators, the device given to patients or caregivers to increase the stimulation voltage (or any other parameter) provides no warning if the stimulation voltage exceeds safe levels. Consequently, you should limit the upper limits of the stimulation parameters, such as voltage, to keep stimulation within safe levels. Again, it is important to recognize that some commercial IPGs make certain assumptions about therapeutic impedance when calculating the electrical current densities (*see Chapter 5—DBS Safety*). You should consult the appropriate manufacturer's manual for information on each IPG.

AN APPROACH TO DBS IN THE VICINITY OF VIM FOR TREMOR

Currently, the primary goal of thalamic DBS is to control tremor. Tremors respond rapidly to changes in DBS stimulation, so you can make small, incremental changes. Begin at the lowest parameters that generally improve symptoms—say, a pulse width of 150 μs, monopolar cathodes (more common practice is to start lower, 60 s for example; however, see discussion of pulse width in Chapter 9), and a stimulation rate of 130 pps. If the patient is taking antitremor medications, begin programming when drug effects are minimal, usually after an overnight fast from the medications or just before the next dose is due. You can ask the patient to postpone taking selected medications until just before DBS programming. However, use this approach with caution. If the patient's symptoms are intolerable or present a safety risk if the medications are not taken as prescribed, advise the patient to continue to take them without interruption, and then observe the patient in the clinic as the time for their next dose approaches. This approach is especially useful for patients with Parkinson's disease. After changing the stimulation parameters, it is also important to observe the patient for about an hour after antitremor medications are taken.

As of the time of this publication, FDA-approved indications for thalamic DBS are idiopathic Parkinson's disease and Essential tremor. Even for these, only unilateral DBS has FDA approval. However, bilateral thalamic DBS often is necessary to control axial tremor, particularly head tremor. Some patients benefit greatly when bilateral tremor is controlled. In such cases, bilateral thalamic DBS would be considered "off-label," not experimental or investigational. As is the case with hyperkinetic disorders, thalamic DBS is effective in treating cerebellar outflow tremor, regardless of the underlying cause, such as multiple sclerosis or trauma. However, acceptance of these off-label indications has been problematic and has been compounded by confusion about what constitutes acceptable outcomes in clinical trials and case reports (Montgomery 2008a).

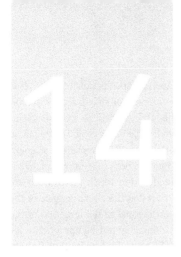

ALGORITHM FOR SELECTING ELECTRODE CONFIGURATIONS AND STIMULATION PARAMETERS

Chapter 9, Approaches to Programming, provided a general discussion regarding the approaches to DBS programming. The focus of Chapter 9 was on the underlying electroneurophysiological principles rather than an explicit algorithm that addressed every possible circumstance. Chapter 11, Approach to DBS in the Vicinity of the Subthalamic Nucleus, Chapter 12, Approach to DBS in the Vicinity of the Globus Pallidus Interna, and Chapter 13, Approach to DBS in the Vicinity of the Thalamic, discussed approaches in the context of specific DBS targets. These approaches emphasized interpreting the DBS responses to visualize the location of the DBS contacts in the unique regional anatomy of the individual patient. For example, the production of paresthesias at stimulation currents insufficient to produce clinical benefit with DBS in the vicinity of the STN indicates that the DBS lead probability is too posterior. By understanding the angle of the DBS lead in the sagittal plane, one can see in their mind's eye how moving the volume of the electrical field to more dorsal contacts also moves the field anteriorly, thereby lessening the risk of paresthesias.

Some programmers find visualization of the regional anatomy and the location and volume of the electrical field difficult. Unfortunately, it is unlikely that neuroimaging will provide the ability to visualize, for reasons that are discussed in *Supplemental essay - Automated Assisted DBS Programming, at http://www.greenvilleneuromodulationcenter.com/ DBS_Programming_essays/*. For these programmers, an attempt to formalize an algorithm was made and is presented here.

Such algorithms, while based on responses to DBS programming, cannot make anatomical inferences that might allow narrowing of the range of electrode configurations, stimulation parameters, and pulse trains that would have to be considered when programming for a particular patient is problematic. Rather, the algorithm provided may allow the programmer to provide adequate clinical benefit in the absence of adverse effects. At the least, it is fairly exhaustive, and programmers can therefore feel more confident that they have exhausted a reasonable number of options in particularly difficult patients. This algorithm is presented with check boxes and spaces for comments in to the *Supplemental Tool - Programming: Algorithm and Check List for Electrode Configurations*, at *http://www.greenvilleneuromodulationcenter.com/DBS_Programming_ forms/*, and can be photocopied as needed (you may want to enlarge the image when photocopying. The algorithm is particularly useful for patients whose parameters are difficult to program. Checking off the various steps helps document and summarize the findings for individual patients, ensuring that every configuration has been tried without duplication.

Many of the steps in the algorithm can be bypassed for greater efficiency by careful analysis of the monopolar survey in light of the regional anatomy surrounding the DBS leads (see *Supplemental Tool-Index to DBS Side Effects, by Side Effect and Site of Stimulation at*

http://www.greenvilleneuromodulationcenter. com/DBS_Programming_forms/which catalogues various adverse effects based on the DBS site. The tool is organized based on the adverse effects and and site, and then directs the reader to the appropriate section in the textbook for a discussion of the side effect and possible means to resolve them).

The numbering conventions for the contacts used here assume that the DBS lead contains four levels of negative contacts (cathodes), based on their position along the long axis of the DBS lead and whether the contact at the level is segmented (Figure 14.1). Unfortunately, there has been an undisciplined proliferation of numbering conventions. For example, one DBS system configuration uses contacts numbered 0, 1, 2, and 3 for the right side DBS lead, and contacts numbered 8, 9, 10, and 11 for the left DBS lead. Other IPGs number the right-sided contacts 1, 2, 3, and 4 and the left-sided contacts as 5, 6, 7, and 8. Rather than risk compounding the confusion, I will refer to the contacts as *mos ventral, ventral, dorsal*, and *most dorsal*

(Figure 14.1). However, introduction of DBS leads with more than four levels of electrodes arrayed on the long axis of the DBS lead will be more problematic. For segmented leads, a suffix capital letter can be added to the level-descriptor for appropriate segmented DBS leads. Note that these suggestions are based on a DBS segmented lead in which the contacts are arranged as sectors around the circumference of the lead in the plane orthogonal to the long axis of the lead. These suggestions may not be appropriate for other segmented DBS lead architectures, but the general principles still may apply. It is important to note that changing from a continuous circumferential contact stimulation to a subset of contacts in a segmented lead can change the surface area of the electrical contacts over which the stimulation is applied. This could change the current densities and thus affect safety (*see Chapter 5—DBS Safety*). These caveats apply to any and all discussions of segmented DBS leads in this book.

Electrode configurations are described as *monopolar* (DBS lead contacts as negative [cathodes] and the IPG as positive [anode]), *wide bipolar* (both positive [anodes] and negative [cathodes] on the DBS

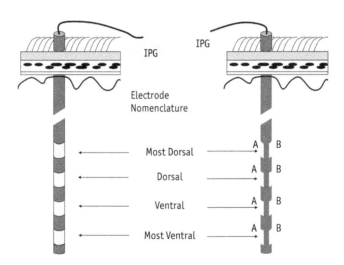

Figure 14.1: One possible electrode nomenclature. With the proliferation of DBS leads of different architectures, establishing a consistent and universally accepted nomenclature is difficult. At least for some architectures (available or anticipated), the basic structures are contacts that span the circumference around the long axis of the DBS lead, hence the terms based on their relative positions along the long axis of the lead. These contacts can be continuous around the entire circumference and are referred to as *circumferential-continuous*. Some potential segmented leads maintain this general architecture, but the contacts are not continuous, but rather segments representing sectors around the circumference. Note that when all contacts at a level are active, this is taken as synonymous with continuous circumferential stimulation. When a subset of contacts at each level is active, this will be denoted by indicating the relative depth and labeling the contact with an uppercase letter.

lead, and there are two inactive contacts between the positive [anodes] and negative [cathodes]), *close bipolar* (both positive [anodes] and negative [cathodes] on the DBS lead, and there is one inactive contact between the active positive [anode] and negative [cathode] contacts), and *narrow bipolar* (both positive [anodes] and negative [cathodes] on the DBS lead, and there is no inactive contact between the active positive [anode] and negative [cathode] contacts).

As discussed in Chapter 9, Approaches to Programming, the choice of DBS frequency and pulse width to start the DBS programming is problematic. Convention had starting at frequencies such as 130 pulses per second (pps) and pulse widths of 60 microseconds. However, it is now clear that, at least as it relates to bradykinesia in patients with Parkinson's disease and within the higher frequency range, patients are somewhat idiosyncratic, and small changes in frequency can have significant impact. For that reason, and generalizing from the experience in patients with Parkinson's, an initial monopolar survey is suggested to identify the optimal DBS frequency for use throughout the DBS programming session. The exception is the presence of adverse effects that cannot be obviated by other adjustments.

Similar concerns attend the initial choice of pulse width. As discussed Chapter 9, Approaches to Programming, it is hard to know where to start and where to end in the titration of pulse width. One method is to start of 150 microseconds and not increase by much, based on careful though limited studies of chronaxie; except in the case of adverse effects. Notable exceptions would be in the case of DBS for dystonia where higher pulse widths have been reported.

Table 14.1 describes the process of adjusting stimulation parameters. The two columns, Conventional method and Alternative method, recognize the extensive experience that has been amassed when using conventional approaches, but also recent studies of the effects of pulse width in chronaxie studies and more precise studies of the effects of DBS frequencies on bradykinesia in Parkinson's disease. The conventional approach typically starts with a DBS frequency of 130 pps and a pulse width of 60 microseconds. Starting with a pulse width of 60 microseconds is based on the presumption that this would cause less drainage of the battery charge. However, based

on chronaxie studies, such as those presented in Chapter 9, Approaches to Programming, any gains by using a shorter pulse width may be offset by required higher stimulation intensities.

The Alternative method column of the table is based on chronaxie studies and more complete studies of DBS frequency. However, these studies have been limited to small numbers of patients with Essential tremor and Parkinson's disease in the chronaxie studies, and limited to measures of bradykinesia limited to hand-opening and -closing in a very small number of patients with Parkinson's disease in the case of studying DBS frequencies. In principle, the alternative approach has much to recommend it, such as simplification of DBS stimulation parameter programming, which can improve the efficiency of postoperative DBS management.

Step 1. Start
  Single cathode (−) monopolar stimulation
  Most-Ventral contact cathode (−); case anode (+)
  Change stimulation parameters as described in
    Table 14.1—Stimulation parameter adjustment
  Adverse effects: go to Step 1.1
  Lack of efficacy: go to Step 1.1

Step 1.1. Single cathode (−) monopolar stimulation
  Ventral contact cathode (−); case anode (+)
  Change stimulation parameters as described in
    Table 14.1—Stimulation parameter adjustment
  Adverse effects: go to Step 1.2
  Lack of efficacy: go to Step 1.2

Step 1.2. Single cathode (−) monopolar stimulation-Dorsal contact cathode (−); case anode (+)
  Change stimulation parameters as described in
    Table 14.1—Stimulation parameter adjustment
  Adverse effects: go to Step 1.3
  Lack of efficacy: go to Step 1.3

Step 1.3. Single cathode (−) monopolar stimulation
  Most-Dorsal contact cathode (−); case anode (+)
  Change stimulation parameters as described in
    Table 14.1—Stimulation parameter adjustment
  Adverse effects: go to Step 2.0
  Lack of efficacy: go to Step 2.0

Step 2.0. Wide bipolar polar stimulation
  Most-Ventral contact cathode (−);
  Most-Dorsal contact anode (+)

Table 14.1 *Stimulation parameter adjustment*: Two approaches to adjustments of the stimulation parameters. Column 1 is an algorithm based on conventional approaches as described in the text. Column 2 is an alternative approach based on studies of DBS frequency and chronaxie as discussed in the text. *Note*: The specific stimulation parameters are suggestions and may vary with different IPGs and different manufacturers. The programmer is advised to consult with the manufacturer's recommendations

Conventional method	Alternative method
Starting with the conventional DBS frequency of 130 pps, pulse width of 60 microseconds, and stimulation intensity of 0 mA (0 volts), go to A1.	Parkinson's disease (and perhaps other disorders): Starting with the optimal DBS frequency defined by the monopolar survey, set pulse width to 150 microseconds, set stimulation intensity to 0, and go to B1.
A1: Increase stimulation intensities by 0.5 mA (0.5 v for constant current/voltage IPGs), assess, and go to A2.	B1: Increase stimulation intensities by 0.5 mA (0.5 v for constant current/voltage IPGs), assess, and go to B2.

A2:
If assessment demonstrates—
a) Insufficient benefit in the absence of adverse effects, go to A1.
b) Sufficient benefit achieved—proceed to exit procedures (*see Chapter 9—Approaches to Programming*).
c) Encounter a limiting adverse effect—reset stimulus intensity to 0, return pulse width and DBS frequency to starting value, and return to algorithm below for possible change in electrode configuration.
d) Reach 4 mA (5 v for constant current/voltage IPGs) without sufficient clinical benefit and absent adverse effects; and
  i) DBS frequency is not at maximum, return stimulation intensity to 0, increase DBS frequency, and return to A1.
  ii) DBS frequency at maximum, proceed to A3.
	B2:
	If assessment demonstrates—
	a) Insufficient benefit in the absence of adverse effects, go back to B1.
	b) Sufficient benefit achieved—proceed to exit procedures (*Chapter 9—Approaches to Programming*).
	c) Encounter a limiting adverse effect—reset stimulus intensity to 0 and return to algorithm for possible change in electrode configuration.
	d) Reach 4 mA (5 v for constant current/voltage IPGs) without sufficient clinical benefit and absent adverse effects, set stimulation intensity to 0 and return to algorithm for possible change in electrode configuration. Alternatively, particularly if reasonable electrode configurations have been exhausted, consider implementing the Conventional method described in this table at left.

A3: a) If DBS pulse width not at maximum, reset stimulation intensity to 0, return DBS frequency to starting value, increase pulse width, and go to A1. b) If DBS pulse width at maximum, reset stimulation intensity to 0, return pulse width and frequency to starting value, and return to algorithm for possible change in electrode configuration.	

Change stimulation parameters as described in *Table 14.1—Stimulation parameter adjustment*
    Adverse effects: go to Step 2.1
    Lack of efficacy: go to Step 2.1

Step 2.1. Wide bipolar polar stimulation
    Most-Ventral contact anode (+); Most-Dorsal contact cathode (–)
    Change stimulation parameters as described in *Table 14.1—Stimulation parameter adjustment*
    Adverse effects: go to Step 3.0
    Lack of efficacy: go to Step 3.0

Step 3.0. Multiple cathodes (–) monopolar stimulation
    Most-Ventral and Ventral contacts cathode (–); case anode (+)
    Check therapeutic impedances
    Change stimulation parameters as described in *Table 14.1—Stimulation parameter adjustment*
    Adverse effects: go to Step 3.1
    Lack of efficacy: go to Step 3.1

Step 3.1. Multiple cathodes (–) monopolar stimulation
    Ventral and Dorsal contacts cathode (–); case anode (+)
    Check therapeutic impedances
    Change stimulation parameters as described in *Table 14.1—Stimulation parameter adjustment*
    Adverse effects: go to Step 3.2
    Lack of efficacy: go to Step 3.2

Step 3.2. Multiple cathodes (–) monopolar stimulation
    Dorsal and Most-Dorsal contacts cathode (–); case anode (+)
    Check therapeutic impedances
    Change stimulation parameters as described in *Table 14.1—Stimulation parameter adjustment*
    Adverse effects: go to Step 4.0
    Lack of efficacy: go to Step 4.0

Step 4.0. Wide multiple cathode (–) bipolar stimulation
    Most-Ventral and Ventral contacts cathode (–)
    Most-Dorsal contact anode (+)
    Change stimulation parameters as described in *Table 14.1—Stimulation parameter adjustment*
    Adverse effects: go to Step 4.1
    Lack of efficacy: go to Step 4.1

Step 4.1. Wide multiple cathode (–) bipolar stimulation
    Most-Dorsal and Dorsal contact cathodes (–)

Most-Ventral contact anode (+)
Change stimulation parameters as described in *Table 14.1—Stimulation parameter adjustment*
    Adverse effects: go to Step 5.0
    Lack of efficacy: Check system for hardware failure; confirm correct DBS lead location. Note that interleaved configurations and parameters have not been recommended at this point in the algorithm, for two reasons. First, there is insufficient experience with this method. Second and based on principle, the most likely use of the interleaved stimulation will be to deal with side effects that are not the issue at this point in the algorithm. Furthermore, monopolar and wide bipolar configurations are most likely to have the highest efficacy and would already have been tested by this point in the algorithm.

Step 5.0. Close single cathode (–) bipolar stimulation
    Most-Ventral contact cathode (–); Dorsal contact anode (+)
    Change stimulation parameters as described in *Table 14.1—Stimulation parameter adjustment*
    Adverse effects: go to Step 5.1
    Lack of efficacy: go to Step 5.1

Step 5.1. Close single cathode (–) bipolar stimulation
    Ventral contact cathode (–); Most-Dorsal contact anode (+)
    Change stimulation parameters as described in *Table 14.1—Stimulation parameter adjustment*
    Adverse effects: go to Step 5.2
    Lack of efficacy: go to Step 5.2

Step 5.2. Close single cathode (–) bipolar stimulation
    Most-Dorsal contact cathode (–); Ventral contact anode (+)
    Change stimulation parameters as described in *Table 14.1—Stimulation parameter adjustment*
    Adverse effects: go to Step 5.3
    Lack of efficacy: go to Step 5.3

Step 5.3. Close single cathode (–) bipolar stimulation
    Dorsal contact cathode (–); Most-Ventral contact anode (+)
    Change stimulation parameters as described in *Table 14.1—Stimulation parameter adjustment*
    Adverse effects: go to Step 7.0
    Lack of efficacy: go to Step 6.0

Step 6.0. Close multiple cathodes (−) bipolar stimulation

Most-Ventral and Ventral contacts cathode (−); Dorsal contact anode (+)

Change stimulation parameters as described in *Table 14.1—Stimulation parameter adjustment*
Adverse effects: go to Step 6.1
Lack of efficacy: go to Step 6.1

Step 6.1. Close multiple cathodes (−) bipolar stimulation

Ventral and Dorsal contacts cathode (−); Most-Dorsal contact anode (+)

Change stimulation parameters as described in *Table 14.1—Stimulation parameter adjustment*
Adverse effects: go to Step 6.2
Lack of efficacy: go to Step 6.2

Step 6.2. Close multiple cathodes (−) bipolar stimulation

Most-Dorsal and Dorsal contact cathodes (−); Ventral contact anode (+)

Change stimulation parameters as described in *Table 14.1—Stimulation parameter adjustment*
Adverse effects: go to Step 6.3
Lack of efficacy: go to Step 6.3

Step 6.3. Close multiple cathodes (−) bipolar stimulation

Dorsal and Ventral contact cathodes (−); Most-Ventral contact anode (+)

Change stimulation parameters as described in *Table 14.1—Stimulation parameter adjustment*
Adverse effects: go to Step 7.0
Lack of efficacy: Check system for hardware failure; confirm correct DBS lead location. Note that interleaved configurations and parameters have not been recommended at this point in the algorithm, for two reasons. First, there is insufficient experience with this method. Second and based on principle, the most likely use of the interleaved stimulation will be to deal with side effects that are not the issue at this point in the algorithm. Furthermore, mon-opolar, wide bipolar, and close bipolar configurations are most likely to have the highest efficacy and would already have been tested by this point in the algorithm.

Step 7.0. Narrow single cathode (−) bipolar stimulation
Most-Ventral contact cathode (−); Ventral contact anode (+)

Change stimulation parameters as described in *Table 14.1—Stimulation parameter adjustment*
Adverse effects: go to Step 7.1
Lack of efficacy: go to Step 7.1

Step 7.1. Narrow single cathode (−) bipolar stimulation
Ventral contact cathode (−); Dorsal contact anode (+)

Change stimulation parameters as described in *Table 14.1—Stimulation parameter adjustment*
Adverse effects: go to Step 7.2
Lack of efficacy: go to Step 7.2

Step 7.2. Narrow single cathode (−) bipolar stimulation
Dorsal contact cathode (−); Most-Dorsal contact anode (+)

Change stimulation parameters as described in *Table 14.1—Stimulation parameter adjustment*
Adverse effects: go to Step 7.3
Lack of efficacy: go to Step 7.3

Step 7.3. Narrow single cathode (−) bipolar stimulation
Ventral contact cathode (−); Most-Ventral contact anode (+)

Change stimulation parameters as described in *Table 14.1—Stimulation parameter adjustment*
Adverse effects: go to Step 7.4
Lack of efficacy: go to Step 7.4

Step 7.4. Narrow single cathode (−) bipolar stimulation
Dorsal contact cathode (−); Ventral contact anode (+)

Change stimulation parameters as described in *Table 14.1—Stimulation parameter adjustment*
Adverse effects: go to Step 7.5
Lack of efficacy: go to Step 7.5

Step 7.5. Narrow single cathode (−) bipolar stimulation
Most-Dorsal contact cathode (−); Dorsal contact anode (+)[3]

Change stimulation parameters as described in *Table 14.1—Stimulation parameter adjustment*
Adverse effects: go to Step 8.0
Lack of efficacy: Check system for hardware failure; confirm correct DBS lead location

Step 8.0. Narrow multiple anodes (+) tripolar stimulation
Dorsal and Most-Ventral contacts anodes (+); Ventral contact cathode (−)

Change stimulation parameters as described in *Table 14.1—Stimulation parameter adjustment*
Adverse effects: go to Step 8.1
Lack of efficacy: go to Step 8.1

Step 8.1. Narrow multiple anodes (+) tripolar stimulation

Most-Dorsal and Ventral contact anodes (+); Dorsal contact cathode (−)

Change stimulation parameters as described in *Table 14.1—Stimulation parameter adjustment*

Adverse effects:

At this point, interleaved configurations and parameters should be tried. The stimulation current/voltage can be apportioned based on the side effect profile and efficacy. For example, if stimulation of the Most-Ventral contact provided greater efficacy but with significant side effects, while the ventral contact produced less efficacy but no side effects, the first step would be to apply the maximum stimulation current/voltage tolerated on the Most Ventral contact and then the maximum stimulation current/voltage tolerated on the Ventral contact and determine whether this resulted in sufficient efficacy without significant side effects. If this fails, check system for hardware failure and confirm correct DBS lead location.

Lack of efficacy: check system for hardware failure; confirm correct DBS lead location.

HELPFUL PROGRAMMING HINTS

USE OF CONSTANT VOLTAGE DBS (TO BE DISCOURAGED)

With constant voltage stimulation, wait at least two weeks after lead implantation before programming the IPG. Starting DBS too soon after implantation could cause marked adverse effects. The relative trauma of implantation can change tissue impedance. For example, if tissue impedance is high immediately after implantation, the patient will require—and will tolerate—higher electrical stimulation currents. However, as the initial tissue reaction subsides, impedance may drop, and the charge density may increase, possibly resulting in adverse effects. Consequently, it is better to postpone programming until tissue reactions have subsided. However, these changes in tissue impedance may not be a factor when using constant current stimulation. The changing impedances acutely following DBS lead implantation are not a problem for constant current IPGs. Programming of constant current IPGs could begin as soon as convenient.

Constant current IPGs have a significant advantage over constant voltage IPGs because the strength of stimulation is the same regardless of changes in the electrode impedances. Even in patients who have had the DBS leads implanted for some time and in whom the variation in electrode impedances is minimal, constant current DBS still is advantageous, for three reasons. First, each electrode may have different impedances; consequently, the same constant voltage applied to a new contact could result in very different

electrical current densities and hence clinical response. Second, because of considerable inter-subject variability in impedances, it is very difficult to generalize one's experience in one patient to predictions of how another patient would respond. This makes learning from experience using constant voltage DBS highly problematic. Thirdly, the DBS pulse waveform is much more efficient at delivering electrical charges.

For patients with implanted segmented DBS leads, it is important to remember when changing for a circumferential continuous stimulation—for example, all the contacts at a certain position on the DBS lead, to a subset of the segmented contacts—the surface area over which the stimulation is applied will change. This could affect the safety of stimulation. Similarly, when changing from fewer to more contacts, the surface area will increase, and the current densities associated with each contact may decrease if the stimulation current is maintained. Note, these suggestions are based on a DBS segmented lead in which the contacts are arranged as sectors around the circumference of the lead in the plane orthogonal to the long axis of the lead. These suggestions may not be appropriate for other segmented DBS lead architectures, but the general principles still may apply. It is important to note that changing from a continuous circumferential contact stimulation to a subset of contacts in a segmented lead can change the surface area of the electrical contacts over which the stimulation is applied. This could change the current densities and thus, affect safety (*see Chapter 5—DBS Safety*). These caveats apply to any and all discussions of segmented DBS leads in this textbook.

CONDUCT A MONOPOLAR SURVEY

The efficacy, and more importantly, the tolerability, of DBS is directly related to the regional anatomy around the active DBS cathodes. Every patient's regional anatomy is potentially different. The monopolar survey can provide a reasonable representation of the regional anatomy unique to each patient. The patient's responses to the monopolar survey also provide important clues to which electrode configurations will be most effective and least likely to cause adverse effects. Not every programmer conducts monopolar surveys, but in my experience, such a survey often makes programming more efficient. An algorithm to facilitate the monopolar survey is described in detail in Chapter 14, Algorithm for Selecting Electrode Configurations and Stimulation Parameters.

ALWAYS INCREASE THE CURRENT/VOLTAGE TO CLARIFY ANY SIDE EFFECTS

The adverse effects from DBS provide important clues about the anatomy around the active DBS cathodes. However, understanding these clues requires clearly assessing the nature of the adverse effects (*see Chapter 10—Clinical Assessments*). For example, a patient may report having a "funny feeling" from a muscle contraction that does not visibly change the muscle's shape or action. This "funny feeling" can be confused with a paresthesia, in turn leading to incorrect inferences about the location of the lead and resulting in incorrect programming. Instead, continue to increase the stimulation current/voltage. If the initial sensation is related to sub-threshold muscle contraction, the contraction will become obvious.

CHECK THERAPEUTIC IMPEDANCES ON IPGS IN ACCORDANCE WITH THE MANFACUTURER'S RECOMMENDATIONS

For constant voltage IPGs, check the therapeutic impedances with each change in electrode configurations, particularly when using multiple active cathodes. Substantial decreases in impedance can increase electrical current densities above safety limits. Note that there have been concerns about the accuracy of measuring

therapeutic impedances, so it is incumbent on the programmer to be thoroughly familiar with the devices being used. Programmers can consult the manufacturer in the event of any questions. Also, some constant voltage IPGs make certain assumptions about therapeutic impedances that may not be warranted, given the patient's unique circumstances (*see Chapter 5—DBS Safety*). You should consult the appropriate manuals to determine stimulation safety and impedance measures.

CONFIRM THAT THE PARAMETERS UNDER PATIENT CONTROL ARE WITHIN SAFE LIMITS

Some IPGs allow the patient or caregiver to increase various DBS stimulation parameters. However, the patient's device may not warn of unsafe stimulation levels. Consequently, if you intend to allow the patient or caregiver to change any parameter, you need to ascertain or test the highest limits under the patient's control to be sure that they are safe.

SYSTEMATICALLY DOCUMENT ALL CLINICAL RESPONSES TO ALL DBS STIMULATION PARAMETERS AND ELECTRODE CONFIGURATIONS

Some programmers document only the final DBS parameters and electrode configurations. This practice may seem efficient in the short term, but in the long term, it may be counterproductive. There are literally thousands of stimulation parameters and electrode configurations. Although relatively few combinations are typically used, some unusual combinations may be required to treat a given patient. You may think that you can determine the most effective combinations in a few programming sessions, but if optimal control is not achieved quickly, you won't remember what combinations you tried. You may miss combinations that would be helpful or that would unnecessarily duplicate the combinations previously found to be ineffective. Should a different programmer assume responsibility for the patient, the new programmer essentially has to start over again, at great cost and with delays in controlling symptoms. The purpose of documentation is not for the convenience of the programmer or for reimbursement, per se. Rather it is to enable others who may assume programming responsibility in the future. Thus, you should document the clinical response to each and every combination of parameters and electrode configurations you try. Examples of forms used to document the clinical response are provided in the *Supplemental Tools - Aid to Programming: Algorithm and Check List for Electrode Configurations, at http://www.greenvilleneuromodulationcenter.com/DBS_Programming_forms/.*

ALWAYS RESET COUNTERS AND TROUBLESHOOT INCONSISTENT RESPONSES

Many DBS systems can be affected by environmental electromagnetic fields. Fields interacting with the DBS leads can generate deleterious electrical current/voltages in the brain. For example, diathermy has resulted in abnormal heating of the DBS contacts, and the resulting tissue destruction has led in some patients to severe neurological impairment and even death. Rarely, electromagnetic fields can also change stimulation parameters and electrode configurations, resulting in undesired stimulation. Unexpectedly turning the stimulator from "on" to "off" could cause sudden worsening of symptoms, or from "off" to "on" could cause undesired adverse effects.

Many sources of electromagnetic fields with the potential to affect IPGs are known, such as metal detectors and MRI scanners, but programmers continue to be surprised by patient encounters with unknown and unanticipated electromagnetic fields. Often, the only evidence of electromagnetic interference is the record of unaccounted activations collected by interrogating the IPG. Frequent rechecking of the number of activations recorded in the IPG and having patients or caregivers frequently check to see if the IPG is on or off and keep diaries of their activities just before they noted the IPG to be off can help identify the source of the interference.

You should also consult the manufacturer's manual for information on possible interfering or dangerous electromagnetic fields.

ADVISE PATIENTS, FAMILY MEMBERS, AND CAREGIVERS TO TAKE THEIR DBS CONTROLLING DEVICES WITH THEM TO EMERGENCY ROOMS OR DOCTOR'S VISITS

Physicians and nurse practitioners who can program DBS systems are in short supply. This shortage may be particularly acute in areas far from where the DBS surgery was performed. However, the shortage of programmers is most acute in emergency situations. The nearest emergency room or the physician's office may not have staff experienced in managing DBS systems. More important, many emergency rooms and physician's offices do not have DBS programming devices. As a consequence, physicians may inappropriately avoid performing tests or procedures that pose no risk or can be conducted following some preparation of the DBS system. Alternatively, the physician may inappropriately perform tests or procedures that expose the patient to risks.

Patients and caregivers should be instructed to take the devices needed to turn the IPGs "off" or "on" to the emergency room or doctor's offices in emergencies. The emergency does not necessarily have to be neurological. For example, patients may require radiological or surgical interventions for any number of reasons, and their evaluation and treatment can be affected by the presence of a DBS system. If the patient or caregiver has the controlling device, local medical staff can be instructed over the telephone as to how to turn the DBS system off. *Importantly, the patient's controlling device may not be able to set the IPG voltages or currents to zero, which is recommended for patients exposed to strong electromagnetic fields such as MRI scans or electrocautery used in surgery.* The increase in the variety of IPGs available and anticipated makes it difficult to discuss every eventuality. Therefore, the programmer should be thoroughly familiar with the DBS systems being used. Generally, it is recommended that centers use a limited number of specific DBS systems so as to maintain proficiency and avoid confusion.

BE PATIENT AND PERSISTENT!

The response of the brain to stimulation is complex and poorly understood. Indeed, the remarkable effectiveness of DBS after failed pharmacological therapies and failed fetal cell transplantation argues for the existence of unique therapeutic mechanisms that are not yet fully understood. In addition, research into the mechanisms of DBS clearly shows that many hypothesized physiological and pathophysiological relationships are untenable and need to be revised. Consequently, the clinical response to DBS is often difficult to predict.

Given the very large numbers of possible combinations of stimulation parameters and electrode configurations, both you and your patients need to be patient and persistent during programming. A common mistake in DBS programming is to give up too soon. Consult with programmers with greater experience, if necessary. You need to be sure that every option has been considered before giving up or scheduling revision surgery.

WHEN IN DOUBT, TURN THE PULSE GENERATOR OFF AND WAIT

Experience with DBS in treating a variety of neurological and psychiatric disorders is increasing rapidly, but you will continually be confronted with novel situations or unusual presentations of more common clinical responses. This uncertainty likely to increase as new devices and new indications emerge.

One of the remarkable and unique features of DBS is its nearly immediate reversibility when stimulation is discontinued. This feature is especially useful when you are trying to determine whether an adverse experience is related to DBS. Suspending stimulation long enough to note changes in adverse events can be a useful strategy. However, do so carefully, because the patient's original symptoms will probably worsen.

TROUBLESHOOTING

The majority of problems with DBS programming relate to poor placement of the DBS leads or a particular patient's unique regional anatomy around the DBS lead. Chapter 11, Approach to DBS in the Vicinity of the Subthalamic Nucleus, Chapter 12, Approach to DBS in the Vicinity of the Globus Pallidus Interna, and Chapter 13, Approach DBS in the Vicinity of the Ventral Intermediate Nuclues of the Thalamus address potential solutions to these problems. This section addresses some approaches to diagnosing hardware and/or electrical problems. Again, these methods are based on the principles covered in Chapter 2, Principles of DBS Electronics, and Chapter 3, Principles of Electrophysiology.

Hardware or electrical problems generally can be of two types: (1) a lack of efficacy despite exhaustive attempts at DBS programming, and (2) adverse

effects. Adverse effects can be caused by stimulating unintended structures but in the presence of normally functioning hardware and electronics. Alternatively, adverse effects can be the result of electrical malfunctions, resulting in unintended stimulation.

Lack of effect because of hardware and/or electronic causes is usually associated with a break in the electrical continuity of the system or the migration of the DBS lead out of the effective target region in the brain. A wire in the extension or DBS lead may have broken. There may be a defect in the implanted pulse generator (IPG) itself. A break in the electrical continuity of the system usually manifests as high impedance and limited current being passed. This can be determined in many IPGs by the electrode impedance test. (Note that the electrode impedance test is different from the therapeutic impedance test for some IPGs.) The electrode impedance test conducts a check of the impedance and electrical current flowing between all possible pairs of DBS lead contacts and the IPG case. A high impedance—for example, in some systems greater than 2000 ohms and a low current—would be less than 15 μa. However, with the increase in the number and types of different DBS systems, it

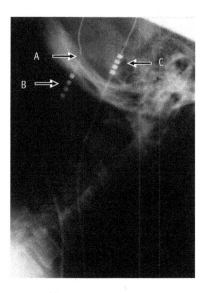

Figure 15.1: X-ray demonstrating a DBS lead fracture (A). A physical discontinuity can be seen in the DBS lead. The extension connection is in the neck (B) as opposed to over the skull (C). Placing the connector in the neck and its migration from the skull to the neck are associated with a high risk of lead fracture.

is important that you check the manufacturer's manual of the specific system or consult directly with the manufacturer. Note that measuring impedances is complicated (see Note Regarding Impedances in *Chapter 2, Principles of DBS Electronics*). You should consult the manufacturer's recommendations about interpreting the electrode impedances and currents.

A break in electrical continuity could be the result of a wire conductor fracture or a disconnection between the DBS lead and the extension wire, or between the extension wire and the IPG. A skull (Anterior-Postereior (AP) and lateral views), neck, and chest X-ray can be used to look for fractures or disconnections (Figures 15.1 and 15.2). We recommend obtaining these X-rays as a matter of routine immediately post-operatively. In addition to demonstrating the physical integrity of the system and its connections, it is also helpful for subsequent comparisons, particularly if a lead migration is anticipated.

Note that placement of the junction between the DBS lead and the extension wire in the neck increases the risk of lead fracture. Most surgeons are aware of this potential problem and place the junction over the skull. However, the junction can migrate with head movement about the neck. It is wise to periodically check the position with routine skull X-rays. If the connector migrates into the neck, some consideration of revision should be given to prevent a lead fracture which would require a revision of the entire DBS system.

Another approach to determine whether electrical current is reaching the DBS lead is to use a small portable AM radio set to the lowest frequency. The AM radio can pick electrical noise or interference when brought close to the DBS lead or extension. Failure to hear the electrical noise suggests that no current is flowing through the DBS lead or extension. *A note of caution: you may need to move the AM radio around to*

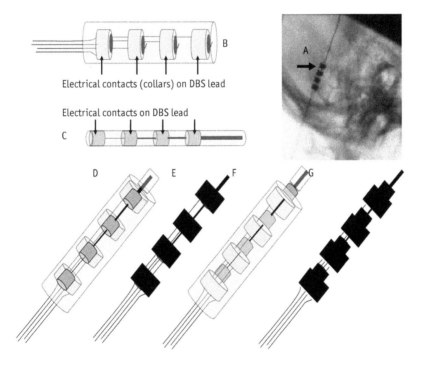

Figure 15.2: Schematic representation of a normal connection and a disconnection between the DBS lead (C) and the extension (B). Figure A shows a normal connection between the DBS lead and the extension on X-ray (reverse image). The extension (B) has a series of metal collars that act to contact the electrical contacts on the DBS lead (C). If there is proper alignment (D), the electrical contacts should be inside the collars. On X-ray, the collars will be seen, while the electrical contacts of the DBS lead will not be seen, as shown in A. If the DBS lead is pulled out of proper alignment (F), then the electrical contacts will not be wholly contained within the electrical collars (F) and will be seen on X-ray (G, reverse image).

obtain the proper orientation of the AM radio antenna to the DBS system. You should perfect your technique on a DBS system that you know is working.

Positive adverse effects associated with a DBS hardware and/or electrical failure usually relate to a short-circuit. But the positive symptoms, usually manifesting as paresthesias, can be frustratingly intermittent. Sometimes it is head position–dependent. Sometimes, asking the patient to position his or her head in various positions can reproduce the symptoms. Sometimes, gentle palpation on the DBS IPG, extension wire, extension wire/DBS lead junction, or DBS lead can reproduce the positive symptoms.

These positive symptoms are often associated with multiple breaks in the extension or DBS lead, allowing the exposed conductor in one wire to electrically contact the broken end of another wire and causing improper stimulation. Sometimes, a short-circuit may be due to electrically conductive fluid entering into the connections. A check of the electrode impedances usually reveals low impedance and a relatively high current. You should consult the manufacturer's recommendations about interpreting the electrode impedances and currents.

Some patients may have unusual sensations over the IPG site. Typically, this occurs with the IPG in monopolar configuration with the metal contact surface of the IPG is electrically active and the anode. This can stimulate peripheral nerves or cause muscle contractions. Routinely, the IPG is placed with the metal contact in contact with the skin rather than the underlying tissue, particularly muscle tissue. Sometimes the IPG can "flip," so that the metal electrical contact surface of the IPG is now in electrical contact with the muscle. Monopolar stimulation with the IPG case as the positive contact could then cause muscle contractions.

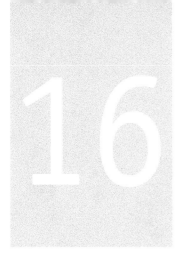

OSCILLATOR BASICS

Increasingly, brain physiology is thought to be based on neural oscillators (Busaki 2006). Several kinds of oscillations can occur: some at the level of individual neurons (*neuronal oscillators*), and others consequent to interactions among neurons connected in closed feedback loops (neural oscillators). Given the increasing importance of neural oscillators, a basic understanding of them would be helpful. Therefore, the following discussion is intended to provide an intuitive sense of these oscillators. Interested readers are encouraged to consult other works for more definitive and, particularly, mathematical discussions (e.g., Strogatz 1994).

The defining feature of oscillatory activity is the recurrence or repetition of a phenomenon, such as the repetitive flashing of a light at a railroad crossing. When this type of repetitive activity recurs at specific time periods, it is called *periodic*. However, not all periodic activity is necessarily oscillatory. What distinguishes oscillatory activity as a subgroup of periodic activities is the presumption that the underlying mechanism of the activity involves a repeating closed process. Some periodic activities can be produced by non-repeating processes. Imagine a line of soldiers passing by in review, saluting the review stand as they pass. The salutes would be a repeating or periodic phenomenon. However, the underlying mechanism is not repeating, because each recurring salute is given by a different soldier. However, if the soldiers were to march in a circle in front of the reviewing stand and

to salute the stand each time they approached it, then the salutes would be oscillatory: the periodic behavior is produced by a repeating process, not by a series of independent processes.

Given this intuitive notion of an oscillator, we can address how oscillators are measured, how they interact, and how they can perform important brain functions. There are many examples of physical oscillatory activity, such as the back-and-forth movement of a pendulum, or racecars traversing a circular racetrack (Figure 16.1). When the racecar is viewed from ground level, the cicular motion will be seen as a back and forth motion, either as a sine or cosine wave. Such back-and-forth motion is considered an oscillation and clearly is appreciated as the racecar traversing the track. The magnitude of the back and forth motion is the amplitude of the sine or cosine wave. As can be appreciated, the amplitude of the sine or cosine wave is directly related to the radius of the race track. The time it takes to make one complete back-and-forth motion from and back to the same starting position is the period of the sine or cosine wave. As can be appreciated, the period corresponds to the time it takes the racecar to may one complete lap on the race track. The number of time of a complete back-and-forth motion or lap per second is the frequency of the oscillation. Note that the sine wave and cosine wave are related to each other because they are just different prespectives of the same racecar on the same track. However, when viewed from position A* in Figure 16.1, the racecar starts at the middle and

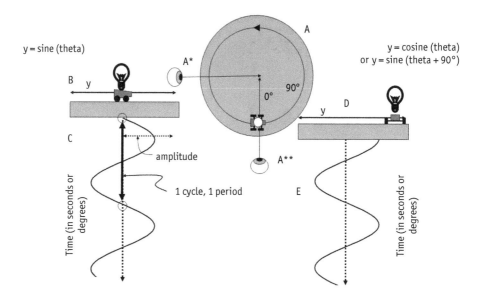

Figure 16.1 An example of an oscillator represented by a racecar moving on a closed, circular track. A light is attached to the top of the car. The importance of the light will eventually be clear, but for the moment, the light is assumed to be constantly on. View A shows the racecar and track from above, and the racecar is seen as moving in a circle. The starting point can be referenced to any arbitrary point, but a point of convenience might be the line of sight from the eye to the center of the racetrack. Thus, two lines—the line of sight to the center of the racetrack, and the line connecting the position of the racecar to the center of the racetrack—create an angle, *theta*. The speed of the racecar can be measured by its ground speed around the track, for example as miles per hour. Alternatively, the speed of the racecar also can be measured by the number of degrees that the angle, theta, changes per unit of time (such as seconds). This alternative description in degrees per second is termed the *angular velocity*.

When the racecar circling the track is viewed from ground level, the appearance is quite different (B and D). Now the racecar is seen as moving back and forth. If we could trace the back-and-forth movement of the car over time, we would have a tracing that looks like a sine wave (C) or cosine wave (E), depending on the viewpoint. We can now define the movement of the racecar as a sine or cosine function. We also can translate certain features of the sine or cosine functions to the angular descriptions when the racecar is viewed from the top (A). The time it takes for the sine or cosine wave to complete both the negative and positive parts of the wave is the *period* of the wave and correlates with the time it takes the racecar to make one circuit around the racetrack. The *frequency* is the number of complete cycles in the sine or cosine function per unit of time (typically seconds) and correlates with the number of times the racecar goes around the track in a unit of time. The frequency and period are related, and the frequency is the inverse of the period (frequency = 1 ÷ period). The maximum distance to the right and then to the left that the racecar moves back and forth in the side view (B and D) would be the *amplitude,* and it corresponds to the radius of the circular track when viewed from above (A).

Note that the initial position of the racecar is different depending on the perspectives A* and A**. The position of the car measured in the degrees from the original line of sight is the *phase*. Note that the perspective of A** in view B shows the initial position to be in the middle of the track in the line of sight. Thus, the initial phase is 0°, and the subsequent tracing of the movement produces a sine wave. From perspective A* in view E, the initial position is at the rightmost edge of the tract, corresponding to the maximum amplitude, and with a phase of 90° and the subsequent back and forth movement traces a cosine wave.

At the start, there is a phase difference between the two perspectives of 90°. This phase difference is maintained as the racecar circles the track. Thus, the views from the side perspectives (B and D) maintain the same phase difference and consequently are *phase-locked*. In addition, each observer would measure the same frequency; consequently, the two observations are *frequency-coherent*. This makes sense because both observers are viewing the same car. However, it does become significant if at the beginning the observers don't know that they are observing the same mechanism.

can be considered starting at angle 0 degrees, which is referred to as the phasae. The racecar starts at the right when viewed from perspective A** and can be said to start at an angle of 90 degress. Thus, the two perspective differ by 90 degrees or their phase difference is 90

degrees. These features are the parameters that characterize oscillatory activities.

Oscillators can be complex, especially when they result from interactions or combinations of other oscillators. Consider the example in Figure 16.2. The

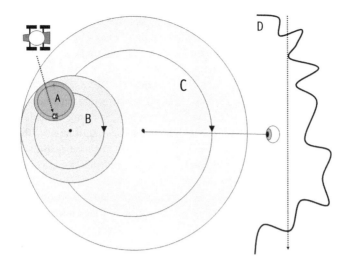

Figure 16.2 In this example, the original racecar track (A) shown in Figure 16.1 is itself circling another, larger racetrack (B), which itself is circling an even larger racetrack (C). When viewed from the perspective represented by the schematic eye, the back-and-forth motion of the racecar will be complicated (D). Tracing D is purely hypothetical and does not actually describe the back-and-forth motion of the racecar, it just shows that the motion is complicated.

back-and-forth motion, when viewed from the level of the racetrack, will be complicated and will depend on the angular velocity, or the speeds (degrees of the arc traversed per second) of the car on track A (w_A), on the angular velocity track A on track B (w_B), and the angular velocity of track B on track C (w_C).

The path of the car depends on the diameters of track A (d_A), track B (d_B), and track C (d_C). Finally, the starting position (measured by the arc between the initial position of the racecar and an arrow from the eye to the center of racetrack A [θ_A], track B [θ_B], and track C [θ_C]) must be considered. However, the complicated motion is really just the sum of the oscillations occurring on each track. The oscillatory activity on the first track (A) is summed with the oscillatory activity on the second track (B), which then is summed with the oscillatory activity on the third track (C), producing the plot of the location of the racecar *over time* (D). Thus, the position (y) of the racecar on the horizontal plane of the racetrack at time t is given by Equation 16.1:

$$y = d_A * sine(\theta_A + w_A * t) + d_B * sine(\theta_B + w_B * t)$$
$$+ d_C * sine(\theta_C + w_C * t) \qquad \text{Eq. 16.1}$$

The term "y" is the position of the racecar in the field of view, and it increases and decreases as the racecar moves back and forth in the observer's view. The term "$d_A * sine(\theta_A + w_A * t)$" represents the position of the racecar on Track A, where "d_A" is the diameter of Track A, "θ_A" is the starting point on Track A measured as an angle when viewed from above, and the change in the position from the initial position and is determined by the product of the angular velocity, "w_A", and time, "t", since the observations began. The other terms for each of the other tracks can be understood similarly.

An unlimited number of racetracks can be constructed by stacking them on top of each other (Figure 16.2). Similarly, the complexity of the movement of the racecar on the horizontal plane of the racetracks in unlimited. But no matter how complicated the movement of the racecar, it can always be understood as the sum of the contributions made by all the racetracks. You only have to know the values of the variables: the diameter, angular velocity, and initial position (phase) of each track. However, most remarkable is the fact that all these values can be determined from the complicated path itself. A mathematical technique, the Fourier transform, can determine the number of oscillators and their values. (*See Strogatz, 1994.*) Consequently, any periodic behavior can be decomposed into a Fourier transform series similar to that shown in Equation 16.2:

$$F(t) = d_A * sine(\theta_A(t)) + d_B * sine(\theta_B(t))$$
$$+ d_C * sine(\theta_C(t)) + ... \text{ and so on} \qquad \text{Eq. 16.2}$$

$F(t)$ is the same as "y" above in Equation 16.1 except the notation including "t" denotes the dependence of "y" over time. The sine of the various angle functions, $\theta_A(t)$, $\theta_B(t)$, $\theta_C(t)$, ..., determines the amplitudes of the components of the signal $F(t)$ through time. In this case, $\theta_A(t)$ takes the place of $(\theta_A + w_A{}^*t)$ to demonstrate the dependence of $\theta_A(t)$. This new $\theta_A(t)$ is simplified from the previous $(\theta_A + w_A{}^*t)$ in Equation 16.2, because all the initial or starting angles are the same and thereby can be dropped from consideration. The value of amplitude of the components will rise and fall from the value of "1," through "0," to "–1" and back again, tracing a sinusoidal wave (Figure 16.1). The rates or speeds by which the amplitudes rise and fall, hence the frequencies, are related to the unique functions, $\theta_A(t)$, $\theta_B(t)$, $\theta_C(t)$, ... Indeed, the change in angles over time that are regular and repeating, such as $\theta_A(t)$, thus tracing a sine wave over time, themselves can be considered a frequency (see below, and Equation 16.3). The values, d_A, d_B, d_C ..., relate to the amplitude (or power) of the specific oscillator, roughly analogous to the diameters of the racetracks. Consequently, the complex movements of the racecar on the horizontal surface can be considered a complex periodic function that itself is merely the sum of the periodic function of each of the component sine waves produced by oscillators of a single frequency. The contribution of each frequency is weighted by the values d_A, d_B, d_C ....

Fourier transforms are used to determine the power spectra that indicate how much power at any one frequency is represented in the complex periodic behavior. The power spectra of any complex periodic behavior are important measures of the complex behavior. Any time-varying signal, particularly repeating or periodic signals, $F(t)$, can be represented as the sum of simple frequencies, f_A, f_B, f_C, ... with their associated magnitude constants, d_A, d_B, d_C .... (Equation 16.3). Likewise, the final complex behavior can be determined from knowing the frequencies and magnitudes (and the phase of the frequencies, not shown, which varies over time).

$$F(t) \propto d_A{}^*f_A + d_B{}^*f_B + d_c{}^*f_c + \dots \quad \text{and so on } \textbf{Eq. 16.3}$$

The concept of building complex periodic behaviors from combinations of simple oscillators of different frequencies and phases (a process called an *inverse Fourier transform*) is an important and powerful concept that can be applied to the complex orchestration of muscle activities that underlie movement. For example, muscle activations for rapid single-joint movements have a characteristic pattern (*see Chapter 7—DBS Effects on Motor Control*). Initially, a burst in the agonist muscle activity is followed by a burst in the antagonist muscle and finally by a third burst in the agonist muscle. The initial agonist burst overcomes the inertial loads of the limb, and the antagonist burst brakes the initial acceleration so that the limb does not go past the target. The final agonist burst brings the limb to the target.

The actual muscle activities are caused by repetitive discharges of the lower motor neurons, which, in turn, are being driven by repetitive discharges of neurons in the basal ganglia–thalamic-cortical system (and also with the input of the cerebellum, although not discussed here, but *see Chapter 7—DBS Effects on Motor Control*). The repetitive discharges of the lower motor neurons can be thought of as reflecting the activities of an oscillator(s), like the racecar on the first track. The goal, then, is to modulate the activity of the first oscillator(s) so as to modulate the number of motor units it (they) recruits. This modulation can be accomplished by other oscillators. The complex pattern of muscle activity described above (called the *triphasic pattern of muscle activity for ballistic movements*) can be understood as the inverse Fourier transform of the activities of the oscillators in the basal ganglia–thalamic-cortical system, as posited in the Systems Oscillators Theory (Montgomery 2008b).

The notion that patterns of increasing and decreasing muscle activity are a consequence of an inverse Fourier transform of oscillator activities in the basal ganglia (and by extension, cerebellum)–thalamic-cortical systems can be extended to complex behaviors and skill acquisition. As described above, any periodic function (within certain assumptions and limiting conditions), including any arbitrarily complex patterns of muscle activities underlying the most complex behaviors, can be decomposed by Fourier transformation into the summed or integrated activities of several oscillators. Mathematically, any arbitrarily complex function can be learned by a network of loosely coupled oscillators, provided there are enough oscillators to cover the range of frequencies in the complex function—for example, the functions, f_A, f_B, f_C ..., in Equation 16.3. Through repeated training, the "coupling strength" between certain oscillators, represented by d_A, d_B, d_C . . . , is strengthened and between others weakened, until entering only the initial part of the original complex function is sufficient for the network of oscillators to produce the entire remaining portion of the complex function (Longuet-Higgins 1968).

We can apply this concept to movement and show that neurons in the basal ganglia–thalamic-cortical system simultaneously entrain many different frequencies (Montgomery 2004a; Montgomery 2008b). Thus, the basal ganglia–thalamic-cortical system can be thought as a set of loosely coupled oscillators. With repeated training, associations between oscillators are created by "strengthening" some and "weakening" others, so that finally, when the neuronal analogue of the intention to produce a behavior is introduced into the basal ganglia (and cerebellum)–thalamic-cortical system, the coupled oscillators can produce the entire motor behavior. This initial intent need not itself specify the subsequent modulation of activity in the ventral lateral thalamic–motor cortical oscillator, but merely trigger the completion of the signal, which is specific to the necessary modulation of the ventrolateral thalamic–motor cortical oscillator. This initial intent could arise internally or be triggered by external events.

Another important implication from the modeling of loosely coupled oscillators is that the same system of oscillators can be trained to produce a variety of outputs in response to different inputs, a concept called *holographic memory* (Longuet-Higgins 1968). Thus, the same piece of anatomy can encode multiple functions. Therefore, a precise one-to-one correspondence between a given region of the brain and a specific function is not necessary. Historically, the efforts of neuroscience have been to establish such one-to-one anatomical–functional correspondences (correlations), but they have not always worked. The principles of holographic memory suggest that this premise of a strict one-to-one correspondence is not necessary (Montgomery 2008b). However, the power of this long-held presumption of a one-to-one correspondence is evident in the results of a study where non-experts were more likely to believe a bad explanation when they were falsely told that the property was localized to a certain brain region (Weisberg et al. 2008).

The oscillators described thus far have been *harmonic oscillators*, which means that their behaviors, graphed as sinusoidal functions, are continuous and everywhere differentiable, in the sense of calculus. Their behaviors are periodic and therefore predictable. However, many oscillators are not harmonic. For example, whereas the waxing and waning of a tornado-warning siren is a harmonic oscillator, the beating of a drum is a discrete oscillator; it is episodic, not continuous. In certain circumstances, a discrete oscillator (*see Chapter 17—Discrete Neural Oscillators*) may be described in the same terms as a "harmonic oscillator," but not always. Discrete oscillators are more likely to be non-linear (not describable in relatively simple mathematics) and consequently, less predictable. However, these non-linear features give these oscillators unique advantages.

Interacting harmonic oscillators have a very large number of important properties that can be exploited in engineering. Examples include the mechanical oscillators that make up clockworks. Indeed, clockworks in the 1700s and 1800s were able to perform very complex and nearly animal- and human-like behaviors (Figure 16.3) through the interactions among gears, which can be viewed as different oscillators. Consider music and speech, which are various oscillations in the air that are translated into first mechanical and then neuronal oscillations in the ear.

Amplitude-modulated (AM) radios and radio stations utilize oscillators to transmit and receive information such as music and speech. The radio station sends out a carrier signal at a specific frequency (Figure 16.4). The information is encoded in the amplitude of the carrier frequency. At the same time, many other AM radio stations are transmitting information. For the radio receiver to select the information from a single specific radio transmission station, the receiver has an oscillator that can be tuned to the frequency of the carrier signal from the desired radio transmission station. The oscillator in the receiver interacts with the oscillator of the carrier signal to amplify that carrier signal above all others and thus, tune in the specific radio station.

The interactions between the harmonic oscillators described above for AM radios are examples of *positive resonance*, where the oscillator in the radio receiver adds to the oscillators received from the radio station. Car mufflers are an example of oscillators interacting to reduce sounds by *negative resonance*. The car muffler takes the sound waves of the engine

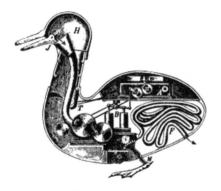 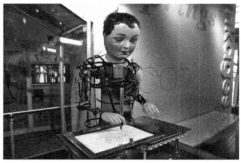

Figure 16.3 Two examples of automatons based on oscillators (gears) demonstrating complex behaviors driven by mechanical mechanisms. The *Canard Digérateur*, or Digesting Duck, invented by Jacques de Vaucanson in 1739 was reported to bite, chew and swallow feed, and to produce and "lay" an artificial egg. More advanced automatons, such as shown in the panel to the right, were humanlike in appearance and could write or draw complex images (see https://www.youtube.com/watch?v=C70SFNKIlaM).

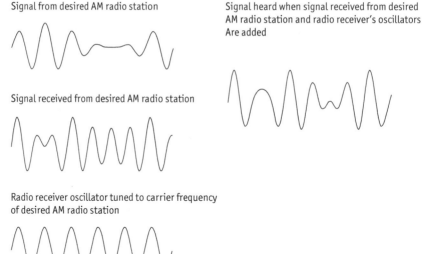

Figure 16.4: Schematic representation of independently encoded information among different oscillators that use the same medium, such as a two radio signals from two radio stations. In this representation, the different oscillators are the electromagnetic waves generated in space at different fundamental frequencies unique to each radio station. The desired AM radio station transmits an electromagnetic wave of a specific frequency. The transmitted information is encoded in the various amplitudes of the same electromagnetic wave (the signal from the desired AM radio station). The antenna of the AM radio receiver receives the signal from the desired AM station along with signals from all the other AM radio stations in the area. The AM receiver has an oscillator tuned to the carrier frequency of the desired AM radio station, which is added to the received signal. The result is then sent to the radio's speaker, which renders the signal audible over the other signals that are not amplified. The result is an acceptable replication of the original signal from the desired AM radio station.

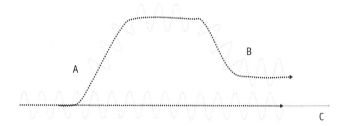

Figure 16.5: Schematic representation of negative resonance, as might be found in a car muffler. The engine noise enters the muffler and is divided into two paths (A). One part continues in a straight line, while the other is diverted to take a longer path. The two paths are brought back together (B), where they interact. However, because of the longer path, the diverted sound waves are phase-delayed relative to the sound waves that passed through. The interaction is such that high pressures of the diverted wave align with the low pressures in the sound wave not diverted, and similarly, the low pressures of the diverted wave match the high pressures of the sound not diverted. As a consequence, the two sound waves cancel each other out (C).

(considered as an oscillator) and routes them back to interact with the other sound waves. However, the timing is adjusted so that a high pressure of the engine sound interacts with the low pressure of the rerouted sound in the muffler, and the sound waves cancel each other out (Figure 16.5).

Continuous harmonic oscillators also display *beat interactions*, where sounds from two different sources interact to produce a wavering quality. For example, a sound at 1000 Hz can interact with a sound of 1050 Hz to produce a sound that wavers at 50 Hz (Figure 16.6). The beat interactions have important implications for

studies of oscillator power in local field potentials. Because of the relatively large surface area of the electrical contacts typical of local field potential recordings, the recordings may reflect beta phenomena among multiple simultaneously recorded oscillators. Thus, a beta oscillation of 20 Hz could be produced by any combination of individual oscillators whose differences in frequencies equal 20 Hz: for example, 100 Hz and 120 Hz or 280 Hz and 300 Hz oscillators. The presence of power in the beta frequencies, such as 20 Hz, does not mean that an oscillator at 20 Hz actually exists.

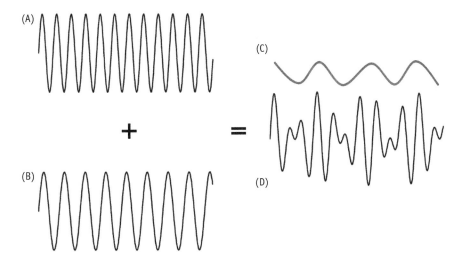

Figure 16.6: Schematic representation of beat interactions between two oscillators of different frequencies (A and B). When these two oscillators are combined (D), there results a complex oscillator whose magnitude (C) oscillates, typically at a frequency that is the difference between the frequencies of the two original oscillators.

The discussion above of the dynamics of continuous harmonic oscillators is not meant to suggest that actual neuronal and neural oscillators operate as continuous harmonic oscillators. Rather, neuronal and neural oscillators are more likely to operate as discrete oscillators (*see Chapter 17—Discrete Neural Oscillators*). However, many of the dynamics just described for continuous harmonic oscillators will be applicable to discrete oscillators as well.

DISCRETE NEURAL OSCILLATORS

IMPORTANCE OF NEURAL OSCILLATORS IN NERVOUS SYSTEM FUNCTION

Research has shown time and again that the therapeutic mechanisms of action of DBS involve neural and neuronal oscillators. A distinction is made here between neural and neuronal oscillators at the level of description, but the physiologies are inextricably linked. *Neural oscillators* relate to a description at the level of closed loop (feedback) multi-neuronal polysynaptic circuits primarily on account of the propagations of action potentials through the circuit. *Neuronal oscillators* relate primarily to periodic fluctuations of electrical potentials across the neuronal membrane, particularly in the soma, which is reflected in an action potential–initiating segment. Because generation of action potentials is determined by the status of the transmembrane electrical potential at the action potential–initiating segment, the two levels are tied. However, the all-or-nothing nature of an action potential becomes shorthand, as it were, for electrical events occurring in the action potential–initiating segment and the axons. Because these phenomena are ultimately electrical, they provide means by which DBS may affect operations of the nervous system. Also, these effects are likely to be best understood according to DBS's effects on neural and neuronal oscillators.

It has been increasingly recognized that, with respect to DBS for movement disorders, the basal ganglia–thalamic-cortical system functions are a network of loosely coupled nonlinear neural oscillators, and that DBS may be regarded as an additional nonlinear oscillator that is embedded among the oscillators of the basal ganglia–thalamic-cortical system (*see Chapter 8—Pathophysiological Mechanisms*). Networks of loosely coupled nonlinear oscillators may be ubiquitous in the central nervous system, intervening between effectors, such as lower motor neurons, and peripheral sensors, such as the retina. Dynamics of systems of oscillators may thus be central to effective post-operative DBS management for any neurological and psychiatric disorder. This will become clearer with further development of technologies that exploit the dynamics of oscillators, such as paired-pulse and interleaved pulse trains of different frequencies. The present writing introduces the concepts of neural oscillators; most importantly, discrete neural oscillators. This chapter builds on information introduced in Chapter 16—Oscillator Basics.

Rafael Lorente de Nó (Lorente de Nó 1933) and Donald O. Hebb (Hebb 1949) suggested that reentrant oscillations formed by closed long chains of neurons served short-term memory and various other neural functions. De Nó went as far as to suggest that abnormal oscillators may underlie Parkinson's disease—related to sustained rest tremor, perhaps—and obsessive-compulsive disorder, the obsessions thereof he may have considered "perseverative behavior." Later scientists discounted these possibilities, arguing

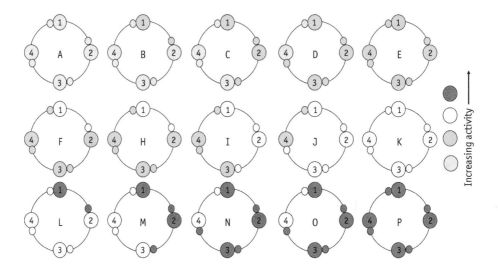

Figure 17.1: Schematic representation of a four-node continuous oscillator in which all interactions are depolarizing and excitatory. In A, activities in neurons of each node are at a minimal discharge frequency. At time B, the neuronal activity of neurons in node 1 increases. The increase in activities then propagates to neurons in each successive node until it reaches the neurons in node 1 at time E. Neuronal activities in the nodes, which have further increased, propagate repeatedly through the oscillator until all neurons in all nodes have reached the maximum neuronal activity, as indicated by the solid red circles. At time P, the oscillator is said to be *saturated*.

that any closed reentrant long chain of neurons with predominantly excitatory interactions would drive oscillators to saturation (Figure 17.1). Also, for certain neurons, which have a baseline frequency of discharge that may be increased or decreased by depolarizing or hyperpolarizing inputs, respectively, any reentrant circuit having an even number of hyperpolarizing neurons would experience an overall net excitatory effect produced by the subsequent neuron, resulting in an overall positive feedback loop (Figure 17.3). For these same types of neurons, all, or an odd number, of neurons that hyperpolarize a subsequent neuron would result in inhibition—that is, in an overall negative feedback loop (Figure 17.2). The prevailing presumption in de Nó and Hebb's time was that such negative feedback oscillators would cease their oscillations, and this was described as "a collapse" of the oscillator (Milner 1996).

It is clear from research on nervous systems of invertebrates that having entirely inhibitory neurons does not lapse into inactivity as the inhibition would shut down all the neurons (Manor et al. 1999). At least one mechanism that prevents collapse is post-inhibitory rebound excitation. The effect is schematically represented in Figure 17.4. As may be appreciated from the hypothetical oscillator represented in Figure 17.4,

neurons are able to increase or decrease their activities without collapse or saturation of the oscillator, and information may thus be continuously processed within it. In many ways, the oscillators of the basal ganglia–thalamic-cortical system are analogous, as the majority of the interconnections are mediated by the hyperpolarizing neurotransmitter, GABA, and at least some of the neurons demonstrate rebound excitation following hyperpolarization.

CONTINUOUS HARMONIC OSCILLATORS

Defined as changes in states (degrees of neuronal activities) over time, *dynamics* in the different oscillators shown in Figures 17.1 depend on effects that are induced at one period and carry to the next time period. There are several mechanisms that prolong the consequent changes, such as the time course of postsynaptic transmembrane electrical potentials, in part determined by the dynamics of ligand-gated ionic conductance channels, as well as by cascading effects in the electrical dynamics such as post-hyperpolarization rebound depolarization (Goaillard et al. 2010). Yet this often is

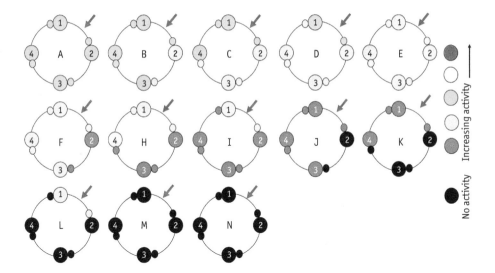

Figure 17.2: Schematic representation of a four-node continuous oscillator in which all but one interaction depolarizes and becomes excited. One interconnection indicated by the red arrow is hyperpolarizing and inhibiting (the distinction between hyperpolarizing and exciting is discussed in the main text: *see Chapter 6—Nervous System Responses to DBS*). Similar dynamics are observed in any oscillator with an odd number of hyperpolarizing and inhibiting interactions. In A, the activities in the neurons of each node are at a moderate discharge frequency. At time B, the activity in neurons of node 1 reduces the activity in neurons in the subsequent node 2, which in turn reduces the activities in subsequent nodes C–L until all neuronal activities have ceased, as indicated by the solid black circles. The oscillator is said to have *collapsed*.

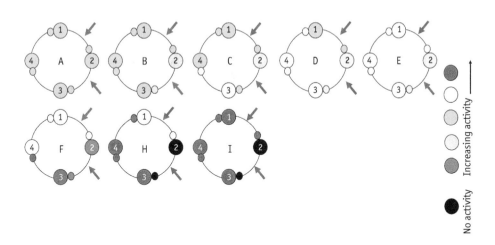

Figure 17.3: Schematic representation of a four-node continuous oscillator in which all but two interactions depolarize and become excited. Two interconnections indicated by the red arrows are hyperpolarizing and inhibiting (the distinction between hyperpolarizing and exciting is discussed in the text and represented in Figure 17.4). There are an even number of nodes whose neurons are thus hyperpolarizing and inhibiting. In A, activities in neurons of each node have a moderate discharge frequency. At time B, activity in neuron in node 1 reduces the activity in subsequent neurons in node 2, which in turn reduces inhibition of neurons in node 3 at time C. At time D, increased activity in neurons in node 3 results in increased activity in neurons of node 4, which at time E increases activity in neurons in node 1. The process continues. By time I, activities in neurons of nodes 1, 3, and 4 have become observably saturated.

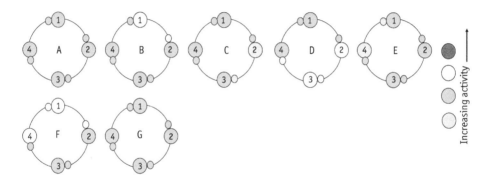

Figure 17.4: Schematic representation of a four-node continuous oscillator in which all interactions hyperpolarize, resulting in an initial reduction of neuronal activity in the subsequent nodes, which then experience rebound excitation. At time A, all neurons in the nodes are moderately active. At time B, an excitation of neurons in node 1 reduces activities of neurons in node 2 at time C. Reduced neuronal activity in node 2 results in increased neuronal activity in node 3 at time D, which in turn results in reduced neuronal activity in node 4 at time E. Rebound neuronal excitation in node 2 reduces the previously greater neuronal activity in node 3 to normal at time E (in this hypothetical case). Decreased neuronal activity in node 4 at time E, which is due to increased neuronal activity in node 3, results in decreased inhibition of neurons in node 1 and subsequent increased activities of neurons in node 1 at time F. Rebounding increased neuronal activity in node 4 at time F reduces the increased neuronal activity in node 1 to normal at time G. The oscillator neither saturates nor collapses.

not the case in discrete oscillators. Thus, in continuous oscillators, the effects in each node's individual neurons are incremental or decremental from the previous time period. In this sense, an oscillator may be described as "continuous." Concepts borrowed from the physics of classically defined continuous harmonic oscillators

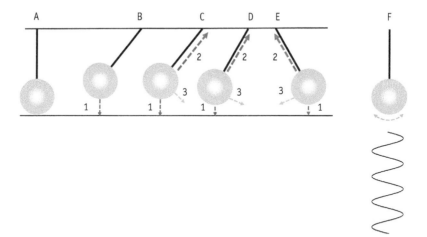

Figure 17.5: Schematic representation of a simple harmonic oscillator consisting of a weight (pendulum) suspended by a cable. At A, the system is at equilibrium (rest). At B, the pendulum is displaced to the left. As a consequence, potential energy is created (translated from the force that displaced the pendulum). It is denoted by vector 1. The potential energy creates force, gravity, to move the pendulum downward (B). The cable creates a restraining force that will not permit the pendulum to fall in a straight line relative to gravitational force (C). A resultant force is created (vector 3) from gravitational and restraining forces that move the pendulum toward the equilibrium position at rest (D). The pendulum gains kinetic energy from the acceleration and creates a force that moves the pendulum past the equilibrium point (E). The consequence is generation of more potential-energy gravitational force, that when combined by the restraining force, moves the pendulum in the opposite direction. And the process repeats. If no energy is lost—owing to friction, for example—the pendulum will continue to sway back and forth. Over time, it will begin to trace a sine wave whose phase is 90 degrees (F).

may help provide a basis of neural and neuronal oscillators, which extends to discrete neural oscillators.

A *harmonic oscillator* is a system whose force displaces it from equilibrium and whose displacement generates an equal counterforce that restores it to equilibrium. Illustrative of this phenomenon is the case of a simple frictionless pendulum (Figure 17.5). The motion of the pendulum over time traces a sine wave whose initial phase is 90 degrees (*see Chapter 16—Oscillator Basics, for definitions of terms*). If one assumes that the nervous system, particularly the brain, is a network of interacting oscillators, one may begin to understand possible interactions in the light of actual interactions, primarily by addition, between continuous harmonic oscillators by combinations of continuous sine waves.

Continuous sine waves and physical systems represented by them interact by addition. Thus, the consequence or result of interactions between any two points on two continuous sine waves, for example, is the addition of the values at each point. This phenomenon is known as *resonance* (Figure 17.6). The result may be increased positive or negative amplitude if the values of the two points are of the same sign (i.e., both are positive or negative), or it may be reduced amplitude if the values of the two points are different. Increasing the amplitude is positive resonance; decreasing the amplitude is negative resonance. If at every point the two sine waves have equal amplitude, the resulting merged wave will simply become amplified. If at every point the two sine waves have opposite signs, the resulting merged wave will become diminished. It must be noted that, in order for the amplification or diminishment to occur, the two sine waves must share both frequency and phase. When some homologous points on the interacting sine waves are a mix of the same sign, then interactions of greater complexity, such as beat interactions, are possible (Figure 17.7).

In neural networks that consist of loosely coupled oscillators of different frequencies, information may be carried independently over different oscillators if the oscillators are incommensurate; that is, unrelated by some common harmonic. (A *harmonic* is a sine wave that is a product of the fundamental frequency and an integer or the quotient of the fundamental frequency divided by an integer.) This phenomenon is fundamental to the operations of AM radio signals. A radio station broadcasts an electromagnetic wave of a single frequency, the information therein encoded in that wave's amplitude (Figure 17.8). A radio receiver's antenna picks up the electromagnetic wave, along with electromagnetic waves broadcast by every other AM radio station in the area. The receiver is able to tune in or select the desired AM radio station signal because it has its own oscillator, whose frequency can

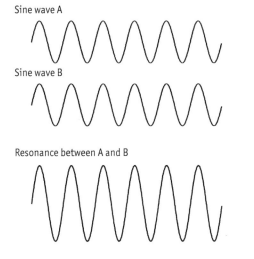

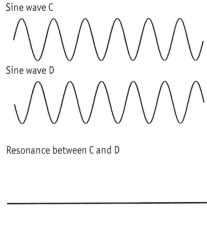

Figure 17.6: Results of resonance interactions between pairs of sine waves. Because the sine waves A and B are of equal frequency and phase, interactions between homologous points increase the amplitude in a purely positive resonance. Because sine waves C and D are of equal frequency but have a phase difference of 180 degrees, the interactions between homologous points decrease the two interacting waves' amplitude to zero, creating purely negative resonance.

Signal from desired AM radio station

Signal heard when signal received from desired AM radio station and radio receiver's oscillators are added

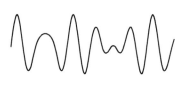

Signal received from desired AM radio station

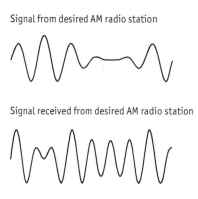

Radio receiver oscillator tuned to carrier frequency of desired AM radio station

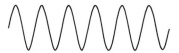

Figure 17.7: Schematic representation of independently encoded information among different oscillators that use the same medium. In this representation, the different oscillators are the electromagnetic waves generated in space at different fundamental frequencies unique to each radio station. The desired AM radio station transmits an electromagnetic wave of a specific frequency. The transmitted information is encoded in the various amplitudes of the same electromagnetic wave. The antenna of the AM radio receiver receives the signal from the desired AM station along with those of all other AM radio stations in the area. The AM receiver has an oscillator tuned to carrier frequency of the desired AM radio station, which is added to the received signal. The result is then sent to the speaker, which renders the signal audible. The result is an acceptable replication of the original signal from the desired AM radio station.

be changed. The receiver's oscillator is tuned to the frequency of the desired radio station and is added to all the electromagnetic waves received. The radio receiver's oscillator enters into positive resonance with the desired radio station's electromagnetic waves and amplifies them above all the other radio stations' signals. The theory, which is presented in Chapter 6, Nervous System Responses to DBS, is that DBS may act like the oscillator in an AM radio receiver to selectively affect information in the network of brain oscillators, either to improve the signal-to-noise ratio (positive resonance) or to suppress misinformation (negative resonance).

It must be noted that, as shown in Figure 17.8, information is encoded in the amplitudes of the carrier frequency. Information quality is highly dependent on the carrier frequency. Higher carrier frequencies provide a more robust representation of the information (Figure 17.8). This is consistent with the Nyquist Theorem, which relates the frequency at which a periodic signal is sampled to the robustness of the representation. Generally, the periodic

signal must be sampled at twice its fastest frequency component. The modulation of the amplitude in the carrier wave may be considered a form of *sampling*, for which the Nyquist theorem applies as described above. Most discussions related to oscillations in the brain—in the basal ganglia–thalamic-cortical systems, particularly—have concerned relatively low frequencies compared to the frequency components of motor unit recruitment and de-recruitment (*see Chapter 7—DBS Effects on Motor Control*). They are therefore unlikely to provide robust representation of the information that must be encoded in the oscillations of the basal ganglia–thalamic-cortical system.

DISCRETE OSCILLATORS

The various modes of interaction between continuous oscillators are also available to discrete oscillators. The interactions among discrete oscillators, however, are far more complex. This complexity of interactions greatly increases the degrees of freedom and thus the

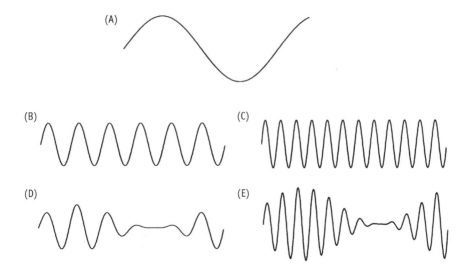

Figure 17.8: Representation of the importance of a carrier frequency that is much higher than frequencies contained in information to be encoded by amplitude modulation. Information is encoded in the signal shown in A. B represents a lower-frequency carrier signal than the carrier signal shown in C. The modulations of the carrier frequency amplitudes are shown in D for carrier frequency B, and in E for carrier frequency C. The high-frequency signal conveys a better representation of the information shown in A.

dimensions over which information may be encoded, processed, and transmitted. Discrete oscillators—neural oscillators, for purposes of the present discussion—are not continuous. Continuous oscillators have only a very short amount of time during which the values of the oscillator is zero and therefore not interacting with other oscillators at those times. The times of zero value in a continuous oscillator are at 0 and 180 degrees of phase. (It must be noted that a phase of 360 degrees is the same as a 0 degree phase in an ongoing oscillator.)

An example of a hypothetical discrete oscillator is shown in Figure 17.9. In this case, a continuous oscillator in the manner of a racecar with a continuously lit lightbulb traveling around a racetrack, which itself is traveling around another racetrack, which in turn is traveling around yet another racetrack. A person observing the racecar would see a complex but continuous periodic function traced by the continuously lit lightbulb. Next consider the situation in which there is a single track but also a barrier that obstructs the view of the racecar (Figure 17.10). Now the observer only sees flashes of light as the car with the lit lightbulb passes in the line of sight (Figure 17.10B). The only information contained in the flashes of light is the speed at which the car traverses the racetrack; in other words, its frequency (Figure 17.10D).

One can extend the scenario described above by allowing the racecar driver to voluntarily control whether the light is on or off. This introduces another degree of freedom and thus more information, such as in Morse code (Figure 17.10E). The difference in the timing of the flashes of light between Figure 17.10D and 17.10E is the new information that the racecar driver has created. Further extend the scenario to a situation in which the switch the racecar driver uses to encode information is faulty, and the electrical current supplied is erratic and at times does not provide enough current to illuminate the light. The result is misinformation (represented by Figure 17.10J). However, the managers of the racetrack bring in a charger (represented by the supply truck in Figure 17.10I) that can charge the battery as needed to illuminate the light. However, the supply truck is stationed only at one point along the track and can only provide a brief pulse of electrical energy. The racecar must pass by that point at the very time the supply truck can deliver the electrical energy to receive the electrical charge. Now the combination of the oscillators formed by the racecar and the supply truck can interact to provide sufficient electrical power, and the result is changing the misinformation to appropriate information (Figure 17.10K). It is proposed that this

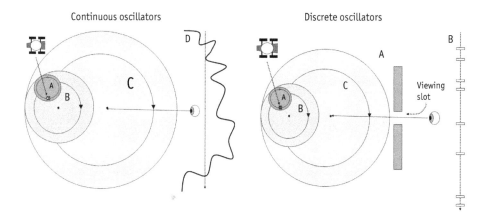

Figure 17.9: An example of a more complex, discrete oscillator. The racecar moving around the track produces a continuous or harmonic oscillation (*see Chapter 16—Oscillator Basics*). However, the flashing light is a discrete process. An observer in the dark will see the light only when it is on. If the light is lit continuously, an observer would see a complex periodic pattern of light (D in the continuous oscillator on the left). If the observer is looking through a slot, she will see a regular pattern of flashes as the racecar passes the viewing slot corresponding to a discrete oscillator in B the right).

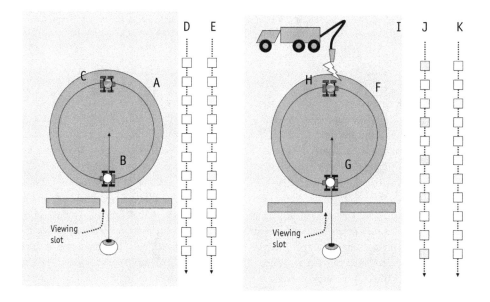

Figure 17.10: Hypothetical description of the interactions between two discrete oscillator. A racecar traverses a single race-track (A). There is a light affixed to the racecar, and each time the racecar passes by the viewing slot in the barrier (B), the observer sees a flash of light (D) corresponding to a discrete oscillator. However, when the light is constantly on, the racecar driver cannot convey any information except the speed of the racecar (D). If the driver can control when the light is on, much more information can be conveyed in the sequence of light flashes (E), a situation analogous to Morse code. A disorder of the light, such as a bad battery, may mean that the light will go on for a while but then fade out. In this case, the information originally encoded in E become degraded as shown in J. The observer could not tell if the information in J is a correct new code or whether it is a faulty version of the code represented in E. Suppose a battery charger recharges the battery each time the racecar completes a cycle (I). Further suppose that the ability of the recharger to recharge the battery depends on the precise timing of the recharging process. For example, say the charger can only give a recharge once per second. In other words, the charger cannot provide a continuous opportunity to recharge the racecar's battery. If the recharger has the same frequency (1 Hz) as the racecar and an appropriate phase (corresponding to the position of the racecar on the track), it will always be able to recharge the battery, and the driver will always be able to correctly convey information (K). In this case, the interaction between the racecar and the recharger is analogous to resonance amplification between two discrete oscillators. Note that if the battery charger has a different frequency from the racecar or the wrong phase (timing of the recharge relative to the position of the racecar on the track such that the racecar is not in position to receive the charge), then there will be a failure to recharge the racecar light bulb and the result will be continued misinformation.

may be one mechanism by which DBS can restore more normal function.

This analogy has important applications in understanding DBS. As shown in Figure 17.10I, a recharger on the other side of the racetrack can deliver electricity, but only in small amounts and at a certain rate. Each charge is sufficient to power the light so that it functions reliably the next time it is supposed to flash. The recharger is analogous to DBS, and each small charge is analogous to a DBS pulse. Clearly, DBS must occur at the same frequency (and phase) so that each charge is delivered just as the car is driving past. This recharging is analogous to a resonant effect that builds (or sustains) the periodic activity of the light flashes. Now the driver can deliver information as usual (Figure 17.10K). One hypothesized mechanism of action of DBS is that DBS restores normal information to the nervous system (Montgomery and Gale 2008).

A discrete oscillator may take a form in which information is encoded in brief departures from zero, thus creating long periods during which the value of an oscillator is zero and therefore will not interact with any oscillators (Figure 17.11). In the discrete or discontinuous oscillator, the brief departures from zero represent the signal. The duration of each signal is given as d_s. The frequency (f) is the number of signals per second. The time between the signals is the period (p), also known as *cycle time*, and is related to the frequency as $\frac{1}{f}$. The duty cycle is the percent of the period (p) composed of the signal and is given by $\left(\dfrac{d_s}{p}\right) \times 100$ (Figure 17.11).

If one has multiple discrete neural oscillators, each oscillator is able to carry different information, such as information contained in the amplitudes of the discrete non-zero signals. Also, there may be a set of neurons receiving information from both oscillators, but the information will remain separate. Though continuous oscillators at non-commensurate frequencies are able to maintain separate channels of information simultaneously, the above-mentioned discrete oscillators of equal frequencies are able to carry separate information, depending on phase differences and duty cycles (Figure 17.12). Neurons in networks of coupled discrete oscillators will carry simultaneously independent channels of information at different time scales. This ability is important in motor control, whose different orders of motor unit recruitment and de-recruitment, though they are simultaneous, are organized at different time scales (*see Chapter 7— DBS Effects on Motor Control*).

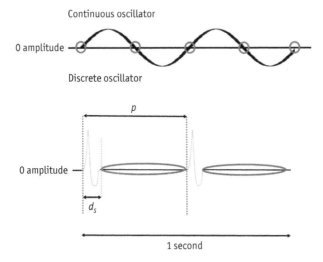

Figure 17.11: Examples of a continuous oscillator and a discrete oscillator. Because the continuous oscillator has amplitudes of zero (shown by the open red circles) for only quite brief times, it is able to interact with other oscillators over quite a large percentage of its duty cycle; that is, the percentage of its period in which a signal is present. The discrete oscillator contains a relatively brief signal (blue line) of duration d_s. Its period (p) is the time between signals. The number of signals per second is the frequency (f), which is related to the period $= \frac{1}{f}$. The ratio of the duration (d_s) to the period (p) determines the duty cycle by $\left(\dfrac{d_s}{p}\right) \times 100$. For a continuous oscillator, the duty cycle is 100%. The discrete oscillator will only interact during the duty cycle, which in this example is only a very brief period of time.

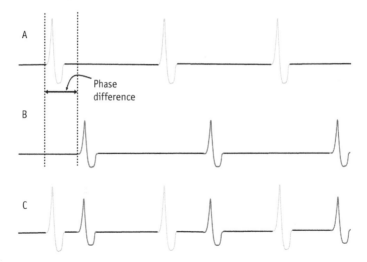

Figure 17.12: Schematic representation of interaction (C) between two discrete oscillators of equal frequency (A and B) in a way that preserves information originally contained in each oscillator. The phase difference between oscillators A and B is longer than the duty cycle. When the two oscillators interact, the signal in one falls at a moment in which the amplitude of the other is zero. The two oscillators therefore will not interact.

SINGLE REENTRANT DISCRETE OSCILLATOR

Rafael Lorente de Nó and Donald O. Hebb believed that reentrant activity could result in a sustained pattern of activity that perhaps represents working memory. The key to sustained activity was an effect that lasted longer than the stimulus. For example, a transient stimulus applied to a closed long chain of neurons would cause reentrant oscillatory activity, thereby providing a type of memory.

The effects of an axon's action potential are of quite limited duration, and they are *biphasic*—a hyperpolarization follows an initial depolarization. The first phase is a depolarization followed by a hyperpolarization, during which an absolute and a relative refractory period occur. These events last a few milliseconds. The mechanisms underlying the action potential are thus unlikely to contribute to evolving activity of closed reentrant long chain neural oscillators. The situation is quite different in the dendrites and cell body. Changes in the electrical potential of the neuronal membrane associated with a postsynaptic event may last from several milliseconds to 50 ms or more. This means that synaptic inputs are arriving at points along the dendrite or cell body that are within the range of spatial summation and only need a frequency ≥ 20 Hz in order to have a cumulative effect.

In other words, this relatively modest rate of synaptic inputs may have lingering effects, causing activities within closed chains of neurons to evolve over time in a manner similar to that which was suggested by de Nó and Hebb. Several factors determine the duration of effect of postsynaptic potentials and thus also determine their capacity to generate reentrant activity that evolves in a single discrete oscillator. These relate to the time course of presynaptic neurotransmitter release, reuptake, or metabolism; the effects of any neuromodulators; the biophysics of the ionic conductance changes; and the membrane characteristics, such as capacitance and resistance, that affect spatial propagation and temporal decay of the postsynaptic potentials.

The role of DBS based on the above-mentioned considerations is interesting and largely unexplored. Admittedly, one of the critical nervous system responses to DBS is apparently generation of action potentials in axons in the vicinity of the electrical field that is generated by a DBS pulse. However, the action potential generated probably has additional significant effects on the dendrites and cell bodies. Action potentials are initially conducted in an orthodromic direction to axon terminals and in an antidromic conduction (Figure 17.13). Those conducted antidromically may invade an axon collaterally and propagate orthodromically to the axon terminals, which will

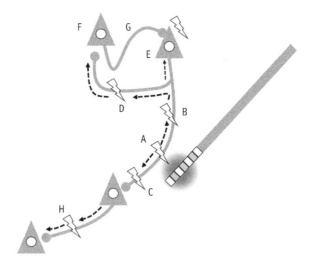

Figure 17.13: Schematic representation of antidromic action potential propagation. Local responses (in the physiological rather than the anatomical sense; see text). In A, the electrical field generated by the DBS electrode excites an action potential in the axon near the electrode. The action potential is propagated antidromically (B) to the neuron from which the axon originated and travels orthodromically (C) to the neuron receiving the axon's synapses. Antidromically traveling action potentials may encounter a branch point to an axon collateral. If this happens, the antidromic action potential is carried orthodromically (D) to another neuron (F), which in turn may send an action potential to other neurons or to the neuron (G) that originates the axon in which the antidromic action potential was initiated. Neuron C, which receives the influences of action potentials generated in the axon at A, may propagate that effect to the next neuron (H). The antidromic action potential may also invade the originating neuron (E), back-propagating into the soma to affect information-processing in that neuron.

affect the postsynaptic potentials of subsequent neurons. In this manner, DBS of even modest frequencies may have a significant impact on reentrant oscillation.

Antidromic action potentials invade the cell body and dendrites in a retrograde manner, causing massive depolarization of the cell body and dendritic membranes. This massive depolarization, it is believed, activates n-methyl-d-aspartate (NMDA) receptors, which could facilitate *Hebbian learning*. Facilitation of Hebbian learning by DBS may help explain the long latencies to symptomatic improvements in such disorders as dystonia and OCD.

It is important to recognize that the action potentials driven by DBS are not normal or physiological. For example, a DBS pulse is thought to generate highly synchronized action potentials that, when propagated initially or subsequently orthodromically, depolarize or hyperpolarize large numbers of presynaptic membranes. This results in highly synchronized postsynaptic potentials that may produce large postsynaptic potentials. Based solely on neuronal membrane capacitance and resistance, these large postsynaptic potentials may persist. Also, as evidence

of microelectrode recordings of extracellular action potentials suggests, the postsynaptic potentials are not precisely synchronized. This dispersion of postsynaptic effects may also contribute to prolonged responses, which in turn may contribute to the evolution of activities in recurrent chains of neurons (Figure 17.14). Neurons typically do not immediately attain one state and remain in it for the duration of DBS. Rather, their responses evolve. Though the precise mechanisms that underlie the evolution of the neuronal responses are unknown, evolving reentrant neural oscillators interacting with the DBS pulse train may be one of those mechanisms.

INTERACTIONS AMONG DISCRETE OSCILLATORS

A DBS pulse train may be regarded as a discrete oscillator (Figure 17.15). For example, DBS at 150 pps per second with a 90-ms pulse width has a duty cycle of 13.5%, which means that, for 86.5% of the time, electrical current is absent from the DBS electrodes. The

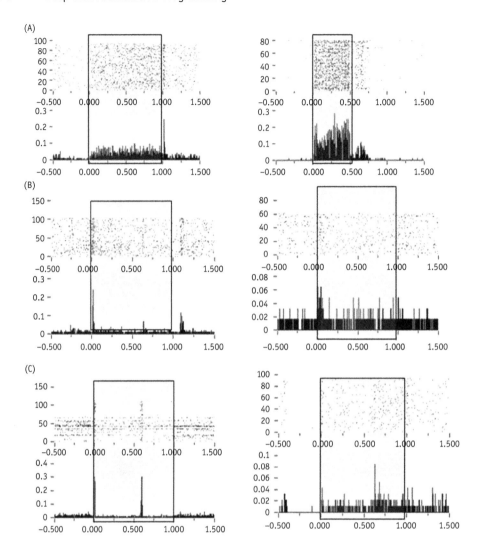

Figure 17.14: Representative examples of peri-event rasters and histograms centered on the onset of a DBS cycle that lasted 500 ms or 1000 ms. The microelectrode recordings were taken from the subthalamic nucleus (STN) during DBS in the vicinity of the contralateral STN. The upper half of each figure displays rows of dots. Each dot represents the discharge of the neuron, and each row represents a single cycle of DBS. The lower half of each figure is a histogram that is constructed by collapsing the rows into columns. Time zero is the onset of the cycle of DBS. The box demarcates the onset and duration of the DBS cycle relative to the neuronal activities. It must be noted that neuronal responses following the cycle foreclose interpretation, because the stimulation did not cease cleanly at the end of the cycle.

discrete oscillator of the DBS pulse train can then interact with neural oscillators (examples of this interaction are discussed in *Chapter 6, Nervous System Responses to DBS*). The following discussion presents the interactions between neural oscillators and a DBS oscillator.

A four-neuron reentrant oscillator interacts with DBS, which is itself an oscillator (Figure 17.16). The results of computational modeling appear in the lower panel of the figure, as do amplitudes over time of a neuron in node 4. In delivery of a DBS pulse every fourth cycle beginning with the third cycle (Figure 17.16C), the frequency of the oscillator is equal to that of the DBS. Also, spontaneous activation of neurons in node 3 occurs at the initial time period A, and it propagates through the remainder

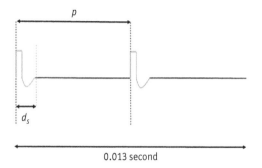

Figure 17.15: Example of the DBS pulse train regarded as a discrete oscillator. The signal has the duration **ds**, and the interpulse interval (**p**) is 0.0067 seconds for a duty cycle of 13.65%. Because two DBS pulses occur in 0.013 seconds, the DBS oscillator's frequency (**f**) is 150 Hz.

those of continuous oscillators. Computer simulations of these conditions appear in Figures 17.17, 17.18, and 17.19.

DISCRETE NEURAL OSCILLATORS

Neural oscillators depend on dynamics of the individual neurons that constitute their nodes. The dynamics of individual neurons are highly nonlinear: The output of neurons does not follow simply as the sum of their inputs. At the very least, significant non-linearity is induced by the need for the electrical potential across the neuronal membrane at the action potential–initiating segment to cross a threshold in order to generate an action potential output. "Non-linear" means that the output of a system is not directly proportional to the inputs. As the electrical potential across the neuronal membrane at the action potential–initiating segment depolarizes, there is no output. With traversal of the membrane comes output, the all-or-nothing nature of the action potential is the only a single output value, (*see Chapter 3— Principles of Electrophysiology*). Depolarization of the membrane by a factor of two may produce no output if the depolarization is subthreshold, but only slightly greater further depolarization may result in the maximal all-or-nothing action potential and any further depolarization will not change the output.

The signal portion of the neuron in the discrete neural oscillator is further complicated by multiple phases during which the neuron goes from relatively unexcitable at rest, to excitable at times of relative depolarization, to absolute refractoriness owing to Na^+ channel inactivation, and finally to relatively refractory, before returning to relatively unexcitable because in a hyperpolarized state. Therefore, the same input to the neuron will thus have starkly different effects, depending on the particular phase of excitability the postsynaptic neuron is at relative to the time of the presynaptic input.

The computer simulations discussed above were based on a model whose oscillators contained only a single neuron. Also, the magnitude of activity in the node was analog in nature, its values continuous, and its range of possible values linear. This last fact means output was directly proportional to the inputs. For the reasons discussed above, the behavior is quite unlike what happens with actual neurons. The problem

of the oscillator with each cycle. The spontaneous activation of neurons in node 4 occurs at time periods B, F, J, and N. The first DBS pulse, which occurs at time period C, drives increased activity in neurons of node 4 at time D. Because this activity propagates through the oscillator and returns to neurons of node 3 immediately prior to the subsequent DBS pulse, the effect of the propagated pulse arrives at neurons in node 4 at the same time that the subsequent DBS pulse arrives at neurons in node 4. The two activations summate, and the increasing activities thereof propagate throughout the oscillator to cause a progressive increase in neuronal activities in node 4 at time periods D, H, L, and P. It must be noted that activities generated by spontaneous activation of neurons in node 3 continue to cycle through the oscillator but do not interact with the DBS effects. Though the oscillator and DBS are of equal frequency, their respective duty times are shorter than the phase delay between the spontaneous and the DBS-induced activities.

The effects of ongoing intrinsic oscillations and interactions with the DBS oscillator reflect the fact that the duty cycle of the signals in both the intrinsic oscillator and the DBS oscillator is a small percent. Also, the phase difference is such that the signals of the two oscillators do not interact. Each oscillator may therefore entrain information independently. Creating a different situation are larger duty cycles whose phase offsets do not sufficiently prevent overlap of discrete signals. For regions of overlap, the interactions between the two oscillators resemble

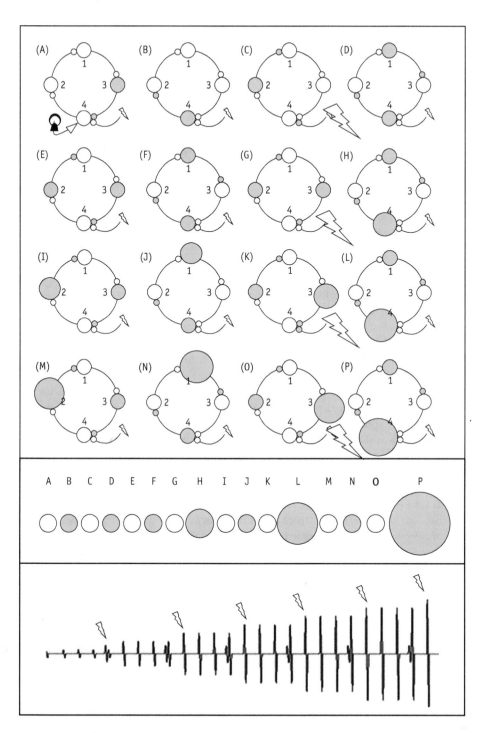

Figure 17.16: Continued

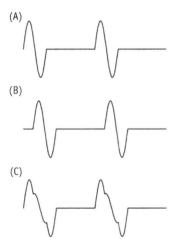

(A)

(B)

(C)

Figure 17.17: Interactions between two discrete oscillators (A, B) and their result (C). Though the two oscillators have equal frequencies, the phase of oscillator B is delayed. Because the phase delay is of shorter duration than the duty cycle of oscillator A, however, a complex interaction results.

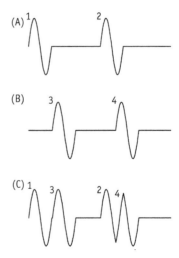

(A) 1   2

(B) 3   4

(C) 1 3   2 4

Figure 17.18: Interactions between two discrete oscillators (A, B) and their result (C). Though its phase is delayed relative to oscillator A, oscillator B has a higher frequency. The duration of oscillator A's duty cycle, however, is shorter than oscillator B's delay; thus waveforms 1 and 3 are preserved. Waveforms 2 and 4, on the other hand, enter into complex interaction.

becomes that of representing activity within a node in light of the fact that the output of all the node's neurons is an all-or-nothing binary signal.

One theory suggests that each node contains multiple neurons (*see Chapter 8—Pathophysiological Mechanisms*). With each cycle of an oscillator, a subset of neurons discharges and thus continues propagation of the oscillation. At any one time, a different set of neurons within each node is activated (Figure 17.20).

Evidence for this phenomenon is presented in Chapter 8, Pathophysiological Mechanisms. If it is assumed that this notion is biologically plausible, then the magnitude of information within reentrant oscillators whose nodes contain multiple neurons may be represented by the proportion of neurons within the node that discharge with each cycle.

Figure 17.16: Continued

Figure 17.16: Upper panel contains a schematic representation of the interaction between DBS and an ongoing four-node neural oscillator. Each node is represented as experiencing no activity (solid pale blue circles) or activity (solid green circles: the larger the circle, the greater the activity). Node 4 shows an activity that occurs independently of the DBS pulse on an ongoing basis—at time B, for example. At time C, a DBS pulse is delivered (lightning bolt symbol), which initiates activity in node 4 at time D. This activity propagates through the oscillator at times E–H, during which reentrant activity coincides at time H with the effects of the next DBS. The interactions are additive and result in greater activity that then propagates through the circuit. In the interim, the original activity propagates, reaching node 4 at time J at the original magnitude. The activity associated with the DBS pulse continues to propagate and reenters node 4 at the same moment as the next DBS pulse, at time L. This process continues, the original oscillatory activity continuing without any change in amplitude, but the activity associated with the DBS pulses continues to increase. The pattern of activities appears in the central panel. There are two separate trains of activity and thus two separate channels of information. The first channel is related to the original oscillations, and the second is related to information that flows from interactions with the DBS pulses. The lower panel shows the result of a computer simulation in which ongoing neuronal activity was established at a frequency of 50 Hz and the signal had a 20% duty cycle. DBS was also initiated at 50 pps but at a phase delay of 0.5 ms relative to the original oscillations, and the DBS pulse's duration was 0.5 ms. The delivery of each DBS pulse is represented by the lightning bolt symbol. The signals are recoded from node 4 (upper panel). The results are consistent with the mechanism and are described in the upper and central panels.

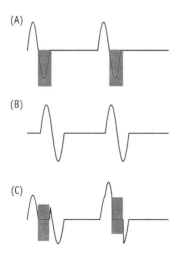

Figure 17.19: Interactions between two discrete oscillators (A, B) and their result (C). Though the two oscillators are of equal frequencies, the phase of oscillator B is delayed, and thus the waveforms interact in C. In this example, preventing any interaction is oscillator A's refractory period, which is indicated by the solid red rectangle. The result is the complex interaction that appears in C.

The theory holds that, though at baseline relatively few neurons within each node discharge during each cycle, they are sufficient for activating a sufficient number of neurons in the subsequent node and thus perpetuating oscillations. With changes in the excitability of neurons within each node, the net number of neurons active with each cycle may vary, creating information within the oscillator. The probability of any particular neuron's discharging with a specific cycle is determined by a number of factors, including the *fan-in ratio*. The fan-in ratio is determined by how many neurons in the previous node synapse on the individual neuron of the subsequent node, and how their mode of synapsing affects spatial and temporal summation in the postsynaptic membrane potentials. Other factors include the efficacy of a presynaptic action potential in generating a postsynaptic potential, and the electrical potential across the neuronal membrane relative to the threshold for generating an action potential.

Changes in the excitability of neurons within a node may change the frequency of action potentials conducted out of any single neuron. For example, a neuron that discharges on average once every 10 cycles may increase or decrease its discharge frequencies tenfold, thus increasing markedly, without collapse or saturation, the information capacity of the neural oscillator whose nodes consist of multiple neurons. This capability answers Milner's objections that such oscillators would saturate or collapse.

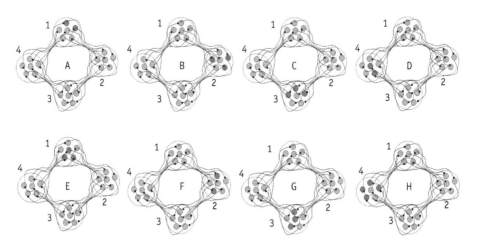

Figure 17.20: Schematic representation of a four-node oscillator (nodes 1–4) whose nodes contain five neurons each. A series of time intervals (A–H) are represented. Neurons become active in node 1 at time A. The activity then propagates to neurons in subsequent nodes. For any part of the cycle, a subset of neurons in each node becomes active, and the specific neurons that are active vary with each cycle. Thus the neurons active at time B in node 2 are different from the neurons active in node 2 at time F. This means that the frequency of any individual neuron will be less than the inherent fundamental frequency of the oscillator. In other words, each neuron will be a rate divider.

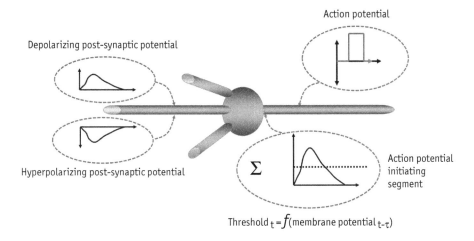

Threshold $_t = f$(membrane potential $_{t-\tau}$)

Figure 17.21: Model neuron that consists of multiple dendritic inputs whose changes in transmembrane electrical potentials are summed at the action-potential-initiating segment. If the summed potentials exceed a dynamic threshold, an action potential is generated and transmitted down the axon to the next neuron. The dendritic potentials are modeled on a decaying exponential function as either depolarizing or hyperpolarizing. The threshold for initiating an action potential varies with the previous transmembrane electrical potential, and in doing so, model changes in Na^+ voltage-gated ionic conductance channel activation and inactivation. In this manner, post-hyperpolarization excitation and depolarization blockade are modeled.

OSCILLATORS WITH MULTIPLE REALISTIC NEURONS

To explore the dynamics of neural oscillators, computer simulations were performed. A version of the integrate-and-fire model of neurons was used (Figure 17.21). The model neuron consisted of dendrites that received inputs from other neurons that produced either depolarizing or hyperpolarizing postsynaptic potentials, which were modeled as a decaying exponential function. The postsynaptic potentials were summed at the action potential–initiating segment. If the sum exceeded the threshold, an action potential was initiated in the axon. The threshold was dynamic, increasing or decreasing according to the time-history of the electrical potential across the neuronal membrane at the action potential–initiating segment. This was meant to reflect inactivation and reactivation of Na^+ voltage-gated ionic conductance channels (*see Chapter 3—Principles of Electrophysiology*). The dynamic threshold also represented absolute and relative refractory periods following action potentials.

The induction of a postsynaptic potential by a presynaptic action potential in each neuron of a node is determined by a probability function and thus reflects synaptic efficiency. Conduction times for action potentials generated at the action potential–initiating segment to reach the presynaptic terminals are modeled as two components, the first accounting for the electrical propagation of action potentials, and the second accounting for neurotransmitters' release, diffusion across the synaptic cleft, and binding to the postsynaptic membrane. Each conduction time is varied by random selection of a conduction time from a predefined distribution.

In one instantiation, a network of oscillators was constructed (Figure 17.22). The network consisted of three oscillators of 4, 5, and 6 nodes. One node in each oscillator connected to the other designated node in all of the other oscillators, thus loosely coupling the individual oscillators. Each node contained 100 neurons that receive input from all the neurons in the previous node and send axons to every neuron in the subsequent node.

The various parameters, such as synaptic efficiency, refractory periods, and conduction times, were adjusted to produce stable neuronal activities in the network. The trains of action potentials (spike trains) were analyzed for their frequency content by use of a circular statistical algorithm that is mathematically equivalent to the Fourier transform but easier to implement (Takeshita et al. 2009). The circular statistical measure used a two-second window

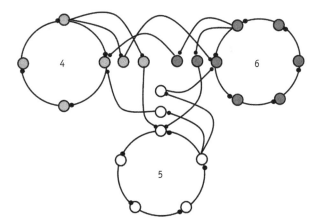

Figure 17.22: One instantiation of the four-oscillator network. There are three oscillators that consist of 4, 5, and 6 nodes, respectively. Each node contains 100 neurons. In each oscillator, a designative node also connects to the corresponding node in the other oscillators, creating a loosely coupled network. The neurons in each node received inputs from all neurons in the previous node and sent outputs to each neuron in the subsequent node.

that was moved through time in 0.2 sec steps to implement a spectrogram. An example appears in Figure 17.23.

Figure 17.23 reveals a remarkable similarity in the spectrograms of neuronal activities that is consistent with, though not proof of, a similarity of underlying mechanisms. In all the spectrograms, the trains of action potentials appear to have a set of specific frequencies that is relatively stable for a period of time prior to shifting rapidly to another discrete set of frequencies. Such a rapid shift is known in Complex Systems science as *bifurcation*. In addition, the specific sets appear to be repeated

over time, which suggests a return to a specific set of dynamics. Example appear in Figures 17.24 and 17.25.

The center panel of Figure 17.24 shows the spectrogram of a neuron recorded in the basal ganglia of a non-human primate. Frequencies appear to cluster over time. An *n*-dimensional, unsupervised, cluster analysis routine was applied (Montgomery et al. 2005), in which each of the 250 frequencies constituted a dimension and each epoch in time was plotted in the 250-dimensional space according to the power at that frequency. The cluster analysis identified four clusters shown in the other panels (Figure 17.24).

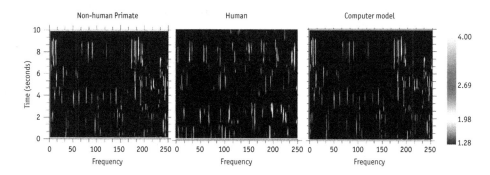

Figure 17.23: Spectrograms showing amount of activities (power) at different frequencies over time. The power is represented as the z-score difference (color scale) over a randomized train of action potentials (spike train). At each epoch in time, the train of action potentials has a specific set of frequencies. Also, the train of action potentials appears to be stable in their frequency content, and then they change (bifurcate) to other sets of frequencies. Shown are spectrograms of actual recordings in the globus pallidus externa of a non-human primate, the subthalamic nucleus in a human, and a neuron in the computer model of the network described in Figure 17.22.

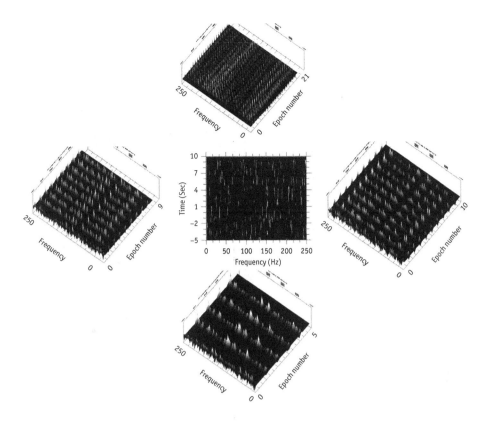

Figure 17.24: The center panel contains a spectrogram of the train of action potentials that was recorded from a neuron in the basal ganglia of a non-human primate. The neuronal activities contain sets of multiple frequencies over time. The train of action potentials appear to bifurcate (shift) among the different sets. A multidimensional cluster analysis was performed (see text for details), and it demonstrated that there were four sets of frequencies.

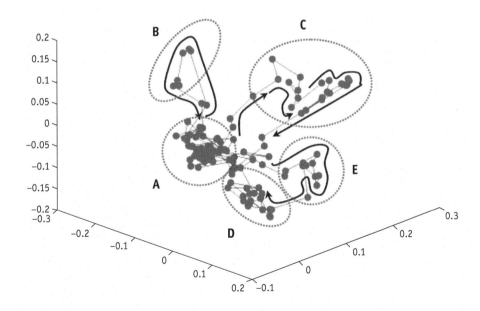

Figure 17.25: Demonstration of transitions between different sets of frequencies in the train of action potentials recorded from a neuron in the basal ganglia of a non-human primate. Multidimensional cluster analysis was conducted. The multidimensional space was reducible to the three dimensions shown by principal components analysis. Evident is the train of action potentials, which appears to have specific sets of frequencies and transitions between them.

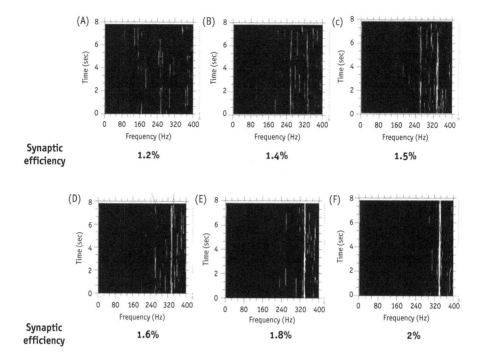

Figure 17.26: Spectrograms of neuronal activities in the computer network model consisting of a single oscillator of four nodes, each node containing 100 neurons. Initial parameters were determined that provided sustained oscillator activity, as shown in spectrogram A where the synaptic efficiency was 1.2%. The synaptic efficiencies were changed to 1.4% (B), 1.5% (C), 1.6% (D), 1.8% (E), and 2% (F). With greater efficiency, frequencies collapsed to a single frequency.

The same analyses were applied to recordings from another neuron, and the multidimensional space was reducible to a three-dimensional space by principal components analysis (Figure 17.25). The sets of neuronal frequency content appears to bifurcate serially: $A \rightarrow B \rightarrow A \rightarrow C \rightarrow A \rightarrow E \rightarrow D$.

The properties of networks of loosely coupled, discrete nonlinear oscillators were studied further. The effects of changes in synaptic efficiency in the computer model are presented in Figure 17.26. The computer model is shown in Figure 17.22. At relatively low synaptic efficiencies, which are characteristic of biological neurons, multiple frequencies appear in the spectrogram, and no single frequency dominates. With increasing synaptic efficiency, the number of frequencies decreases, and one dominant frequency emerges. The frequencies are said to collapse to a fundamental frequency of some small number of oscillators or a single oscillator. It must be noted that the frequency that becomes dominant is higher than the fundamental frequency of any single oscillator. This demonstrates that numerous action potentials may be carried simultaneously in any single cycle, because the duty time is quite brief relative to the cycle time.

Figure 17.27 shows the effects of progressively prolonged refractory periods in a computer model. With increasing refractory periods, the frequencies collapse to just two frequencies or a single frequency. The increasing refractory periods prolong the duty cycle relative to the cycle time, which leads to increased interactions between modeled presynaptic inputs with the refractory period of a postsynaptic neuron. The interactions with inputs and the refractory period may be considered a form of negative resonance. This interaction acts as a filter, and at different refractory periods different oscillators are affected. For example, at a refractory period of 2.5 ms, the predominant frequency is approximately 250 Hz. At a refractory period of 3.5 ms, the predominant frequency shifts to approximately 170 Hz.

THE SYSTEMS (DISCRETE) OSCILLATORS THEORY

An alternative theory, the Systems Oscillators Theory, posits that the basal ganglia–thalamic-cortical system

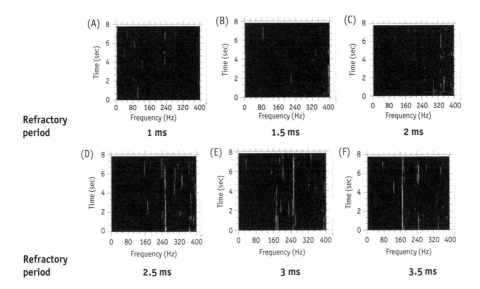

Figure 17.27: Spectrograms of neuronal activities in the computer network model described in Figure 17.26. In this case, the refractory periods were systematically varied. With refractory periods of greater duration, the frequencies collapsed to a single frequency.

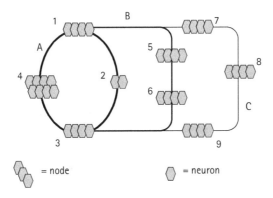

Figure 17.28: A hypothetical reentrant discrete oscillator and a set of nested reentrant oscillators. The oscillators are labeled A, B, and C. Oscillator A contains nodes 1, 2, 3, and 4; Oscillator B contains nodes 1, 5, 6, 3, and 4; and Oscillator C contains nodes 1, 7, 8, 9, 3, and 4. Assuming a transmission time between nodes of 4 ms, the fundamental frequency is about 63 Hz for the four-node Oscillator A, 50 Hz for the five-node Oscillator B, and about 42 Hz for the six-node Oscillator C. Each node contains several neurons. All but nodes 2 and 4 contain four neurons, whereas node 2 contains two neurons, and node 4 contains eight neurons. According to the Systems Oscillator Theory, each neuron does not discharge with each cycle of oscillation. Thus, the minimum average discharge rate of individual neurons is determined by the fundamental frequency divided by the number of neurons in each node. For neurons in node 2 of Oscillator A, the minimum average discharge frequency of each neuron would be about 21 Hz. For neurons in node 4, when they participate in Oscillator A, the average discharge frequency would be about 8 Hz. The theory holds that several high-frequency oscillators in the basal ganglia–thalamic-cortical system have frequencies much greater than the average discharge rate of the individual neurons within each node. The actual discharge frequencies of all the neurons are complex because the oscillators are nested. In this example, all oscillators share nodes 1 and 3. Thus, oscillations in Oscillator A will spill over into Oscillators B and C, and vice versa. Indeed, the interactions could result in oscillations much faster than the 63 Hz fundamental frequency of Oscillator A and frequencies much slower than the 42 Hz fundamental frequency of Oscillator C.

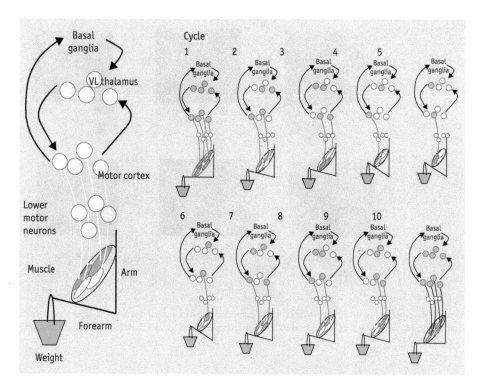

Figure 17.29: Representation of the relationship of the Vop-cortical oscillator to the basal ganglia and motor units in the muscle, according to the Systems Oscillators Theory. The figure on the left illustrates the various components. Active neurons and motor fibers are filled in yellow. The Vop (labeled VL in this figure) and motor cortex form a positive feedback loop, whereas the motor cortex projects to the motor units (a combination of lower motor neurons and muscle fibers). The activity of the motor units is sustained by ongoing reentrant activity within the Vop-cortical oscillator, while the number of Vop and motor-cortical neurons active through each cycle of the oscillations is regulated by the basal ganglia (and cerebellum, not shown) side loops. The series of smaller figures represent the generation of a muscle force to elevate and lower a weight. The transition from no motor units active (cycle 1) to the beginning of the muscle contraction (cycle 2) is caused by an increase in the excitability of Vop neurons, in response to influences of the basal ganglia. This influence is represented by two hypothetical neurons being activated in Vop, two hypothetical neurons in the motor cortex, and two hypothetical motor units in the muscle. Likewise, the increase in motor unit recruitments (represented by three hypothetical motor units) is caused by an increase in the number of neurons active in the Vop thalamus during cycle 4 that, in turn, activates three neurons in the motor cortex. The ongoing reentrant activity in the Vop-cortical circuit, under the influence of the basal ganglia side loops, sustains the increased motor unit activities (cycles 2–3, 4–6, and 7–8). The process is reversed to lower the weight, again under the influence of the basal ganglia (and cerebellum, not shown).

is organized as sets of nested or interconnected discrete oscillators representing many different frequencies. The oscillators are made up of nodes connected in a reentrant architecture (Figure 17.28). Activity traverses the entire circuit. The number of nodes determines the length of the circuit, and the number of nodes determines the fundamental frequency of that oscillator. For example, if activity takes 4 ms to travel between nodes and there are four nodes, then the total time required for activity to make one transit around the oscillator is 16 ms, or about 63 Hz

(= 1/0.016 s), and a two-node oscillator would have a fundamental frequency of 125 Hz.

The Systems Oscillators Theory posits that the main oscillator is the reentrant circuit consisting of the thalamic-cortical system (Figure 17.29). With respect to motor function, the main circuit is the Vop-motor cortex system. This disynaptic circuit has a high fundamental frequency estimated to be about 143 Hz. The Vop-motor cortex oscillator is responsible for driving lower motor neurons and, subsequently, muscle activity. The number of motor units recruited is a

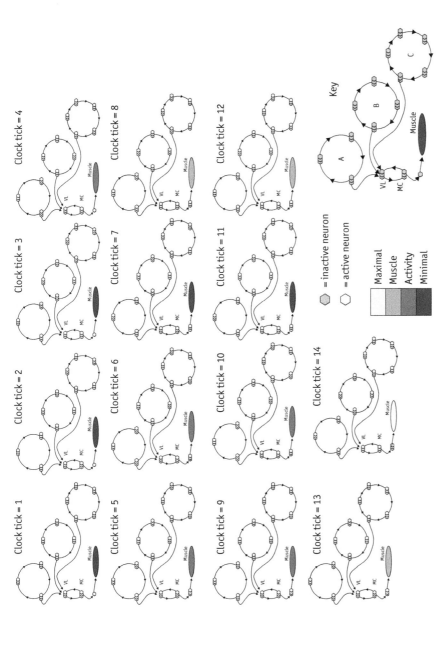

Figure 17.30: Representation of the interactions between the main oscillator, the Vop (labeled VL in this figure) motor cortex circuit, and the other side loops through the basal ganglia. Building on the concepts illustrated in Figure 17.28, the purpose of Figure 17.30 is to show how the interactions among the oscillators in the basal ganglia–thalamic-cortical system can modulate the motor unit activity over time. Three hypothetical basal ganglia side loops are represented by Oscillators A, B, and C, each containg a different number of nodes (see key). Oscillator A is a three-node loop, B is a four-node loop, and C is a five-node loop. The main oscillator, the Vop–motor cortex circuit, is responsible for motor unit recruitment by the connections of the motor cortex to the bulbar and spinal motor neurons, as illustrated in Figure 17.29. The side loops determine the percentage of motor cortex neurons active with each cycle through connections from Oscillators A, B, and C to Vop neurons. The recruitment process begins with the activation of a single neuron in the Vop and Oscillators A, B, and C. With each clock tick, the activation from the previous node is conveyed to the subsequent node. The number of neurons activated in the subsequent node equals the number of neurons activated in the previous node during the previous clock tick. Over time, the interactions between the Vop–motor cortex loop and the other oscillators gradually increase muscle force.

function of the percentage of motor cortex neurons activated with each cycle of the Vop-motor cortex oscillator. The theory also proposes that the percentage of motor cortex neurons activated with each cycle is determined by inputs from the basal ganglia (and other structures such as the cerebellum) side loops. Thus, the basal ganglia side loops determine the magnitude of motor unit recruitment and, therefore, the orchestration of muscle forces necessary to produce movement (Montgomery 2007b). Figure 17.30 depicts how the multiple side loops in the basal ganglia operate over lower frequencies to control the longer time scale of motor unit recruitment that is necessary to orchestrate the synergistic muscles to carry out a normal movement.

For a resonance effect, the frequencies of the DBS must match the fundamental frequencies in the targeted oscillator in the basal ganglia–thalamic-cortical system (*see Chapter 7—DBS Effects on Motor Control*). High-frequency DBS applied primarily to the lower-frequency basal ganglia side loops could have deleterious effects. In this case, the high-frequency DBS does not match the lower fundamental frequencies of the basal ganglia side loops, resulting in an abnormal pattern of neuronal activity in these loops. This abnormal neuronal activity affects the ability of the basal ganglia side loops to modulate the excitability in the Vopl–motor cortical oscillator necessary to orchestrate the muscle activity, that in turn, is necessary for such highly complex movements as speech, gait, and balance. Lower-frequency DBS, primarily in the basal ganglia side loops, and particularly when it is equal to the fundamental frequencies of the side loop oscillators, has a very different effect. In this case, the pattern of neuronal activity in the basal ganglia side loop disrupted by disease could be restored. The restored patterns of neuronal activity in the basal ganglia side loops would improve the modulation of excitabilities within the Vop -motor cortical loop, leading to improved orchestration of motor unit activities and more normal behavior (Montgomery 2007b).

The Systems Oscillators Theory (as described in the figures above) has several important properties (*see* Montgomery 2004a). Not only are the predictions of the theory consistent with empirical observations, the theory also suggests potential explanations for a range of important observations, such as the different effects of high- and low-frequency DBS on speech in patients with Parkinson's disease (*see Chapter 7—DBS Effects on Motor Control*), the "U-shaped" response to increasing DBS, and the variability in latencies to clinical effects.

APPENDIX OF SUPPLEMENTAL MATERIAL

Two types of additional materials are available via the Internet. The first is a set of materials containing several essays on matters that may be of interest to some readers: Deep brain stimulation, and for its future; DBS and pharmacotherapies; a discussion on the central role of antidromic activation of axons; description of what an ideal DBS system might look like; lessons we have learned from past failures; and current DBS paradoxes. These essays can be found here: http://www.greenvilleneuromodulationcenter.com/DBS_Programming_essays/.

In addition to the essays described above, we have also included access to various downloadable tools to assist in post-operative DBS programming. These tools include an index that relates symptoms and signs that might be encountered during programming to anatomical structures that may be in the vicinity of the DBS electrodes. There is also an algorithm and check list for electrode configurations and tools useful for the documentation of electrode configurations, stimulation parameters, and clinical responses during the programming sessions. And finally, an inventory useful for the review of systems in patients with implanted DBS systems is available. These downloadable forms can be found here: http://www.greenvilleneuromodulationcenter.com/DBS_Programming_forms/.

GLOSSARY

ACTION POTENTIAL: a specific change in the electrical potential of the neuronal membrane that is propagated down the axon of one neuron to affect subsequent neurons. The action potential is a basic unit of information, such as the "o's" and "1's" of a computer or the "dots" and "dashes" of Morse code. Information is encoded in the sequence of action potentials. This information from one neuron is translated into postsynaptic depolarizing or hyperpolarizing synaptic potentials in the next set of neurons. These receiving neurons then integrate the postsynaptic potentials (information processing) and translate the results to another set of action potentials, which are relayed further through the network of neurons.

ACTION-POTENTIAL-INITIATING SEGMENT: the region of the neuron at which an action potential is generated. Typically, but not necessarily, the action-potential-initiating segment is at the axon hillock that is the point of origin of the axon from the neuronal cell body.

AMPERAGE (CURRENT): a measure of electrical current; the number of electrons moving past a point in a given period of time.

ANODAL: adjective referring to the electrically positive component of the stimulation pulse or current.

ANODE: the electrically positive contact.

ANTIDROMIC: nerve impulses conducted in a direction opposite to the usual one, typically towards the soma rather than away.

AXON HILLOCK: the junction of the axon and the cell body of the neuron.

CAPACITIVE REACTANCE: a physical phenomenon that occurs when energy, electrical for example, approaches a change in the conductivity of the energy. In electronics, electrons flowing in a conductor will start to "stack up" when

the electrons encounter a region of decreased conductivity. The "stacking up" of the electrons resists further flow of electrons.

CATHODAL: adjective referring to the electrically negative component of the stimulation pulse or current.

CATHODE: the electrically negative contact.

CHARGE DENSITY: the amount of electrical charge delivered during the cathodal (negative) or anodal (positive) phase of the stimulation pulse, divided by the surface area of the electrical contact.

COULOMBS: the total amount of electrical charge delivered over time.

CURRENT (AMPERAGE): the number of electrons flowing per second.

DISCRETE OSCILLATORS: oscillators that are discontinuous as compared to continuous harmonic oscillators. An example of a discrete oscillator may be the intermittent flashing of a firefly.

ELECTRODE: a structure, typically metal, for delivering electrical current. An electrode should not be confused with the DBS lead, which is an arrangement of electrodes, some or all of which may be active in delivering electrical current.

ELECTRODE CONFIGURATION: the specific combination of active contacts (anodes and cathodes) in the DBS lead and IPG case. This does not include the stimulation parameters such as current/voltage, pulse width, stimulation frequency (rate), or pulse train pattern.

ELECTRODE IMPEDANCE: generally, the opposition to the flow of electrical charges through a conduction that results from the combination of resistance, capacitive reactance and inductive reactance. As applied specifically to DBS systems, it is the opposition to the flow of electrical charges measured in ohms when each contact is used in monopolar or bipolar configurations. Typically used to test the electrical integrity of the DBS system. It is not to be confused with therapeutic impedance which is specific electrode configurations and stimulation parameters being used therapeutically.

ELECTROLYSIS: a process in which water molecules are broken down into hydrogen and oxygen gas bubbles; a mechanism by which DBS can damage brain tissue.

ELECTROMOTIVE FORCE OR VOLTAGE: this is another term for *voltage* and represents the amount of potential energy that can move electrical charges.

EXCESSIVE BURSTING THEORY: a theory that posits abnormal bursting neuronal activity as a pathophysiological mechanism causing Parkinson's disease.

EXCESSIVELY HIGH BETA OSCILLATIONS THEORY: a theory that posits abnormal excessive periodic neuronal activity in the beta frequencies—for example, 20 Hz—as a pathophysiological mechanism causing Parkinson's disease.

EXCESSIVE SYNCHRONIZATION OF NEURONAL ACTIVITIES: a theory that posits abnormal excessive synchronization of neuronal activity as a pathophysiological mechanism causing Parkinson's disease.

FAN-IN RATIO: the number inputs to a single neuron from other neurons—for example, a fan-in ratio of 5 means that a single neuron receives inputs from five other neurons.

FOURIER TRANSFORM: a mathematical method for relating any complex periodic function, such as sound, into a sum of weighted components at single frequencies as sine or cosine functions.

GLOBUS PALLIDUS INTERNA RATE THEORY: a theory that posits abnormal excessive neuronal activity in the globus pallidus interna as a pathophysiological mechanism causing Parkinson's disease, and abnormal reduced activity as causal to involuntary movement disorders.

HARMONIC OSCILLATORS: oscillators, graphed as sinusoidal functions, that are continuous and everywhere differentiable, in the sense of calculus. These oscillators are different from discrete oscillators.

HEBBIAN LEARNING: a form of neuronal plasticity where repeated coinciding postsynaptic transmembrane potentials increase synaptic efficiency, such as increasing the probability that a single postsynaptic potential may be sufficient to generate an action potential.

HERTZ: a measure of frequency; here, of electrical waveforms.

HOLOGRAPHIC MEMORY: a type of physical or mathematical system that can be trained to model a number of complex periodic functions so that when a segment of the original complex function is added to the model, the subsequent complete periodic function is created. Typically, these are based on an inverse Fourier transform where the system contains a range of oscillators of different frequencies that can be coupled.

IMPEDANCE: the opposition to the flow of electrical charge, measured in ohms, typically associated with a varying voltage or current source. For example, in direct current (DC) circuits, the opposition is in the form of resistance. For alternating current (AC) circuits, the opposition includes resistance, capacitive reactance and inductive reactance.

INDUCTIVE REACTANCE: a physical phenomenon that occurs when electrical energy in the form of flowing electrical charges through a conductor, for example, generates a magnetic field that "falls back" onto the conduction and counters the flow of the electrical charges.

INVERSE FOURIER TRANSFORM: a mathematical method for creating any complex periodic function, such as sound, by the sum of weighted components at single frequencies as sine or cosine functions.

LEAD: an arrangement of electrodes, some or all of which may be active in delivering electrical current. An *electrode* should not be confused with the DBS *lead*.

LOCAL FIELD POTENTIALS: a method of recording electrical fields generated by neurons. Typically, the potential recording is the sum, representing an average, of all the potentials within a certain radius of the contact. The radius depends on the size of the contact. In the case of a typical DBS contact, the radius may be several millimeters. Typically, the local field potentials recorded are the electrical potential differences generated in the dendrites of a neuron relative to the soma and are therefore thought to represent dendritic activity.

MICROCOULOMBS: a measure of the total amount of electrical charges delivered by stimulation; 1 microcoulomb is 1 one-millionth of a coulomb.

MILLIAMPERES (MA): a measure of the amount of electrical charges delivered each second by stimulation; 1 milliamp is 1 one-thousandth of an amp.

NEURAL OSCILLATOR: a circuit made up of multiple neurons interconnected in such a way that activations continue to circulate within the network thereby producing oscillations of neuronal activities.

NEURONAL OSCILLATOR: neurons that have oscillations specific to the electrical potential across the neuronal membrane referable to mechanisms intrinsic to the neuron, as in contrast to neural oscillators.

NON-LINEAR: typically refers to a system, either physical or mathematical, in which the output is not proportional to the input. For example, the equation $y = x$ is linear because doubling x doubles y. However, the equation $y = x^2$ is nonlinear, because a doubling of x quadruples y. The input/output function of a neuron can be said to be non-linear because the transmembrane potential has to be depolarized to a threshold before an action potential is generated. For example, a depolarization of x millivolts that still is below the threshold will not generate an action potential. However, if the same depolarization spans the threshold, an action potential would be generated. If the voltages associated with the depolarization are all above the threshold, there will not be any change in the action potential, but there may be more repeated action potentials.

OHMS: a measure of the opposition to the flow of electrical charges.

OHM'S LAW: a law that describes the relationship between the flow of electrical charges (measured in amps) and the electromotive force (measured in voltage) that moves the charges, and the opposition to the flow of charges (measured in ohms).

ORTHODROMIC: nerve impulses conducted in the usual direction, typically away from the soma.

PERIODIC: a descriptor of any recurrent activity, such as a flashing light at a railroad crossing.

PHASE: In relation to DBS systems, it is a component of the DBS pulse associated with one polarity of electrical current. The negative (*cathodal*) phase is associated with negative electrical charges flowing *from* the electrical contact. A positive (*anodal*) phase is associated negative electrical charges flowing *into* the contact. In relation to periodic or oscillatory signals, it is the angular degree of some point on the signal. For example, a sine wave at zero time may have an amplitude of zero hence a phase equal to zero. For the cosine wave, the value may be the positive maximum value which corresponds to a phase of 90 degrees.

PHOSPHENES: bright, flashing lights in the visual fields that are not caused by external light sources.

POWER SPECTRA: a manner of representing the amount of energy or power of different frequencies in any signal. For example, any complex varying signal can be decomposed into a series of sine waves, each with a specific frequency (see **Fourier transform**). The amount of each component frequency in the original complex signal is represented in the power spectra.

PULSE TRAIN: refers to the time series (sequence) of pulses of electrical stimulation.

PULSE WIDTH: the duration of an electrical pulse. In many DBS systems, the pulse width is associated with the first phase of the pulse which typically is the phase with the greatest amplitude.

RESISTANCE: a form of opposition to the flow of electrical charges measure in ohms. Resistance is related to the degree an atom binds the electrons orbiting in the outer shell. In direct current (DC) circuits, resistance determines the total opposition. In alternating current (AC) circuits, opposition results from a combination of resistance, capacitive reactance and inductive reactance.

RESONANCE: the phenomenon where several periodic functions, such as individual sounds, interact. These interactions can result in a larger signal through positive resonance or a smaller signal through negative resonance.

SOMA: an anatomical term related to the dendrites and the cell body of a neuron.

STIMULATION PARAMETER: the specific combination of parameters such as current/voltage, pulse width, or stimulation frequency (rate). This does not include the electrode configuration of active contacts (anodes and cathodes) in the DBS lead and IPG case.

SYSTEMS OSCILLATORS THEORY: a theory that posits that the basal ganglia–thalamic-cortical system is composed of loosely coupled, non-linear, polysynaptic, reentrant oscillators in which different oscillators have different fundamental frequencies. Thus, the set of oscillators can interact collectively to produce any periodic signal, such as those that ultimate drive behaviors—both normal and abnormal.

THERAPEUTIC IMPEDANCE: the opposition to electrical flow for the specific stimulation parameters and electrode configurations that are currently in use to treat the patient. Therapeutic impedance is particularly relevant to safe DBS.

VENTRAL THALAMUS PARS ORALIS: the nucleus within the thalamus, which is the basal ganglia's relay to the cortex.

VOLTAGE: a measure of the electromotive force that moves electrical charges through a conductor.

VOP: abbreviation for the *ventral thalamus pars oralis* which is the basal ganglia relay to the cortex.

REFERENCES

Alberts JL, Elder CM, et al. (2004). "Comparison of pallidal and subthalamic stimulation on force control in patients with Parkinson's disease." Motor Control 8:484–499.

Aldewereld ZT, Huang H, et al. (2012). "Effects of Deep Brain Stimulation on M-wave Size in Parkinson's Disease: Evidence of Increased Synchronization." International Motor Unit Conference, Sydney, Australia.

Aldewereld ZT, Huang H, et al. (2012). "Reversal of Size Principle in Parkinson's Disease and Normalization with Deep Brain Stimulation." International Motor Unit Conference, July 23 – 26, 2012, Sydney, Australia.

Alexander GE, DeLong MR, et al. (1986). "Parallel organization of functionally segregated circuits linking basal ganglia and cortex." Annu Rev Neurosci 9:357–381.

Ashby P, Rothwell JC. (2000). "Neurophysiologic aspects of deep nervous system stimulation." Neurology 55:S17–S20.

Baker K, Montgomery EBJr, et al. (2002). "Subthalamic nucleus deep brain stimulus evoked potentials: physiology and therapeutic implications." Mov Disord 17:969–983.

Bekar L, Libionka W, et al. (2008). "Adenosine is crucial for deep brain stimulation–mediated attenuation of tremor." Nat Med 14:75–80.

Bleuse S, Delval A, et al. (2011). "Effect of bilateral subthalamic nucleus deep brain stimulation on postural adjustments during arm movement." Clin Neurophysiol 122:2032–2035.

Busaki G. (2006). Rhythms of the Brain. Oxford, UK: Oxford University Press.

Butson CR, McIntyre CC. (2015). "The use of stimulation field models for deep brain stimulation programming." Brain Stim 8: 976–8

Ceballos-Baumann AO, Boecker H, et al. (1999). "A positron emission tomographic study of subthalamic nucleus stimulation in Parkinson disease: enhanced movement-related activity of motor-association cortex and decreased motor cortex resting activity." Arch Neurol 56:997–1003.

Chomiak T, Hu B. (2007). "Axonal and somatic filtering of antidromically evoked cortical excitation by simulated deep nervous system stimulation in rat nervous system." J Physiol 579:403–412.

Coombs SJ, Curtis DR, Eccles JC. (1957). "The interpretation of spike potentials of motoneurons." J Physiol (London) 39:198–231.

Cooper IS, Upton AR, et al. (1980). "Reversibility of chronic neurologic deficits. Some effects of electrical stimulation of the thalamus and internal capsule in man." Appl Neurophysiol 43:244–258.

Eisenstein SA, Koller JM, et al. (2014). "Functional anatomy of subthalamic nucleus stimulation in Parkinson disease." Ann Neurol 76:279–295.

Gale JT. (2004). "Basis of periodic activities in the basal ganglia-thalamic-cortical system of the rhesus macaque." Biomedical science Ph.D. thesis, Kent State University—Kent, OH.

Goaillard JM, Taylor AL, et al. (2010). "Slow and persistent postinhibitory rebound acts as an intrinsic short-term memory mechanism." J Neurosci 30:4687–4692.

Goetz CG, Tilley BC, et al. (2008). "Movement Disorder Society UPDRS Revision Task Force. Movement Disorder Society–sponsored revision of the

Unified Parkinson's Disease Rating Scale (MDS-UPDRS): scale presentation and clinimetric testing results." Mov Disord 23:2129–2170.

Grill WM, Cantrell MB, et al. (2008). "Antidromic propagation of action potentials in branched axons: implications for the mechanisms of action of deep brain stimulation." J Comp Neurosci 81–93.

Grill WM, Snyder AN, et al. (2004). "Deep brain stimulation creates an informational lesion of the stimulated nucleus." Neuroreport 15:1137–1140.

Groppa S, Herzog J, et al. (2014). "Physiological and anatomical decomposition of subthalamic neurostimulation effects in essential tremor." Brain 137:109–121.

Hebb DO. (1949). The Organization of Behavior. New York: Wiley.

Heimer G, Rivlin M, et al. (2006). "Synchronizing activity of basal ganglia and pathophysiology of Parkinson's disease." J Neural Transm, Suppl 70:17–20.

Hodgkin AL, Huxley AF. (1952). "A quantitative description of membrane current and its application to conduction and excitation in nerve." J Physiol (London) 117:500–544.

Holsheimer J, Dijkstra EA, et al. (2000). "Chronaxie calculated from current-duration and voltage-duration data." J Neurosci Meth 97:45–50.

Huang H, Watts RL, et al. (2012). "Role for Basal Ganglia in Motor Unit Recruitment: Effects of Parkinson's Disease (PD) and Deep Brain Stimulation (DBS) of Subthalamic Nucleus (STN)." International Motor Units Conference, July 23 – 26, 2012, Sydney, Australia.

Huang H, Watts RL, et al. (2014). "Effects of deep brain stimulation frequency on bradykinesia of Parkinson's disease." Mov Disord 29:203–206.

Johnson MD, Miocinovic S, et al. (2008). "Mechanisms and targets of deep brain stimulation in movement disorders." Neurotherapeutics 5:294–308.

Johnson-Laird PN. (2006). How We Reason. New York: Oxford University Press.

Kim Y, Zieber HG, et al. (1990). "Uniformity of current density under stimulating electrodes." Crit Rev Biomed Eng 17:585–619.

Korpel A, Chatterjee M. (1981). "Nonlinear echoes, phase conjugation, time reversal, and electronic holography." Proc IEEE 69:1539–1556.

Larkum ME, Nevian T, et al. (2009). "Synaptic integration in tuft dendrites of layer 5 pyramidal neurons: a new unifying principle." Science 325:756–670.

Llinas RR, Terzuolo CA. (1964). "Mechanisms of supraspinal actions upon spinal cord activities. Reticular inhibitory mechanisms on alpha extensor motoneurons." J Neurophysiol 27:579–591.

Longuet-Higgins HC. (1968). "Holographic model of temporal recall." Nature 217:104.

Lopiano L, Torre E, et al. (2003). "Temporal changes in movement time during the switch of the stimulators in Parkinson's disease patients treated by subthalamic nucleus stimulation." Eur Neurol 50:94–99.

Lorente de Nó R. (1933). "Vestibulo-ocular reflex arc." Arch Neurol Psychiatry 30:245–291

Manor Y, Nadim F, et al. (1999). "Network oscillations generated by balancing graded asymmetric reciprocal inhibition in passive neurons." J Neurosci 19:2765–2779.

McCairn KW, Turner RS. (2009). "Deep nervous system stimulation of the globus pallidus internus in the parkinsonian primate: local entrainment and suppression of low-frequency oscillations." J Neurophysiol 101:1941–1960.

McCairn KW, Turner RS. (2015). "Pallidal stimulation suppresses pathological dysrhythmia in the parkinsonian motor cortex." J Neurophysiol. 113:2537-48.

McIntyre CC, Grill WM. (1999). "Excitation of central nervous system neurons by non-uniform electric fields." Biophys J 76:878–888.

Milner PM. (1996). "Neural representations: some old problems revisited." J Cogn Neurosci 8:69–77

Miocinovic S, Lempka SF, et al. (2009). "Experimental and theoretical characterization of the voltage distribution generated by brain stimulation." Exper Neurol 216:166–176.

Montgomery EBJr (2012). "The epistemology of deep brain stimulation and neuronal pathophysiology." Front Integr Neurosci 6:78.

Montgomery EBJr, Gale JT. (2008). "Mechanisms of action of deep brain stimulation (DBS)." Neurosci Biobehav Rev 32:388–407.

Montgomery EBJr, Gorman DS, et al. (1991). "Motor initiation versus execution in normal and Parkinson's disease subjects." Neurology 41:1469–1475.

Montgomery EBJr, Huang H, et al. (2005). "Unsupervised clustering algorithm for N-dimensional data." J Neurosci Meth 144:19–24.

Montgomery EB Jr, Huang H, et al. (2012). "Interaction of Subthalamic Nucleus Antidromic Action Potentials and Intrinsic Oscillators." Society for Neuroscience, October 13 – 17, 2012, New Orleans, LA.

Montgomery EB Jr, Sillay K. (2008). "Nested Probabilistic Oscillators in DBS and Basal Ganglia Function." Movement Disorders Society 12th Annual Meeting, June 22 – 26, 2008, Chicago, IL.

Montgomery EBJr, Turkstra LS. (2003). "Evidenced based medicine: let's be reasonable." J Med Speech Lang Pathol 11:ix–xii.

Montgomery EBJr. (2004a). "Dynamically coupled, high-frequency reentrant, non-linear oscillators embedded in scale-free basal ganglia-thalamic-cortical networks mediating function and deep brain stimulation effects." Nonlinear Stud 11:385–421.

Montgomery EBJr. (2006a). "Effects of GPi stimulation on human thalamic neuronal activity." Clin Neurophysiol 117:2691–2702.

Montgomery EBJr. (2007a). "Basal ganglia physiology and pathophysiology: a reappraisal." Parkinsonism Relat Disord 13:455–465.

Montgomery EBJr. (2007b). "Deep brain stimulation and speech: a new model of speech function and dysfunction in Parkinson's disease." J Med Speech-Lang Pathol 15:ix–xxv.

Montgomery EBJr. (2008a). "Theorizing about the role of the basal ganglia in speech and language: the epidemic of miss-reasoning and an alternative." Commun Disord Rev 2:1–15.

Montgomery EBJr. (2008b). "Thalamic Stimulation for Other Tremors." In: Tarsy D, Vitek J, Starr PA, Okun MS, eds. Deep Brain Stimulation for Neurological and Psychiatric Disorders. New York: Humana Press: 215–228.

Montgomery EBJr. (2015a). Intraoperative Neurophysiological Monitoring for Deep Brain Stimulation: Principles, Practice and Cases. New York: Oxford University Press.

Montgomery EBJr. (2015b). Twenty Things to Know About Deep Brain Stimulation. New York: Oxford University Press.

Moro E, Esselink RJ, et al. (2002). "The impact on Parkinson's disease of electrical parameter settings in STN stimulation." Neurology 59:706–713.

Moro E, Poon YY, et al. (2006). "Subthalamic nucleus stimulation: improvements in outcome with reprogramming." Arch Neurol 63:1266–1272.

Percheron G, Filion M, et al. (1993). "The role of the medial pallidum in the pathophysiology of akinesia in primates." Adv Neurol 60:84–87. Review.

Quencer K, Okun MS, et al. (2007). "Limb-kinetic apraxia in Parkinson disease." Neurology 68:150–151.

Ranck JBJ. (1975). "Which elements are excited in electrical stimulation of mammalian central nervous system: a review." Brain Res 98:417–440.

Rizzone M, Lanotte M, et al. (2001). "Deep nervous system stimulation of the subthalamic nucleus in Parkinson's disease: effects of variation in stimulation parameters." J Neurol Neurosurg Psychiatry 71:215–219.

Rosen AD. (1981). "Nonlinearity in the generation of antidromic activity during evoked cortical activity." Exp Neurol 71:269–277.

Schaltenbrand G, Wahren W. (1977). Atlas for Stereotaxy of the Human Brain. Stuttgart, Germany: Thieme.

Schettino LF, Van Erp E, et al. (2009). "Deep brain stimulation of the subthalamic nucleus facilitates coordination of hand preshaping in Parkinson's disease." Int J Neurosci 119:1905–1924.

Schüpbach M, Gargiulo M, et al. (2006). "Neurosurgery in Parkinson disease: a distressed mind in a repaired body?" Neurology 66:1811–1816.

Steriade M, Deschenes M, et al. (1974). ". I. Background firing and responsiveness of pyramidal tract neurons and interneurons." J Neurophysiol 37:1065–1092.

Strogatz SH. (1994). Nonlinear Dynamics and Chaos. Cambridge, MA: Perseus Publishing.

Sturman MM, Vaillancourt DE, et al. (2010). "Effects of five years of chronic STN stimulation on muscle strength and movement speed." Exp Brain Res 205:435–443.

Swash M. (2007). "Limb-kinetic apraxia in Parkinson disease." Neurology 69:810–811.

Takeshita D, Gale JT, et al. (2009). "Analyzing spike trains with circular statistics." Am J Physics 77:424–429.

Vaillancourt DE, Prodoehl J, et al. (2004). "Effects of deep brain stimulation and medication on bradykinesia and muscle activation in Parkinson's disease." Brain 127:491–504.

Villardita C, Smirni P, et al. (1982). "Mental deterioration, visuoperceptive disabilities and constructional apraxia in Parkinson's disease." Acta Neurol Scand 66:112–120.

Vitek JL, Zhang J, et al. (2012). "External pallidal stimulation improves Parkinsonian motor signs and modulates neuronal activity throughout the basal ganglia thalamic network." Exp Neurol 233:581–586.

Vyas S, Huang H, Gale J, et al. (2015). "Neuronal Complexity in Subthalamic Nucleus is Reduced in Parkinson's Disease." IEEE Trans Neural Syst Rehabil Engineer 24:36–45.

Walker HC, Guthrie BL, et al. (2008). "Subthalamic Neuronal Activity Is Altered by Contralateral Subthalamic Deep Brain Stimulation in Parkinson Disease." Poster 318. 12th International Congress of Parkinson's Disease and Movement Disorders, June 22 – 26, 2008, Chicago, IL.

Walker HC, Watts RL, et al. (2011). "Activation of subthalamic neurons by contralateral subthalamic deep nervous system stimulation in Parkinson disease." J Neurophysiol 105:1112–1121.

Wang Z, Jensen A, Baker KB, et al. (2009). "Neurophysiological changes in the basal ganglia in mild Parkinsonism: a study in the non-human primate model of Parkinson's disease." Program No. 828.9. Neuroscience Meeting Planner. Chicago, IL: Society for Neuroscience, 2009. Online.

Watson P, Montgomery EBJr. (2006). "The relationship of neuronal activity within the sensori-motor region of the subthalamic nucleus to speech." Brain Lang 97:233–240.

Weisberg DS, Keil FC, et al. (2008). "The seductive allure of neuroscience explanations." J Cogn Neurosci. 20:470–477.

Zimnik AJ, Nora GJ, et al. (2015). "Movement-related discharge in the macaque globus pallidus during high-frequency stimulation of the subthalamic nucleus." J Neurosci 35:3978–3989.

INDEX

Note: page numbers followed by *f* and *t* refer to figures and tables.

Absolute refractory period, 23
Action potential(s)
  antidromic
    definition, 205
    and interactions of pulses with neuronal
      oscillators, 71–73
    orthodromic vs., 28, 30, 30*f*–33*f*
    propagation of, 55–56, 56*f*
    and reentrant discrete oscillators, 188–189, 189*f*
  biphasic effects of, 188
  as DBS network effect, 55–57, 56*f*
  definition, 205
  electronics at, 17–19
  orthodromic
    antidromic vs., 28, 30, 30*f*–33*f*
    definition, 207
    synchronization of, 65, 66*f*, 67, 68*f*
  and programming for optimal benefit, 106
  and voltage-gated ionic conductance channels, 22–24,
    22*f*–23*f*
Action-potential-initiating segment(s)
  definition, 205
  responses to DBS in, 54–55, 54*f*
Adverse effects
  causes of, 51
  clarifying, 130, 166
  and hardware/electrical failures, 170
  late-occurring, 120
  and lead positioning
    GPi DBS, 143–146
    STN DBS, 131–136
    Vim DBS, 149–154
  monopolar surveys of, 112–114

  of neural network activation, 48
  programming to prevent
    electrical field in, 2
    programming for optimal benefit vs., 105–107
    steps in, 117–119
  and site, 158
Algorithms for DBS programming, 2, 49, 157–163
  electrode configurations in, 158, 159, 161–163
  and electrode nomenclature, 158, 158*f*
  function of, 157–158
  pulse width in, 159
  stimulation parameters in, 159, 160*t*, 161–163
Amperage, 12, 205. *See also* Current
Amplitude, of oscillation, 171
AM radio signals
  information encoding in, 96, 97*f*, 98
  testing electrical continuity with, 169–170
Anion, 10
Anodal (term), 205
Anodal current
  and DBS safety, 45, 46
  definition, 11, 12
Anode, 12, 205
Anterior location, lead in
  for GPi DBS, 146
  for STN DBS, 133, 136*f*, 137*f*
Antidromic action potential(s)
  definition, 205
  and interactions of pulses with neuronal
    oscillators, 71–73
  orthodromic vs., 28, 30, 30*f*–33*f*
  propagation of, 55–56, 56*f*
  and reentrant discrete oscillators, 188–189, 189*f*

Apraxias, 86–87

Ataxia, 131, 132

Axon hillocks, 17, 205

Axons
  in DBS mechanism, 3
  diameter of, 30, 31
  synchronization in, 65, 66f, 67, 68f

Balance, loss of, 131

Basal ganglia–thalamic-cortical system
  circuitry of, 50, 50f, 81, 82f
  excessive synchronization of activities in, 90, 91, 93
  in Globus Pallidus Interna Rate theory, 91f
  neuronal dynamics in, 75, 75f, 76
  oscillators in models of, 174–175, 179
  in Systems Oscillators theory, 94f–96f, 97, 98, 198,
    200, 200f

Battery life, 99–100

Beat interactions, 177

Behavior
  intrinsic neuronal dynamics related to, 73, 74f–76f, 75–77
  of neurons vs. discrete neural oscillators, 191, 193, 194, 194f
  synchronization of neurons for, 67–68, 69f
  See also Motor control

Bifurcation, of oscillator frequency, 196, 196f, 197f

Bilateral thalamic DBS, 156

Biphasic effects of action potentials, 188

Bipolar electrode configurations
  close, 118, 159, 161–162
  current in, 35, 36
  current intensity in, 36–38, 37f–41f, 40–41, 43
  definition, 32, 33
  electrical charge in, 34
  and electrical field, 33, 34f, 106
  in GPi DBS, 143
  narrow
    current in, 36, 36f
    current intensity in, 36, 37
    definition, 118, 159
    electrical fields in, 34–35, 35f
    stimulation parameters for, 162–163
    in STN DBS, 132–135
    in Vim DBS, 152, 154
  in programming for optimal benefit, 115–116
  for STN DBS, 133–135
  wide
    current in, 36, 36f
    current intensity in, 37
    definition, 118, 158, 159
    electrical fields in, 34–35, 35f
    stimulation parameters for, 159, 161
    in STN DBS, 132–135
    in Vim DBS, 152, 154

Bradykinesia, 122–123, 122f

Brain
  as electronic device, 1
  oscillators in models of brain function, 174–175

Brain injuries, electricity-related, 45–47

Breaks, in electrical continuity, 116, 168–170, 168f

Capacitance, 5, 7f, 8f

Capacitive reactance, 5, 10, 205

Carrier frequency, 184, 185f

Cathodal (term), 205

Cathodal charges, nervous system responses to, 51

Cathodal current
  and DBS safety, 45, 46
  definition, 10–12

Cathode(s)
  definition, 12, 205
  multiple
    GPi DBS with, 145
    increasing volume of electrical field with, 106–107
    in programming for optimal benefit, 116
    selecting stimulation parameters for, 161–163
    STN DBS with, 132, 134–136, 134f
    Vim DBS with, 150

Cations, 10

Cell body (neuron)
  definition, 17
  responses to DBS in, 54–55, 54f

Cerebellar outflow tremor
  clinical assessment of, 124–125, 124f–125f
  Vim DBS for, 156

Charge
  in bipolar electrode configurations, 34
  cathodal, nervous system responses to, 51
  total, 45
  See also Flow of electrical charge

Charge density, 45, 205

Clinical assessment(s), 121–130
  of corticospinal and corticobulbar stimulation, 128–129,
    128f, 129f
  of disease symptoms, 121–129
    dystonia, 125–126, 126f, 127f
    essential tremor and cerebellar outflow tremor,
      124–125, 124f–125f
    hyperkinetic disorders, 127, 128
    Parkinson's disease, 122–124, 122f, 123f
    tic disorders, 128
  hints for conducting, 130
  of speech, language, and swallowing, 129–130

Clinical responses
  detection of, 114
  documenting, 166–167
  inconsistent, 167

Close bipolar electrode configuration(s)
  definition, 118, 159
  stimulation parameters for, 161–162
Cognitive changes, with GPi DBS, 143
Cognitive symptoms of Parkinson's, STN DBS for, 137
Constant current DBS
  constant voltage DBS vs., 12, 13*f*, 165
  definition, 7, 8*f*
  and IPG battery life, 100
Constant voltage DBS
  constant current DBS vs., 12, 13*f*, 165
  definition, 7, 8*f*
  and impedance, 14, 33, 47
  programming for, 165–166
Contact(s)
  changing, to prevent adverse effects, 117–118
  nomenclature for, 100–102, 101*f*–103*f*
  segmented
    effect of changing to subset of, 102, 115, 158, 165
    GPi DBS for patients with, 143, 145, 147*f*
    monopolar surveys with, 108, 109*f*, 110*f*, 113, 114
    nomenclature for, 100–102, 102*f*, 103*f*
    STN DBS for patients with, 133, 135*f*, 136, 137*f*, 140*f*
    Vim DBS for patients with, 150, 152, 153*f*, 154*f*, 155
Continuous circumferential stimulation, 108–109
Continuous oscillators, 95, 185. *See also* Harmonic
    oscillators
Control
  of IPGs, by patients (*See* Patient-controlled IPGs)
  satisfactory, 119–120
Controlling devices (DBS), 120, 167
Corticobulbar stimulation, 128–129, 128*f*, 129*f*
Corticospinal stimulation
  clinical assessment of, 128, 129, 129*f*
  symptom suppression due to, 121, 125, 126
Coulombs, 11, 205
Counters, resetting, 120, 167
Current, 15, 45
  anodal, 11, 12, 45, 46
  cathodal, 10–12, 45, 46
  clarifying adverse effects with, 166
  definition, 205
  and electrode configuration, 35–36, 36*f*
  intensity of, 36–38, 37*f*–41*f*, 40–41, 43
  in programming for optimal benefit, 116
  See also Constant current DBS
Cycle time, oscillator, 187

DBS. *See* Deep brain stimulation
DBS controlling devices, 120, 167
DBS programming, 99–120, 165–170
  battery life as consideration in, 99–100
  clarifying adverse effects in, 166

complexity of, 1
conceptual approaches to, 105–107, 108*f*
and constant voltage DBS, 165–166
contact nomenclature for, 100–102, 101*f*–103*f*
documenting clinical responses in, 166–167
effective and efficient, 2–3
exiting programming sessions, 119–120
and inconsistent responses, 167
limits on patient-controlled parameters in, 166
for monopolar surveys, 107–109, 108*f*, 111*f*, 112–114, 113*f*, 166
for optimal benefit, 111*f*, 114–117
  electrical field in, 2
  programming to prevent adverse effects vs., 105–106
  steps in, 111*f*, 114–117
patience and persistence in, 167–168
to prevent adverse effects, 2, 105–107, 117–119
  electrical field in, 2
  programming for optimal benefit vs., 105–107
  steps in, 117–119
recording parameters, configurations, and features
    before, 102, 103, 104*f*
resetting counters in, 167
and response detection, 114
suspending stimulation in, 168
and therapeutic impedances, 166
timing of, 103, 105
troubleshooting in, 167–170, 168*f*, 169*f*
See also Algorithms for DBS programming
Deep brain stimulation (DBS)
  basis of effects from, 3
  downstream effects of, 24–26, 24*f*–25*f*
  efficiency of, 57, 70
  fundamentals of, 2
  medical complications with, 47–48
  network effects of, 53*f*, 54*f*, 55–57, 56*f*
  psychosocial consequences of, 48
  safety concerns with, 45–48
  therapeutic mechanism of, 2, 15, 16*t*, 49–51, 50*f*, 87–88, 97–98, 187
  See also specific entries
Dendrite(s)
  definition, 17
  responses to DBS in, 54–55, 54*f*
  voltage-gate ionic conductance channels in, 51–52
Depolarization
  definition, 20
  downstream effects of, 24–25
  at voltage-gated ionic conductance channels, 22–24, 23*f*
Depolarization blockade, 52, 54*f*
De-recruitment, motor unit, 83, 85–87, 86*f*
Dexterity, loss of, 129
Dimpling, skin, 129, 129*f*
Diplopia, 131, 132
Disconjugate gaze, 131

Discrete neural oscillators, 179–202
    behavior of neurons vs., 191, 193, 194, 194f
    and characteristics of discrete oscillators, 184–185,
        186f–188f, 187
    harmonic oscillators vs., 180, 182–184, 182f–185f
    and interactions among discrete oscillators, 189–191,
        191f–194f
    with multiple realistic neurons, 195–196,
        195f–199f, 198
    in nervous system function, 179–180, 180f–182f
    and reentrant discrete oscillators, 188–189, 189f, 190f
    and Systems Oscillators Theory, 198, 199f–201f,
        200, 202
Discrete oscillator(s)
    characteristics of, 184–185, 186f–188f, 187
    continuous vs., 95
    definition, 205
    harmonic vs., 175
    interactions of, 184, 185, 186f, 189–191, 191f–194f
    reentrant, 188–189, 189f, 190f
Disynaptic propagation, of action potentials, 56–57
Doctor's visits, DBS controlling devices at, 167
Documentation
    of clinical responses, 166–167
    prior to DBS programming, 102, 103, 104f
Downstream effects of DBS, 24–26, 24f–25f
Dyskinesias
    GPi DBS for, 146, 147
    STN DBS for, 137
Dystonia
    clinical assessments of, 125–126, 126f, 127f
    and corticobulbar stimulation assessments, 129
    globus pallidus interna DBS for, 148

Edge effects, 43, 43f
Electrical charge. *See* Charge
Electrical current. *See* Current
Electrical field(s)
    and electrode configurations, 31–34, 34f, 35f
    varying intensity vs. shape, size, and location of, 2
    volume of, 27, 106–107, 118
Electrical force lines, orientation of, 27–28, 28f–30f
Electrical principles of DBS, 5, 6f–10f, 7–10
Electricity, injury secondary to, 45–47, 46f
Electrode(s)
    definition, 205
    nomenclature of, 158, 158f
Electrode configuration(s)
    algorithm for selecting, 158, 159, 161–163
    definition, 99, 117, 205
    documenting, prior to programming, 102
    documenting responses to, 166–167
    and flow of electrical charges, 31–36, 34f–36f

monopolar
    current in, 35
    current intensity in, 36–38, 37f–41f, 40–41, 43
    definition, 32, 158
    electrical charge in, 34
    electrical field for, 33, 34f
    in GPi DBS, 143
    reducing adverse effects with, 107
    stimulation parameters for, 158, 161
    in STN DBS, 134, 135
    in Vim DBS, 152, 153f, 154
multipolar, 32
for prevention of adverse effects, 117
See also Bipolar electrode configurations
Electrode impedance
    assessing, 14
    breaks in electrical continuity and, 168–169
    definition, 205–206
Electrolysis, 46–47, 206
Electromagnetic fields, 167
Electromotive force, 12, 206. *See also* Voltage
Electronic (gap) junctions, 21
Electronic principles of DBS, 10–12, 11f, 13f
Electronics
    definition, 10
    of neurons, 17–18, 18f–21f, 20–21
Electrophysiological principles of DBS, 2, 15–26
    and downstream effects, 24–26, 24f–25f
    neuronal architecture, 16–17, 16f
    neuronal electronics, 17–18, 18f–21f, 20–21
    and therapeutic mechanism of medication vs. DBS, 15, 16t
    voltage-gated ionic conductance channels and action
        potentials, 22–24, 22f–23f
Electrostatic forces, 5, 6f
Emergency rooms, DBS controlling devices in, 120, 167
Envelopes of motor unit activity, 87
Essential tremor
    clinical assessment of, 124–125, 124f–125f
    pulse width for suppression of, 112, 113f
Excessive bursting theory, 91, 93, 206
Excessively High Beta Oscillations theory
    definition, 206
    and interpreting nervous system responses to
        DBS, 58–59
    and pathophysiology of Parkinsonism, 90, 92f
Excessive synchronization of neuronal activities, 90, 91, 93, 206
Exhaustion, neurotransmitter, 52, 53

Fallacy of Confirming the Consequence, 55
Fallacy of Pseudotransitivity, 89
Fan-in ratio, 194, 206
Flow of electrical charge, 27–44
    and axon diameter, 30, 31

and current intensity, 36–38, 37*f*–41*f*, 40–41, 43
definition, 11
and electrode configurations, 31–36, 34*f*–36*f*
in monopolar and bipolar electrode configurations, 36–38, 37*f*–41*f*, 40–41, 43
and orientation of electrical force lines, 27–28, 28*f*–30*f*
in orthodromic and antidromic action potentials, 28, 30, 30*f*–33*f*
in segmented DBS leads, 42*f*–43*f*, 43–44
Fourier transforms, 173–174, 206
Frequency
 carrier, 184, 185*f*
 DBS
  in programming for optimal benefit, 115–116
  in programming to reduce adverse effects, 107, 118–119
  selecting initial frequency, 159
  testing, in monopolar surveys, 109, 111*f*, 112
 oscillator, 171
  bifurcation of, 196, 196*f*, 197*f*
  and refractory period, 198, 199*f*
  and synaptic efficiency, 198, 198*f*
Funny feelings, 114, 129, 170

Gap junctions, 21
Gaze, disconjugate, 131
General Review of Systems for Patient's with Implanted DBS Systems, 103
Globus pallidus interna (GPi)
 adverse effects related to, 143–146
 lead position relative to, 143–146
  anterior location, 146
  lateral location, 146
  posterior location, 145, 146*f*, 147*f*
  ventral location, 38, 38*f*, 143, 144*f*, 145
 regional anatomy of, 143
 symptoms and stimulation of, 121
Globus pallidus interna DBS (GPi DBS), 143–148
 adverse effects of, 143–146
 for dystonia, 148
 for hyperkinetic disorders, 148
 lead positioning, 143–146
  anterior location, 146
  lateral location, 146
  posterior location, 145, 146*f*, 147*f*
  ventral location, 38, 38*f*, 143, 144*f*, 145
 network effects of, 56–57
 for Parkinson's disease, 146, 147
 regional anatomy of GPi, 143
 U-shaped response in, 70
Globus Pallidus Interna Rate theory, 90, 91*f*, 206
GPi. *See* Globus pallidus interna
GPi DBS. *See* Globus pallidus interna DBS
Groups (pulse train), 40, 41

Harmonic oscillators, 175, 176*f*–177*f*, 177–178
 definition, 175, 183, 206
 discrete neural oscillators vs., 180, 182–184, 182*f*–185*f*
 interactions of, 175, 177
Harmonics, 183
Heat damage, to brain, 47
Hebbian learning, 189, 206
Henneman Size Principle, 83
Hertz, 206
Holographic memory, 97, 175, 206
Hyperkinetic disorders
 clinical assessment of, 127, 128
 and Globus Pallidus Interna Rate theory, 90
 GPi DBS for, 148
Hyperpolarization
 definition, 23
 effects of, 24, 52
 post-hyperpolarization rebound excitation, 52, 53*f*, 54*f*, 182

Impedance
 definition, 10, 206
 electrode, 14, 168–169, 205–206
 of implanted pulse generators, 14, 33, 47, 166
 and resistance, 11
 therapeutic, 14, 166, 207
Implanted pulse generators (IPGs)
 constant current vs. constant voltage, 165
 in GPi DBS, 147
 impedance of, 14, 33, 47, 166
 patient-controlled, 47, 120, 155, 166
 rechargeable, 99–100
 in STN DBS, 141
 suspending stimulation from, 168
 technological advances in, 49
Induction, 7, 8, 9*f*
Inductive reactance, 10, 206
Inertia, motor unit orchestration and, 84, 85
Information ablation, 73
Integrate-and-fire model of neurons, 195, 195*f*
Intensity
 current, 36–38, 37*f*–41*f*, 40–41, 43
 electrical field, 2
 stimulation, 115–116, 119
Inverse Fourier transform, 174, 206
Ionic conductance channel(s)
 definition, 20
 ligand-gated, 21
 voltage-gated
  and action potentials, 22–24, 22*f*–23*f*
  depolarization blockade in, 52
  in neuronal electronics, 20–21, 21*f*
  responses to DBS in, 51–52

Ions, 17–18, 18*f*, 19*f*, 20
IPGs. *See* Implanted pulse generators

Joint rotations, 83–85, 86*f*

Lack of effect, 116, 168–170
Language
    clinical assessment of, 129–130
    and Vim DBS, 154, 155
Lateral location, lead in
    in GPi DBS, 146
    in STN DBS, 134, 135, 139*f*
    in Vim DBS, 152, 153*f*, 154*f*
Lead(s)
    definition, 206
    evaluating location of, 119
    with poor orientation, 150, 151*f*, 152
    positioning of, 38
        in globus pallidus interna, 38, 38*f*, 143–146
        in subthalamic nucleus, 131–136
        in ventral intermediate nucleus of thalamus, 149–154
    spacing of, 33
    See also Contact(s)
Lead migration, 116–117, 169
Learning, Hebbian, 189, 206
Lenz effect, 8, 9, 10*f*
Ligand-gated ionic conductance channels, 21
Local field potentials, 57–58, 206
Low-frequency DBS, 109

ma (milliamperes), 11, 206
Medial location, STN DBS leads in, 131–133, 133*f*–135*f*
Medical complications with DBS, 47–48
Medications
    adjusting, at end of programming session, 119–120
    and DBS for dystonia, 148
    and DBS for tremor, 156
    documenting, 102, 103
    and GPi DBS, 146, 147
    and STN DBS, 136–137, 139
    synergies of DBS and, 47–48
    therapeutic mechanism of DBS vs., 15, 16*t*
    and timing of DBS programming, 105
Membranes, neuronal
    orientation of electrical force lines and, 27–28, 28*f*–30*f*
    responses to DBS in, 51–52
Memory, holographic, 97, 175, 206
Microcoulombs, 11, 45, 206
Milliamperes (ma), 11, 206
Monopolar electrode configurations
    current in, 35
    current intensity in, 36–38, 37*f*–41*f*, 40–41, 43
    definition, 32, 158

electrical charge in, 34
electrical field for, 33, 34*f*
    in GPi DBS, 143
    reducing adverse effects with, 107
    stimulation parameters for, 158, 161
    in STN DBS, 134, 135
    in Vim DBS, 152, 153*f*, 154
Monopolar survey(s)
    conducting, 166
    and DBS programming algorithm, 157–158
    and initial DBS frequency, 159
    programming, 107–109, 108*f*, 111*f*, 112–114, 113*f*
Motor control, 81–88
    DBS effects on, 50–51
    DBS mechanisms related to, 87–88
    discrete oscillators for, 187
    orchestration of motor unit activities in, 81–87, 84*f*–86*f*
    and Systems Oscillators theory, 97
    and time scales for motor unit recruitment/
        de-recruitment, 86*f*, 87
Motor cortex, synchronization in, 63, 63*f*, 64*f*
Motor nerve axons, synchronization in, 65, 66*f*, 67, 68*f*
Motor unit(s)
    DBS effects on dynamics in, 73–75, 74*f*, 77
    definition, 81
    de-recruitment of, 83, 85–87, 86*f*
    orchestration of activities in, 81–87, 84*f*–86*f*
    recruitment of
        definition, 82–83
        in Parkinson's disease, 83, 84*f*, 85, 85*f*
        synergy in, 86
        time scales for, 86*f*, 87
    temporal responses in, 79, 79*f*
Movement disorders, DBS for, 81
Movement Disorders Society–Unified Parkinson's Disease
    Rating Scales Part III, 122
Multiple cathodes
    GPi DBS with, 145
    increasing volume of electrical field with, 106–107
    in programming for optimal benefit, 116
    stimulation parameters for, 161–163
    STN DBS with, 132, 134–136, 134*f*
    Vim DBS with, 150
Multipolar electrode configurations, 32. *See also* Bipolar
    electrode configurations
Muscle contractions, tonic. *See* Tonic muscle contractions

Narrow bipolar electrode configurations
    current in, 36, 36*f*
    current intensity in, 36, 37
    definition, 118, 159
    electrical fields in, 34–35, 35*f*
    stimulation parameters for, 162–163

in STN DBS, 132–135
in Vim DBS, 152, 154
Negative current. *See* Cathodal current
Negative resonance, 175, 177, 183
Nervous system, function of, 179–180, 180f–182f
Nervous system response(s), 49–79
in action-potential-initiating segments, 54–55, 54f
and behaviorally related intrinsic neuronal dynamics, 73, 74f–76f, 75–77
in cell bodies, 54–55, 54f
in dendrites, 54–55, 54f
depolarization blockade as, 52, 54f
interpretation of, 57–59
knowledge of DBS therapeutic mechanisms vs., 49–51, 50f
and network effects of DBS, 53f, 54f, 55–57, 56f
neurotransmitter exhaustion as, 52, 53
post-hyperpolarization rebound excitation as, 52, 53f
and pulse interactions with neuronal oscillators, 71–73, 72f, 73f
and reentry propagations of pulse, 59–62, 60f–62f
synchronization-related, 62–63, 63f–64f, 65, 66f–71f, 67–68, 70–71
temporal evolution of, 77–79, 77f–79f
in voltage-gated ionic conductance channels of neuronal membrane, 51–52
Neural networks
effects of DBS on, 53f, 54f, 55–57, 56f
information in, 183–184, 187
safety concerns with activation of, 48
Neural oscillator(s)
definition, 206
neuronal vs., 171, 179
pulse train interactions with, 189–191, 191f–194f
See also Discrete neural oscillators
Neurological disorders, 81, 141
Neuron(s)
architecture of, 16–17, 16f
behaviorally-related intrinsic dynamics of, 73, 74f–76f, 75–77
behavior of discrete neural oscillators vs., 191, 193, 194, 194f
discrete neural oscillators with multiple realistic, 195–196, 195f–199f, 198
electronics of, 17–18, 18f–21f, 20–21
excessive synchronization of activities in, 90, 91, 93, 206
integrate-and-fire model of, 195, 195f
neural oscillators and dynamics in, 191, 193, 194, 194f
Neuronal membranes
orientation of electrical force lines and, 27–28, 28f–30f
responses to DBS in, 51–52

Neuronal oscillator(s)
definition, 206
neural vs., 171, 179
pulse interactions with, 71–73, 72f, 73f
Neuron Doctrine, 16, 54, 55
Neurotransmitter exhaustion, 52, 53
Newton's First Law of Motion, 84
Noisy synchronization, 67, 68, 68f, 69f
Non-linear systems, 191, 206–207
Nyquist theorem, 184

Off-label use of DBS, 125, 128, 156
Ohms, 12, 207
Ohm's Law, 11, 207
Optimal benefit, DBS programming for
electrical field in, 2
programming to prevent adverse effects vs., 105–106
steps in, 111f, 114–117
Orthodromic action potentials
antidromic vs., 28, 30, 30f–33f
definition, 207
synchronization of, 65, 66f, 67, 68f
Oscillator(s), 171–178
continuous, 95, 185
discrete
characteristics of, 184–185, 186f–188f, 187
continuous vs., 95
definition, 205
harmonic vs., 175
interactions of, 184, 185, 186f, 189–191, 191f–194f
reentrant, 188–189, 189f, 190f
harmonic, 175, 176f–177f, 177–178
definition, 175, 183, 206
discrete neural oscillators vs., 180, 182–184, 182f–185f
interactions of, 175, 177
information encoded in, 95–97, 97f
interactions of, 87, 172–174, 173f
measuring movement of, 171–172, 172f
modeling brain function with, 174–175
neural
definition, 206
neuronal vs., 171, 179
pulse train interactions with, 189–191, 191f–194f
neuronal
definition, 206
neural vs., 171, 179
pulse interactions with, 71–73, 72f, 73f
reentrant
discrete, 188–189, 189f, 190f
and network effects of DBS, 57
and Parkinson's disease, 179, 180, 180f, 181f
See also Discrete neural oscillators; Systems Oscillators theory

Oscillatory movement
  features of, 171
  measuring, 171–172, 172f

Parameters, stimulation. *See* Stimulation parameter(s)
Paresthesias
  and STN DBS, 131, 135
  and Vim DBS, 149, 150
Parkinson's disease
  clinical assessment of, 122–124, 122f, 123f
  globus pallidus interna DBS for, 146, 147
  motor unit orchestration in, 83, 84f, 85–87, 85f
  and reentrant oscillations, 179, 180, 180f, 181f
  subthalamic nucleus DBS for, 136, 137, 139, 141
  therapeutic mechanisms of medication vs. DBS for, 15
Pathoetiology, 89–90
Pathophysiological mechanisms of Parkinsonism, 89–98
  excessive bursting activities in, 91, 93
  Excessively High Beta Oscillations theory, 58–59,
    90, 92f
  excessive synchronization of neuronal activities, 90, 91
  Globus Pallidus Interna Rate theory, 90, 91f
  Systems Oscillators theory, 93–98, 93f–97f
Pathophysiology
  importance of, 89
  pathoetiology vs., 89–90
Patience, in DBS programming, 167–168
Patient-controlled IPGs
  configuring, 120
  reducing speech and swallowing complications
    with, 155
  safety warnings about impedance in, 47
  stimulation parameters for, 166
Period, oscillation, 171
Periodic activities, 171, 207
Persistence, in DBS programming, 167–168
Persistent paresthesias, 135
Personality changes, with GPi DBS, 143
Phase, 45, 172, 207
Phase delay, 40, 41
Phosphenes, 38, 143, 207
Positive current. *See* Anodal current
Positive resonance, 98, 175, 183
Posterior location, DBS lead in
  for GPi DBS, 145, 146f, 147f
  for STN DBS, 135, 136, 140f
  for Vim DBS, 149, 150f, 151f
Post-hyperpolarization rebound excitation, 52, 53f,
  54f, 182
Post-inhibitory rebound excitation, 180, 182f
Postsynaptic effects of DBS, 189, 195
Power spectra, 174, 207
Psychiatric disorders, 81, 141
Psychiatric symptoms of Parkinson's, STN DBS for, 137

Psychological adverse effects, 136
Psychosocial consequences, of DBS, 48
Pulse train(s)
  definition, 99, 207
  as discrete oscillators, 189, 190
  documenting, prior to programming, 102
  interleaving of, 107, 118
  intrinsic neuronal oscillators and, 71–73, 72f, 73f
  nervous system responses to, 77–79
  neural oscillators and, 189–191, 191f–194f
  reentry propagations of, 59–62, 60f–62f
Pulse width
  definition, 207
  initial, 159
  in monopolar surveys, 112
  in programming for optimal benefit, 115, 116
  in programming to reduce adverse effects, 118
  for STN DBS, 112, 113f
  and volume of electrical field, 106

Reactance, 12
  capacitive, 5, 10, 205
  inductive, 10, 206
Rechargeable IPGs, 99–100
Recruitment, motor unit
  definition, 82–83
  in Parkinson's disease, 83, 84f, 85, 85f
  synergy in, 86
  time scales for, 86f, 87
Reentrant oscillators
  discrete, 188–189, 189f, 190f
  and network effects of DBS, 57
  and Parkinson's disease, 179, 180, 180f, 181f
Reentry propagations, of pulse trains, 59–62, 60f–62f
Refractory period
  absolute, 23
  and oscillator frequency, 198, 199f
Resistance, 10, 11, 207
Resonance
  definition, 207
  and flow of electrical charges, 30
  negative, 175, 177, 183
  as nervous system response, 59, 60f
  of oscillators, 183
  positive, 98, 175, 183
Rigidity, clinical assessment of, 123–124, 123f

Safety concerns, 45–48
  injury secondary to electricity, 45–47, 46f
  medical complications with DBS, 47–48
  with neural network activation, 48
  psychosocial consequences of DBS, 48
Sampling, 184
Satisfactory control, 119–120

Segmented contacts
  effect of changing to subset of, 102, 115, 158, 165
  flow of electrical charges in, 42*f*–43*f*, 43–44
  GPi DBS for patients with, 143, 145, 147*f*
  monopolar surveys with, 108, 109*f*, 110*f*, 113, 114
  nomenclature for, 100–102, 102*f*, 103*f*
  STN DBS for patients with, 133, 135*f*, 136, 137*f*, 140*f*
  Vim DBS for patients with, 150, 152, 153*f*,
    154*f*, 155
Short-circuits, 170
Side effects. *See* Adverse effects
Soma, 17, 207
Somatosensory cortex, synchronization in, 63, 63*f*
Spatial summation
  and downstream effects of DBS, 25–26, 25*f*
  optimizing, 106
Speech
  adverse effects of DBS on, 117
  clinical assessment of, 129–130
  clinical responses related to, 114
  and Vim DBS, 154, 155
Stimulation
  corticobulbar, 128–129, 128*f*, 129*f*
  corticospinal
    clinical assessment of, 128, 129, 129*f*
    symptom suppression due to, 121, 125, 126
  effects of, on disease symptoms, 121
  suspending, 168
Stimulation intensity
  and electrode configuration, 119
  in programming for optimal benefit, 115–116
Stimulation parameter(s)
  algorithm for selecting, 159, 160*t*, 161–163
  definition, 207
  documenting, prior to programming, 102
  documenting responses to, 166–167
  for GPi DBS, 147
  for patient-controlled IPGs, 166
  for STN DBS, 137
Stimulation partitioning, 143, 154
STN DBS. *See* Subthalamic nucleus DBS
Subthalamic nucleus (STN)
  adverse effects related to, 131–136
  lead position relative to, 131–136
    anterior location, 133, 136*f*, 137*f*
    lateral location, 134, 135, 139*f*
    medial location, 131–133, 133*f*–135*f*
    posterior location, 135, 136, 140*f*
    ventral location, 134, 138*f*
  oscillator neurons in, 72–73, 73*f*
  post-hyperpolarization rebound excitation in,
    52, 54*f*
  regional anatomy of, 131, 132*f*
  symptoms and stimulation of, 121

Subthalamic nucleus DBS (STN DBS), 131–141
  adverse effects of, 131–136
  lead positioning, 131–136
    anterior location, 133, 136*f*, 137*f*
    lateral location, 134, 135, 139*f*
    medial location, 131–133, 133*f*–135*f*
    posterior location, 135, 136, 140*f*
    ventral location, 134, 138*f*
  for movement disorders, 81
  network effects of, 55–56, 56*f*
  for neurological disorders, 141
  for Parkinson's diseases, 136, 137, 139, 141
  for psychiatric disorders, 141
  pulse width for, 112, 113*f*
  and regional anatomy of STN, 131, 132*f*
Swallowing
  clinical assessment of, 130
  and Vim DBS, 154, 155
Symptoms Without Evidence of Dopamine Depletion
    (SWEDD), 90
Synaptic efficiency, 198, 198*f*
Synchronization
  excessive, of neuronal activities, 90, 91, 93, 206
  nervous system responses related to, 62–63, 63*f*–64*f*, 65,
    66*f*–71*f*, 67–68, 70–71
  noisy, 67, 68, 68*f*, 69*f*
  of orthodromic action potentials, 65, 66*f*, 67, 68*f*
  in somatosensory cortex, 63, 63*f*
  and Systems Oscillators theory, 70–71
  and U-shaped response, 68, 70–71, 70*f*, 71*f*
Systems Oscillators theory
  definition, 207
  and discrete neural oscillators, 193, 194*f*, 198, 199*f*–201*f*,
    200, 202
  and modeling of brain function, 174
  and pathophysiology of Parkinsonism, 93–98, 93*f*–97*f*
  and synchronization in neurons, 70–71

Temporal summation
  and downstream effects of DBS, 24*f*, 25, 26
  optimizing, 106
Therapeutic impedance, 14, 166, 207
Therapeutic window, 112–114
Tic disorders, 128
Time frame
  for appearance of adverse effects, 117
  for DBS programming, 103, 105, 121
  for motor unit recruitment/de-recruitment, 86*f*, 87
  for nervous system responses, 77–79, 77*f*–79*f*
Tissue activation
  and prevention of adverse effects, 118
  in programming for optimal benefit, 115
  shaping, 107
  volume of, 27, 32, 106, 107

Tonic muscle contractions
    and GPi DBS, 143, 145
    and STN DBS, 131, 133, 134
    and Vim DBS, 149, 152, 154, 155
Total electrical charge, 45
Transient paresthesias, 135
Transmembrane voltage, 22
Tremor
    clinical assessment of, 123–125, 124f, 125f
    Vim DBS for, 155–156
Triphasic pattern of muscle activity for ballistic
        movement, 174
Tripolar configurations, 40f, 43, 118

Unified Parkinson Disease Rating Scales (UPDRS), 114
U-shaped response, 68, 70–71, 70f, 71f

V (volts), 12
Ventral intermediate nucleus of thalamus (Vim)
    adverse effects related to, 149–154
    lead position relative to, 149–154
        lateral location, 152, 153f, 154f
        poor orientation of lead, 150, 151f–153f, 152
        posterior location, 149, 150f, 151f
        ventral location, 154, 155f
    regional anatomy of, 149
Ventral intermediate nucleus of thalamus DBS (Vim DBS),
        149–156
    adverse effects of, 149–154
    lead positioning, 149–154
        lateral location, 152, 153f, 154f
        poor orientation of lead, 150, 151f–153f, 152
        posterior location, 149, 150f, 151f
        ventral location, 154, 155f
    and regional anatomy of Vim, 149
    and speech, language, swallowing, 154, 155
    symptoms and stimulation of, 121
    for tremor, 155–156
Ventral location, DBS lead in
    for globus pallidus interna DBS, 38, 38f, 143,
        144f, 145
    for subthalamic nucleus DBS, 134, 138f
    for ventral intermediate nucleus of thalamus DBS,
        154, 155f

Ventral thalamus pars oralis (VOP)
    definition, 207
    post-hyperpolarization rebound excitation in, 52, 53f
Ventrolateral thalamus (VL), 149
Vim. *See* Ventral intermediate nucleus of thalamus
Vim DBS. *See* Ventral intermediate nucleus of
        thalamus DBS
Visualization, for DBS programming, 2, 157
VL (ventrolateral thalamus), 149
Voltage
    constant voltage DBS
        constant current DBS vs., 12, 13f, 165
        definition, 7, 8f
        and impedance, 14, 33, 47
        programming for, 165–166
    definition, 12, 207
    increasing, to clarify adverse effects, 166, 170
    transmembrane, 22
Voltage-gated ionic conductance channels
    and action potentials, 22–24, 22f–23f
    depolarization blockade in, 52
    in neuronal electronics, 20–21, 21f
    responses to DBS in, 51–52
Volts (V), 12
Volume
    of electrical field
        changing, 106–107, 118
        volume of tissue activation vs., 27
    of tissue activation
        changing, 106, 107
        defined, 32
        volume of electrical field vs., 27
Vop. *See* Ventral thalamus pars oralis
Vop-motor cortex oscillator, 200, 200f, 201f, 202

Wide bipolar electrode configurations
    current in, 36, 36f
    current intensity in, 37
    definition, 118, 158, 159
    electrical fields in, 34–35, 35f
    stimulation parameters for, 159, 161
    in STN DBS, 132–135
    in Vim DBS, 152, 154
Width, pulse. *See* Pulse width

CPSIA information can be obtained
at www.ICGtesting.com
Printed in the USA
BVHW011121230820
586405BV00012B/3